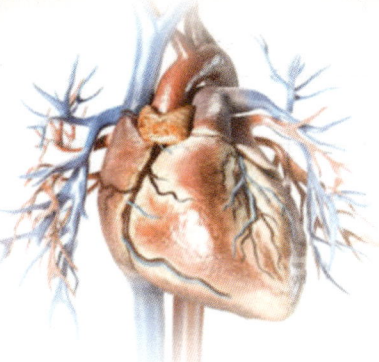

Heart Rate

Is it a Missing Link

Dr. JC Mohan
Dr. Monotosh Panja
Dr. I Sathyamurthy
Dr. Rajeev Agarwala
Dr. Brian Pinto
Dr. CK Ponde
Dr. A Sreenivas Kumar
Dr. Bijay Kumar Mahala

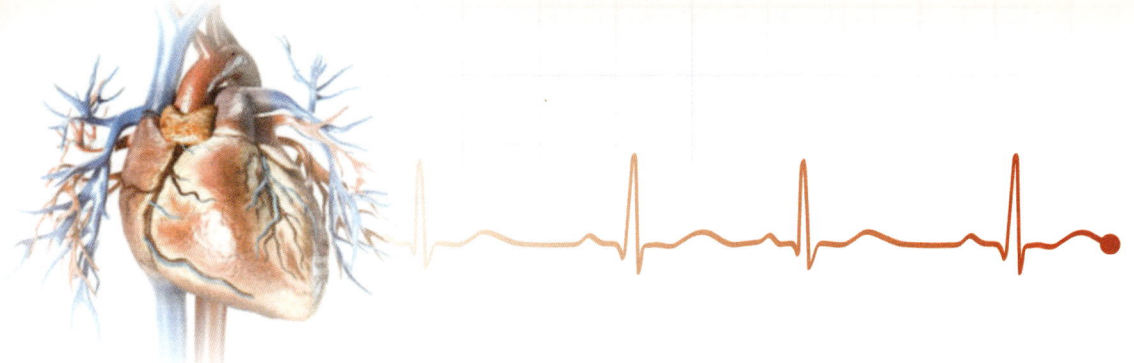

Heart Rate

Is it a Missing Link

Contributors

Dr. JC Mohan

Dr. Monotosh Panja

Dr. I Sathyamurthy

Dr. Rajeev Agarwala

Dr. Brian Pinto

Dr. CK Ponde

Dr. A Sreenivas Kumar

Dr. Bijay Kumar Mahala

Editor

Dr. R Gulshan

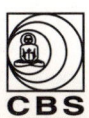

CBS

CBS Publishers & Distributors Pvt Ltd

New Delhi • Bengaluru • Chennai • Kochi • Kolkata • Mumbai

Hyderabad • Jharkhand • Nagpur • Patna • Pune • Uttarakhand

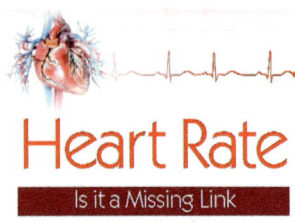

Heart Rate
Is it a Missing Link

ISBN: 978-93-90709-03-8

First Edition: 2021

Published by Satish Kumar Jain and produced by Varun Jain for

CBS Publishers & Distributors Pvt Ltd

4819/XI Prahlad Street, 24 Ansari Road, Daryaganj, New Delhi 110 002, India
Ph: 011-23289259, 23266861, 23266867   Website: www.cbspd.com
Fax: 011-23243014   e-mail: delhi@cbspd.com; cbspubs@airtelmail.in
Corporate Office: 204 FIE, Industrial Area, Patparganj, Delhi 110 092

Ph: 011-4934 4934   Fax: 011-4934 4935   e-mail: publishing@cbspd.com; publicity@cbspd.com

Branches

- **Bengaluru:** Seema House 2975, 17th Cross, K.R. Road,
  Banasankari 2nd Stage, Bengaluru 560 070, Karnataka
  Ph: +91-80-26771678/79   Fax: +91-80-26771680   e-mail: bangalore@cbspd.com
- **Chennai:** 7, Subbaraya Street, Shenoy Nagar, Chennai 600 030, Tamil Nadu
  Ph: +91-44-26680620, 26681266   Fax: +91-44-42032115   e-mail: chennai@cbspd.com
- **Kochi:** 42/1325, 1326, Power House Road, Opp KSEB Power House, Ernakulam 682 018, Kochi, Kerala
  Ph: +91-484-4059061-65   Fax: +91-484-4059065   e-mail: kochi@cbspd.com
- **Kolkata:** No. 6/B, Ground Floor, Rameswar Shaw Road, Kolkata-700014 (West Bengal), India
  Ph: +91-33-2289-1126, 2289-1127, 2289-1128   e-mail: kolkata@cbspd.com
- **Mumbai:** PWD shed, Gala No. 25/26, Ramchandra Bhatt Marg, Next JJ Hospital Gate No. 2,
  OPP. Union Bank of India, Noorbaug, Mumbai-400009, Maharashtra
  Ph: +91-22-66661880/89   e-mail: mumbai@cbspd.com

Representatives

- **Hyderabad** 0-9885175004   • **Jharkhand** 0-9811541605   • **Nagpur** 0-9421945513   • **Patna** 0-9334159340
- **Pune** 0-9623451994   • **Uttarakhand** 0-9716462459

Printed at Nutech Print Services, Faridabad, India

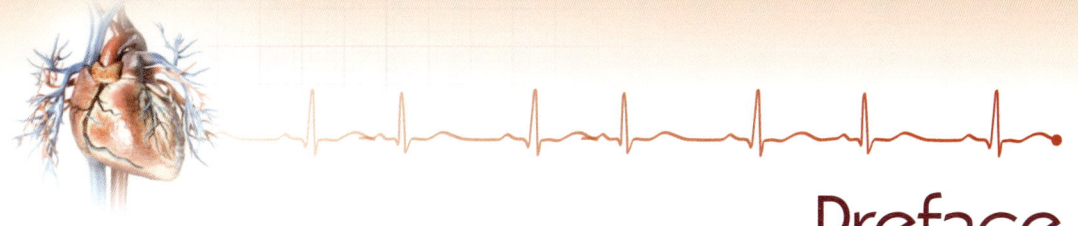

Preface

Science and technology by the way of intentions and innovations have made life easier for everybody in all spheres of life. The doctors in today's world use complex and sophisticated devices to diagnose and manage various diseases in their clinical practice. Palpation and auscultation have become less important over a period of time. One of the most important parameters that are not given due importance in such instances is the measurement of heart rate (HR). HR evaluation has been a prognostic marker of health and disease for centuries. Evidence that RHR may be a marker or even a risk factor for CV morbidity and mortality has been growing since the last two decades. It differs according to sex, age, weight/BMI, and rest. Our insights to determine the importance of HR in health and disease are still evolving. These advances are driving the application of new therapeutic strategies directed at recently discovered molecular targets.

Heart rate variability (HRV) is becoming an increasingly important disease marker. It is the difference in time between the peaks of the heart in RR spans, which are the result of continuous interaction between two arms of the autonomic nervous system (ANS). A high HRV is a sign that the heart is healthy as it shows greater adaptability to respond to any pressure. On the contrary, decreased HRV can be a result of medical problems and can influence immune capacities, self-regulation, and mental abilities. Understanding these key parameters are essential for progress beyond the current standard approaches of using HR as a marker or factor. It has been seen in several epidemiological studies that elevations in RHR are related to increased risk of CVD and total mortality. Elevated RHR is related to diminished artery compliance, endothelial dysfunction and distensibility and subsequently increased arterial wall stress and increased PWV, which is further associated with increased after burden and ultimately systemic HTN. Elevated HR also frequently coexist with CV risk factors such as dyslipidemia, glucose intolerance, obesity, and together they are associated with target organ damage such as chronic kidney disease (CKD), albuminuria, atrial fibrillation, and diabetic retinopathy.

Thus, the treatment of elevated HR may need to be individualized, employing a combination of pharmacological maneuvers. This book provides a "toolkit" in the context of an evidence-based cardiovascular practice in the midst of rapidly evolving scientific knowledge and guidelines. This book fills an important niche for all involved in elevated HR management to help ensure that we implement the variety of available treatments in the most effective and efficient manner and thereby help our patients live better and, ideally, longer lives.

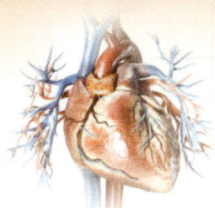

Acknowledgements

We would like to thank the following doctors who provided their valuable opinions for the development of the book:

Dr. Mukul Kumar	Dr. R Sundar
Dr. Aijaz Hussain Mansoor	Dr. AL Narayanan
Dr. Rakesh Kumar Jaswal	Dr. Sivaramakrishnan Manoj
Dr. Amar Singal	Dr. Sanjiv Agarwal
Dr. Parveen Chandra	Dr. Janakiraman Ezhilan
Dr. Manish Bansal	Dr. Prasant KR Sahoo
Dr. Sumeet Sethi	Dr. Hrudananda Mishra
Dr. Rishi Kumar Gupta	Dr. Satyanarayan Routray
Dr. Aditya Batra	Dr. Soumyajit Ghosh
Dr. Jitendra Pal Singh Aawhney	Dr. Prabhat Kumar
Dr. Bharat Bhushan Chanana	Dr. Rajiv Krishana
Dr. Parneesh Arora	Dr. Ritesh Kumar
Dr. Randheer Pal	Dr. Chinmoy Mazumder
Dr. Pramod Joshi	Dr. Kashi Nath Ghosh Hazra
Dr. Yogenra Singh	Dr. Arindam Pande
Dr. Praveen Kumar Jain	Dr. Kanak Kumar Mitra
Dr. Vineet Jain	Dr. Suvro Banerjee
Dr. Deepesh Agarwal	Dr. Khawer Naveed Siddiqui
Dr. Pankaj Rastogi	Dr. Subhendu Bikash Bhattacharyya
Dr. Anil Kumar Trivedi	Dr. Anjan Lal Dutta
Dr. Gaurav Narain Gupta	Dr. Manotosh Panja
Dr. Hosdurg Ramdas Nayak	Dr. Kuntal Bhattacharya
Dr. Somanathan C	Dr. TR Raghu
Dr. SS Binu	Dr. KH Srinivasa
Dr. Krishna Kumar B	Dr. Shreekanth B Shetty
Dr. Pathiyil Balagopalan Jayagopal	Dr. Prabhakar C Koregol
Dr. Arun Gopi	Dr. Tom Devasia
Dr. Saji Jose	Dr. Anand R Shenoy
Dr. Subramanian R	Dr. Pradeep Haranahalli
Dr. Aravindakumar	Dr. Srikanth KV
Dr. Sivakumar	Dr. Sadanand KS

Dr. Dhiren Shah
Dr. G P Ratnaparkhi
Dr. Vivek Mehan
Dr. Pravin Kahale
Dr. Anand Rao
Dr. Nitin Gokhale
Dr. Sharukh Golwalla
Dr. Rahul Gupta
Dr. Bhaskar Shah
Dr. Hasmukh Ravat
Dr. Vidhut Kumar Jain
Dr. Girish Kawthekar
Dr. Anand Mohan Tiwari
Dr. Smit Shrivastava
Dr. Prashant Advani
Dr. Prashant Manohar Jagtap
Dr. Rajiv Sethi
Dr. Hiralal Pawar
Dr. Prashant Pawar
Dr. Dharmesh Ramakant Solanki
Dr. Sumit Sinha
Dr. Nirmal Kumar
Dr. Gokul Reddy Mandala

Dr. Yerra Shiva Kumar
Dr. PA Jiwani
Dr. Rajendra Kumar Premchand
Dr. Rama Kumari Nuthalapati
Dr. Ravinder Reddy Kasturi
Dr. K Purnachandra Rao
Dr. Battina Venkateswara Rao
Dr. C Sesha Srinivasa Raju
Dr. Eric Borges
Dr. Anil Damle
Dr. Sadanand Shetty
Dr. VT Shah
Dr. Chetan Shah
Dr. Rajiv Karnik
Dr. Bharat Shivdasani
Dr. Bhupen Desai
Dr. Ajit Desai
Dr. Sharad Jain
Dr. Ajit Mehta
Dr. Rajdatt Deore
Dr. Kishor Pabitwar
Dr. M Viswanathan

Scientific Support:

Dr. V V Kolapkar
Dr. Lokesh Kumar

Editor

Dr. R Gulshan

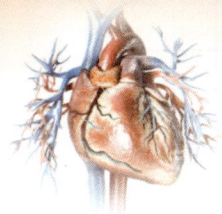

Contents

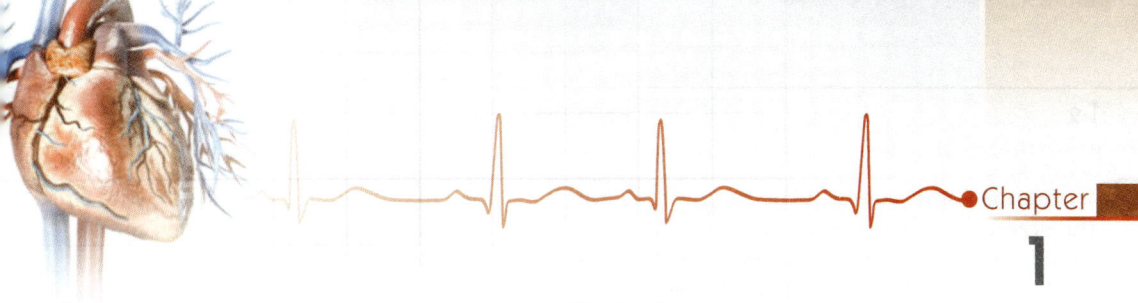

Importance of Heart Rate in Health and Disease

Dr. BK Mahala

Learning Objectives

At the end of this chapter one should be able to:

- Heart rate and its epidemiology
- Regulation of heart rate and significance of I_f channel
- Factors affecting HR and HRV
- Genetic influences on HR and longevity
- High RHV and its association with adverse clinical and cardiovascular outcomes

HEART RATE (HR) AND ITS EPIDEMIOLOGY

Resting heart rate (RHR) is one of the simplest accessible parameters and the most basic indication of life.[1,2] According to the American Heart Association (AHA), the ordinary sinus HR lies in the range of 60 and 100 beats per minute (bpm).[3] Usually, lower HR demonstrated lower all-cause and cardiovascular (CV) mortality.[1] In several studies, it has been shown that low RHR is connected with well-being and increased life span, and on the contrary, a high RHR is related to illness and unfavorable events.[4]

Historical Perspective of HR

HR evaluation has been a prognostic marker of health and disease for centuries. It has been used in a wide range of ancient societies and till now it is being utilized as a health indicator. In 3000–1600 BC, Egyptian papyri composed a portrayal of how to measure the pulse rate.[4] In 600 BC, Sage Kanada, an Indian doctor and logician expressed the assortment of heartbeats during various physiological and pathological conditions in his book, "Science of Sphygmica". In 500 BC, Ayurveda began in the Indian subcontinent, and since that time evaluation of the heartbeat is an indispensable part of Ayurvedic medicine.[5] In 129–200 AD, Greek doctor and Sphygmologist, Galen was well-known for his prophecy established on HR. According to Galen, the pulse has around 27 features which assume a significant role in determining well-being. However, he considered HR as the most significant feature.[4]

Demographic Determinants of HR

HR differs according to sex, age, weight/BMI, and rest. The normal grown-up male pulse is somewhere in the range of 70 and 72 bpm, while the normal for grown-up women is somewhere in the range of 78 and 82 bpm. This distinction is mainly due to the size of the heart, which is ordinarily smaller in females than males. The smaller female heart, pumping less blood with each beat, needs to beat at a faster rate to match the larger male heart's output. Further, women have alternate intrinsic rhythmicity to the pacemaker of their hearts, which makes their heartbeat faster.[6]

As age progresses, there is an expansion in both septal and wall thickness in both genders; however, the left ventricular diameter increases only in males.[6] Autonomic influences on HR are also impacted by aging. With aging in man, decreased HR responses to β-adrenergic agonists and exercise are seen. A parasympathetically mediated respiratory change in pulse diminishes with maturing, and muscarinic parasympathetic blockade with atropine brings about lesser increments in HR in healthy elderly *vs* younger people. The beat-to-beat variation in HR is utilized as an indicator of cardiac autonomic reactions. From childhood to adulthood, a significant distinction in HR is seen. Many investigations have shown a decrease in regions of high-frequency peaks from ages 9 to 30 and diminished low-frequency peaks from childhood through middle-age.[7]

Devoted athletes are known to have slower HR than non-athletes. The heart, like a muscle, boosts its strength because of exercise training, especially with aerobic training. The HR in female athletes and regular exercisers will be lower than that of an amateurish untrained male; anyway, it will, in any case, beat at a quicker rate than a similarly skilled male athlete or regular exerciser.[6] It is likewise seen that overweight and obese individuals have a higher HR than individuals with normal weight, due to their higher metabolic rate and a lesser proportion of body surface to body weight, contrasted with individuals with ordinary weight. A strong connection between HR and wet bulb globe temperature (WBGT) has been further observed. As per an investigation directed to decide the impacts of work environment heat on laborers showed that, HR increases by 1 bpm when the ecological temperature increases by 1°C.[8]

There is a strong correlation between sleep and HR. During sleep, the routine physiological demands are reduced and temperature and blood pressure (BP) drop. One of the potential benefits of sleep is to allow the heart to rest from the steady requirements of wakefulness. As compared to awakening, during non-rapid eye movement (REM) sleep, the overall HR and BP are reduced. During REM sleep, however, there is a more pronounced change in CV activity, with overall increases in BP and HR.[9]

Photoplethysmography (PPG) allows quantifying real-world HR related to age, time, socioeconomic profile, comorbidities, and chronotropic medication use. In the Health eHeart Study, a total of 66,788 patients contributed 3,144,332 HR-PPG estimations between 1st April 2014 and 30th April 2018, leading to a formation of a "full HR-data set". From this data, information was collected relating to mean age, sex, BMI, and average steps per day, as estimated by their smartphone. Results showed that the real-world HR was 79.1 bpm ± 14.5. Females had a normal HR-PPG 4.4 bpm higher than men. As age increased, the 95% confidence interval (CI) of HR estimated by PPG values narrowed in women more than men. The 95th percentile of real-world HR was ≤110 in people aged 18–45, ≤100 in 45–60 age group and ≤95 bpm in those whose age was over 60 years. The 95th percentile of real-world HR was consistently under 100 bpm in people above 45 years old reaching approximately 95 bpm at 61 years old. Asian females revealed the most elevated HRPPG, which was 79.2 ± 14.3 bpm. The number of medical ailments, female gender, increasing BMI, and being Hispanic were the factors related to an increased HR. Thus, it can be concluded from the result that age, height, and numbers of steps are negative indicators of pulse, while female gender, BMI, Asian race, and multi-nationality are indicators of a higher HR.[3]

Estimating a person's HR is a standard part of a clinical assessment, yet no action has been taken based on this finding unless it is well outside a population-based typical range. Quer G *et al.* during a period from March 2016 to Feb 2018, led a retrospective, longitudinal cohort study by including 92,457 people who wore a pulse wrist-worn tracker for a minimum of 20 hours/day. Individual daily RHR and its association with age, BMI, sex, sleep duration, and its variation over time were reported. The results revealed that the mean RHR for all people over the monitored days was 65.5 ± 7.7 bpm, with a minimum and maximum RHR for every individual extending somewhere in the range of 39.7 and 108.6 bpm, respectively. It was likewise observed that women had an essentially higher RHR in all age groups. Across age groups, normal RHR showed an increase until around 50 years and afterward started a descending pattern. RHR and BMI showed a U-shaped relationship. The most reduced RHR was related to a BMI of 21 for women and 23 for men. Normal day-to-day sleep length was additionally connected with RHR, with the minimum RHR registered for people who slept an average of 7–7.5 hours per night. Differences in RHR as a function of age, BMI, and sleep duration were all statistically significant ($p < 0.01$).[10]

Likewise, sex alone was liable for 4% of the difference in the normal RHR among people, while sex and age together represented 6% of the fluctuation, sex and BMI for 7%, and sex and sleep duration for 5%. Sex, age, BMI, and sleep duration together were responsible for no more than 10% of total inter-individual variability.[10]

Take Home Pearls

- RHR is one of the easiest accessible parameters, and AHA defines the normal sinus HR as between 60 and 100 bpm.
- HR may vary with sex, age, weight/BMI, and sleep.
- Women generally have higher HR compared with men.
- Aging alters autonomic influences on HR regulation.
- Overweight and obese people have a higher HR than people with normal weight, because of their higher metabolic rate and a smaller ratio of body surface to body weight, compared to people with normal weight.

REGULATION OF HR AND SIGNIFICANCE OF I_f CHANNEL

Regulation of HR

HR is controlled by the sympathetic and parasympathetic processes of the autonomic nervous system (ANS) (Fig. 1.1). The parasympathetic system works under relaxed situations while the sympathetic system needs the energy to alert the body in an emergency or stressful condition, i.e. fight or flight state. The sympathetic nervous system (SNS) discharges norepinephrine (NE), enhances the HR and myocardial contractility, and is initiated during exercise, emotional excitement, or pathological conditions, for example, heart failure. The parasympathetic nervous system (PNS) discharges acetylcholine (ACh) and reduces HR.[11]

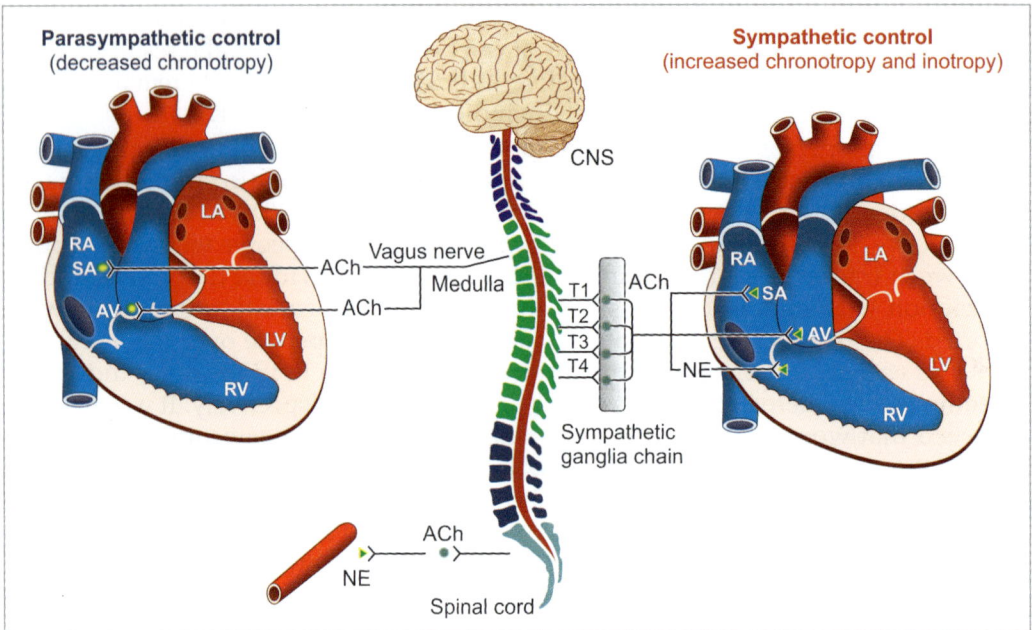

Fig. 1.1: ANS regulation of the heart function. The ANS affects the rate and force of heart contraction. CNS: Central nervous system; RA: Right atria; LA: Left atria; RV: Right ventricle; LV: Left ventricle; SA: Sinoatrial node; AV: Atrioventricular node; NE: Norepinephrine; ACh: Acetylcholine

Cardiac Conduction System

During the normal lifespan, the human heartbeats around 2.5 billion times, an accomplishment achieved by cells of the cardiovascular conduction system (CCS). The functional elements of the CCS can be extensively separated into the impulse-generating nodes (SA node and AV node) and the impulse-propagating His-Purkinje system.[12,13]

Cardiac Action Potential (CAP)

Electrical impulses are the results of the action potential, which is initiated by the sinoatrial (SA) node. This electrical impulse then goes through the heart's electrical conduction system to cause myocardial contraction. The SA node persistently creates electrical impulses, in this way setting the ordinary rhythm and rate in a healthy heart. In the SA node cells, numerous ion channels are present, which help to maintain the ions flow through the channels like sodium channel, HCN channel, calcium channel, and potassium channel.[14]

Channels from the SA Node and CAP Perspective

Hyperpolarization-activated Cyclic Nucleotide-gated (HCN) Channel

HCN channels are additionally called pacemaker channels because of their assumed impact on HR. It has a place with the superfamily of voltage-gated ion channels, and shows increased activation in response to the binding of cyclic adenosine monophosphate (cAMP) to a domain in the C-terminus called the Cyclic Nucleotide-

Binding Domain (CNBD).[15] The activities of the pacemaker start and sustain the electric activity of the heart, independent of the underlying innervations.[16]

Sodium Channel

The sodium channel is a voltage-gated ion channel that looks like an arch-type and consists of 4 homologous domains, arranged in a manner of 4-fold circular symmetry to form the channel. Each sodium channel opens quickly (<1 ms) during over 99% of depolarization. The sodium channel of the cardiac system has consent destinations for phosphorylation by Protein Kinase A (PKA), Protein Kinase C (PKC), and Ca-calmodulin kinase.[16]

Calcium Channel

Calcium channels regulate excitation-contraction coupling, emission, and the activity of many proteins and ion channels. They are the main gateway of the passage of calcium into the cells, a system of intracellular storage sites, and transporters such as the sodium-calcium exchanger. In cardiac muscle, two types of calcium channels are present in the SA node, L-type (low threshold type) and T-type (transient-type).[17] Both these calcium channels differ significantly in their electrical and chemical characteristics and also in the location of these channels in tissues. The L-type channel is responsible for typical myocardial contractility and vascular smooth muscle contractility, and it is commonly found in all cardiac cell types, whereas the T-type channel is found principally in a pacemaker, atrial, and Purkinje cells. It helps in regulating vascular tone, cardiac pacemaking, signal conduction, and also helps in the discharge of certain intercellular transmitters.[17]

Potassium (K⁺) Channel

The cardiac K^+ channel is broadly categorized into three categories: Voltage-gated, internal rectifier channels, and the background K^+ currents. They are also highly regulated and are the basis for the change in action potential configuration in response to variation in HR.[18] Potassium conductance through the potassium channel during the moderate diastolic depolarization will expand the most extreme diastolic potential and moderate the pace of pacemaker depolarization prompting a slower HR.[17]

The Cardiac Rhythm: Ion Channels

The cardiovascular activity expected outcomes from the progression of ions through ion channels, which are the membrane-bound proteins that structure the basic machinery behind heart electrical edginess. Because of changes in electrical potential over the cell membrane, ion channels open and permit particles to go inside the cell and outside the cell along their electrochemical slopes.[19] Ca channel T-type, Ca channel L-type, K channel, I_f channel are the four primary diverts that are engaged with the electric impulse of SA node (Fig. 1.2).[15]

Phases of the Normal Action Potential

Phase 4 is the unconstrained depolarization (pacemaker potential) that triggers the action potential once the membrane potential arrives at a limit between –40 and –30 mV. At the point when the membrane likely is negative (about 60 mV), ion channels open that lead a low, inward (depolarizing) Na^+ current. These currents are classified as "funny" current and truncated as I_f. These depolarizing currents prompt the

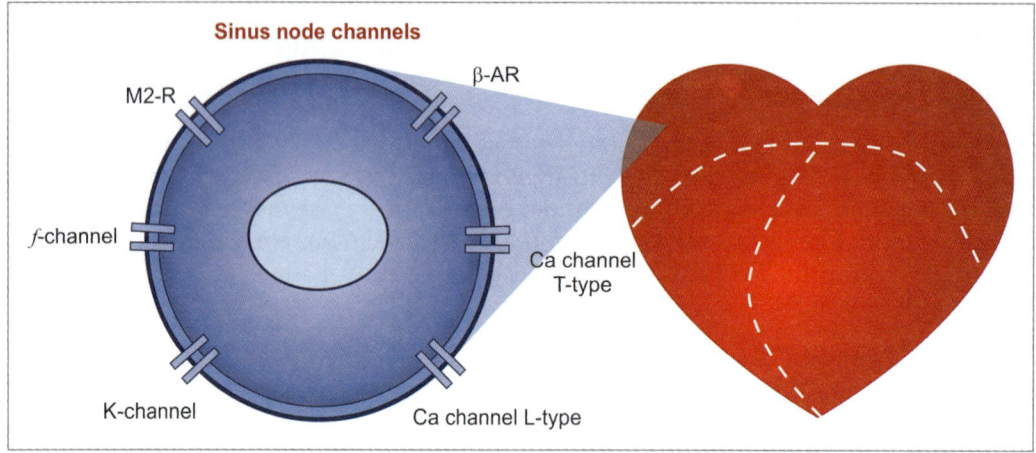

Fig. 1.2: Sinus node and its channel

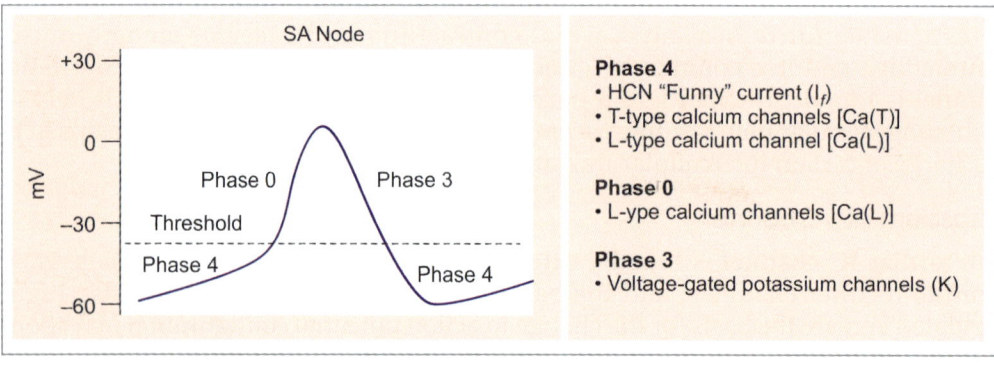

Fig. 1.3: Membrane potentials and ion movement in cardiac conductive cells

membrane potential to start and spontaneously depolarize and thereby starting Phase 4. As the membrane potential reaches about –50 mV, another kind of channel opens. This channel is called transient or T-type Ca^{++} channel. As Ca^{++} enters the cell through these channels down its electrochemical inclination, the inward-directed Ca^{++} flows further depolarize the cell. At the point when the membrane depolarizes to about –40 mV, the second kind of Ca^{++} channel opens. These are the so-called long-lasting or L-type Ca^{++} channels (Fig. 1.3). The opening of these channels causes more Ca^{++} to enter the cell and to additionally depolarize the cell until an activity potential limit is reached (normally between –40 and –30 mV).

Phase 0 depolarization is mainly caused by enhanced Ca^{++} conductance (gCa^{++}) via the L-type Ca^{++} channels that started to open at the end of Phase 4. The "funny" currents and Ca^{++} currents through the T-type Ca^{++} channels decline during this phase as their respective channels remain close. Since the movement of Ca^{++} through these channels into the cell is not quick, the pace of depolarization (slope of Phase 0) is much slower than found in other heart cells (e.g. Purkinje cells).

Phase 3 repolarization happens as K^+ channels open (increased gK^+) in this way increasing the outward-directed, hyperpolarizing K^+ flows. Simultaneously, the L-type Ca^{++} channel become inactivated and close, which decreases gCa^{++} and the inward depolarizing Ca^{++} currents.[20]

I_f Channels and their Significance in Regulation of HR

The pacemaker current, I_f, is vital in the initiation and control of HR. Its dynamic activity begins towards the finish of the repolarization. This channel is activated by intracellular cAMP.[21,22] I_f plays a significant function in the generation of pacemaker action and the regulation of HR. I_f is named 'funny' because of its two peculiar properties: (1) It is a blended sodium-potassium inward current actuated upon hyperpolarization (conversely with most voltage-gated flows), (2) it is directly regulated by cyclic nucleotides.[23]

The f-channels are comprised of the tetrameric relationship of protein subunits coded by the HCN gene channels, which convey the I_f are assigned as HCN channels.[21] HCN channels are actuated by hyperpolarization in the normal range of diastolic membrane potentials. The flows through HCN channels in the SA node are called I_f. It plays a significant key role in the generation of diastolic depolarization and redundant action, as it is enacted by hyperpolarization rather than depolarization.

HCN channel family has four members: HCN1–4, of which the most prevalent family member is HCN4, present in the SA node. cAMP enhances the probability of HCN channel opening (specifically of HCN4, the cardiac pacemaker isoform) and is therefore directly involved in f-channel gating (Fig. 1.4).[21]

The SA node of mammalians is innervated densely with autonomic nervous filaments, controlling heart chronotropic. Sympathetic β-adrenergic stimulation acts by increasing and parasympathetic muscarinic by slowing CV rate. When SA node cells are combined with solutions containing low concentrations of adrenergic agonists, acceleration of unconstrained rate is related to a more extreme slant of diastolic depolarization, with small alteration of action potential duration and shape.

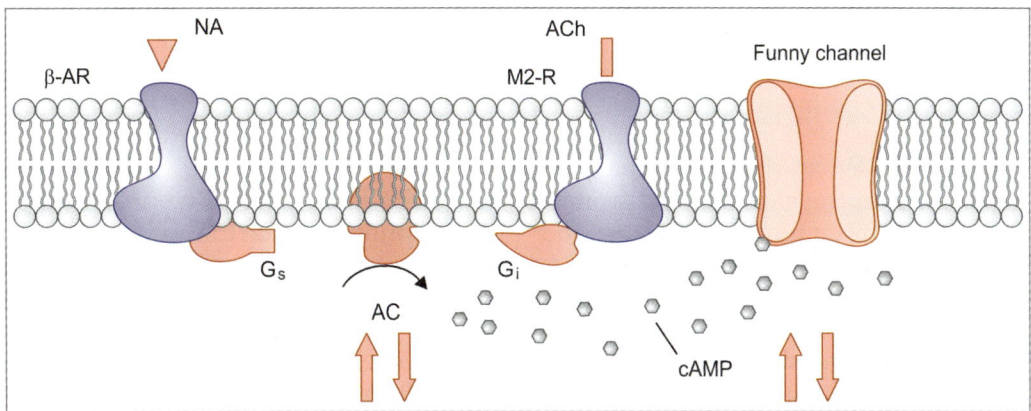

Fig. 1.4: SA node myocyte membrane showing modulation of native funny channels. **ACh:** Acetylcholine; **AC:** Adenylate cyclase; **β-AR:** β-adrenergic receptor; **G$_i$:** Inhibitory G-protein (inhibits AC); **G$_s$:** Stimulatory G-protein (stimulates AC); **M2-R:** Type-2 Muscarinic receptor; **NA:** Noradrenaline (norepinephrine); cAMP: Cyclic adenosine monophosphate

Several additional observations give a definite portrayal of I_f features and more evidence supporting its significance to pacemaker generation and rate control. It has been shown, for example, that β-AR incitement increments I_f by moving the actuation bend of the current to more positive voltages, without alteration of the conductance. The depolarizing shift of the I_f initiation curve is attributable to the β-AR-dependent increment of intracellular cAMP, the second messenger in I_f adjustment. As I_f is controlled by intracellular cAMP and is therefore initiated and repressed by β-AR and M2-R incitement. It represents an essential physiological mechanism intervening autonomic regulation of HR.[24]

I_f channels actuate the diastolic depolarization periods of the SA node activity potential and enhance the rate actuation caused by sympathetic incitement. It also mediates the cAMP-dependent modulation of HR by sympathetic (positive chronotropic, β-adrenergic) and parasympathetic (negative chronotropic, muscarinic cholinergic) stimuli (Table 1.1).[21]

Table 1.1: I_f mediates sympathetic and parasympathetic stimuli

Sympathetic stimuli	Parasympathetic stimuli
β-adrenoceptor stimulation	Muscarinic cholinoceptor stimulation
Activation of adenylate cyclase	Inhibition of adenylate cyclase
Increased local cAMP concentration	Decreased local cAMP concentration
Increased cAMP binding to HCN channels	Decreased cAMP binding to HCN channels
Increased likelihood of channel opening during diastole	Decreased likelihood of channel opening during diastole
Increased rate of diastolic depolarization	Decreased rate of diastolic depolarization
↓ Increased heart rate	↓ Decreased heart rate

cAMP: Cyclic adenosine monophosphate; **HCN:** Hyperpolarization-activated cyclic nucleotide-gated.

Heart Rate Variability (HRV)

HRV is the difference in time between the peaks of the heart in RR spans, which are the result of continuous interaction between two arms of the ANS.[25] Because of the impact of many factors, for example, mental or physical pressure, cardiovascular or non-cardiovascular disease, or pharmacological or invasive treatment, the heart fails to keep up to the same tempo from one heartbeat to the next. By enhancing or diminishing its tempo, the heart responds to any stimulus, so that the body can adjust to any changes. HRV can likewise be recognized in terms of amplitude: Powerless, ordinary, or high. A high HRV is a sign that the heart is healthy as it shows greater adaptability to respond to any pressure (physiological or environmental). On the contrary, decreased HRV can be a result of medical problems and can influence immune capacities, self-regulation, and mental abilities.[26]

Take Home Pearls

- HR is regulated by the sympathetic and parasympathetic input of the autonomic nervous system.

- The human heartbeats 2.5 billion times during a normal lifespan, a feat accomplished by cells of the CCS.
- The SA initiates an action potential that results in an electrical impulse and Ca channel T-type, Ca channel L type, K channel, and I_f channel are the four main channels involved in the electric impulse of the SA node.
- Out of all these channels, I_f plays a major role in the generation of pacemaker activity and the regulation of HR. It both initiates the diastolic depolarization phases of the SA node action potential and accelerates the rate initiation caused by sympathetic stimulation.
- The fluctuations in the time intervals between adjacent heartbeats are termed HRV.
- A high HRV is a sign that the heart is healthy since it has more flexibility to react to any stress, and on the other hand, a reduced HRV is a symptom of health problems and can affect immune functions, self-regulation, and psychological abilities.

FACTORS AFFECTING HR AND HRV

I. Physiological and Pathological Factors

Immune dysfunction leads to low HRV because of incompetent cholinergic reflexes using proinflammatory cytokines. In the long term, this leads to inflammation and cardiovascular disease (CVD). Pathophysiological factors that can affect the HRV are endocrine, respiratory, CV, and neurological factors.[26]

- **Endocrine factors:** Thyroid hormone influences the myocardium by increasing its contractility, but also on the ANS by modifying the sympathetic response. On another side, estrogen levels are connected with HRV measures in healthy women, hence affirming the cardio defensive impact of feminine sexual hormones. Masculine androgens have an advantageous impact (parasympathetic) on the heart autonomous modulation (higher HRV with high testosterone levels) while estradiol tends to incite a parasympathetic action.[26]

- **Neurological factors:** Heart and brain have numerous neural connections between them. If any single structure is impacted HRV will, likewise, be influenced. Neurological disorders associated with brain damage are linked with an HRV decrease: Parkinsonism, spinocerebellar degeneration, Shy-Drager syndrome, multiple sclerosis, Guillain-Barré syndrome. An increase in HRV might, in turn, beneficially affect the symptoms or the pace of the neurological disease.[26,27]

- **Respiratory factors:** Thoracic respiration greatly impacts HRV. A physiological phenomenon happens at every respiration: The respiratory sinus arrhythmia (RSA) where the heartbeat increases with inspiration and decreases with every expiration. Two mechanisms describe RSA: involving tonic and phasic chemo- and barometric reflexes, heart, and lung stretching reflexes, some local metabolic factors, central generators of heart rhythm, and the corresponding nerves (X particularly). RSA is also influenced by other factors, including age, gender, ethnicity, posture, and cardiopulmonary function. These variables can also, in turn, affect the HRV.[26,28]

- **CVD:** HRV is lower for subjects with high BP rather than for subjects with normal BP. A comparative relationship could be built up with an elevated level of blood cholesterol or glucose (diabetes) and a diminished HRV, in this way a reduced HRV can indicate the development of CVD.[26]

- **Other factors:** Many parameters influence HRV, for example, body temperature. If the temperature of the body diminishes enough, it can initiate bradycardia. Alternatively, when the temperature of the body increases as in fever, the heart rate accelerates. The change in HR with these parameters show that ANS and CNS are not by any means the only controllers of HRV; other physiological components are additionally involved.[26]

II. Lifestyle Factors

Lifestyle factors which can influence the HR variation are physical activity, alcohol, tobacco, and drug consumption and meditation, etc.[26]

- **Physical activity:** Physical activity, which can vary from one individual to another, is known to change HRV by diminishing sympathetic activation. According to the Whitehall study, HRV was found to be higher (and cardiac rhythm lower) in subjects having physical activity from moderate-to-vigorous levels. Also, supervised and non-supervised exercise therapy could increase HRV in patients affected by CVDs and diabetes mellitus.[26] Exercise training studies have shown a significant rise in HRV after significant improvements in aerobic capacity. Meersman found that routine aerobic exercise seems to play a role in the maintenance of increased HRV in active men when compared with age- and weight-matched in active individuals. This phenomenon suggests the beneficial role of long-term aerobic exercise in mitigating the age-dependent loss of HRV in physically active persons. There is evidence to suggest that low-pressure cardiopulmonary and high-pressure baroreceptor reflexes might be involved in this.[29]

- **Alcohol, tobacco, and drug consumption:** Utilization of tobacco and alcohol additionally affects HRV. Chronic smokers and alcohol consumers have low HRV; however, this impact is reversible when they quit drinking alcohol or smoking. Alcohol incites an HRV decrease by sympathetic activation or a parasympathetic inhibition.[26] Both active and passive smoking leads to an increase in HRV. Regular consumption of excessive alcohol reduces HRV; while moderate alcohol consumption does not change the HRV drugs can likewise impact HRV. A few drugs (e.g. β-blockers, ACE inhibitors, and psychotropic drugs) have been found to have a direct or indirect influence on HRV.[30] Tricyclic antidepressant medication significantly decreased HRV. Furthermore, results from a study conducted by Dikariyanto *et al.* reveal that snacking on whole almonds instead of typical snacks may reduce the risk of CVD partly by ameliorating the suppression of HRV during periods of mental stress.[31]

- **Meditation:** HRV can be utilized as an indicator of a meditative state. In a transversal study, it was discovered that autogenic meditation (also called "Schultz's autogenic training") prompts an increase of cardiac coherence (CC) score, and of alpha, beta, and gamma brainwaves, and it indicates an improved structural or functional connection between cortical and thalamic regions. This increase is related to an increased attention span and reinforced autonomous regulation (ANS).[26]

III. Non-modifiable Factors

- **Age:** Although RHR is not directly related to increasing age, there is a reduction in HRV as age progresses, which might be a biological marker of the aging process. The impact of aging on HRV has been attributed to a decrease in efferent vagal cardiac tone and diminished β-adrenergic responsiveness. Autonomic derailments can be responsible for increasing cardiovascular degeneration in the aging population, moving the autonomic balance toward sympathetic dominance.[29]

- **Gender and ethnicity:** It has been known that there is a distinction among people in the way the ANS is controlled and thus in the sympathetic–parasympathetic balance and this shows itself in varying HRVs. This contrast between the sexes diminishes as individual approach the age of 50, a fact that is ascribed to the postmenopausal hormonal changes that occur in women.

  In the systemic review, Thayer *et al.* mentioned that ethnicity affects BP and subsequently on HRV. The ethnic origin appears affect HRV. In a meta-analysis including 17 studies and a sum of 11,162 test subjects, Hill *et al.* established a fundamentally higher short-term resting HRV in the Afro-American people than in American people of European origin.[26,30]

IV. Environmental Factors

Apart from environmental conditions and profession related influences, some harmful substances can also affect HRV.[30] These factors include environmental particulate matter, several chemical components, electromagnetic fields (EMF), vibrating tools, psychosocial charge, working time, fatigue, etc. Long-term exposure to these factors causes a decline in HRV.[26] Environmental factors prompt changes in HRV due to the physiological reaction of the vegetative sensory system. SNS activity is increased by heat, which reduces HRV. However, long-term exposure to cold (e.g. at work or throughout winter) has not been found to affect HRV because of adaptation effects. Exposure to the commotion, induced pain decreases HRV due to its impact on SNS activity. Night shift works over numerous years have a lower HRV due to the chronodisruption.[30]

V. Neuropsychological Factors

HRV is not linked to the only personality but a list of psychological considerations, for example, stress, depression, and negative emotions.[26]

- **Stress:** Stress is a very important factor that impacts HRV. Many stressful conditions can lead to low HRV, for example, anxiety, hostility, depression, and work stress. Many analyzed studies uncovered a noteworthy connection between a significant level of work pressure and low HRV. Stress also corresponds with a greater risk of CVD and a high HR.[26]

- **Depression:** The low HRV value, even if depression is not correlated with a CVD, remains an indicator of poor health. A meta-analysis by Kemp showed a significant correlation between depression and a low HRV.[31]

- **Negative emotions:** Many negative emotions like outrage, tension, dissatisfaction, and worry can lead to a diminished HRV.[26] A transversal study on healthy subjects affirmed the significant correspondence between weak neuroticism (negative emotions) and diminished HRV and the inverse as well. Kemp and Quintana also concluded that HRV holds significant functional importance on social conduct, self-regulation, and mental adaptability against life stressors.[32]

Measuring HR and HRV

Monitoring and analysis of HR give important data concerning well-being status and have been widely researched in various activities of healthy subjects as well as in patients experiencing different diseases.[33] To limit the impacts of various confounding factors, the estimation of HR ought to be carefully standardized.[34] According to the Consensus Panel of the European Society of Hypertension, the accompanying data ought to be given in considers detailing HR information: (1) Resting period before estimation; (2) ecological conditions; (3) strategy for estimation; (4) number of estimations; (5) span of measurement; (6) body position; and (7) nature of the observer. The following are the suggestions given by the board concerning how HR ought to be measured.[35]

Procedures for HR Measurement[35]

- The patient ought to be permitted to sit for at least 5 minutes in a quiet room at an agreeable temperature.
- HR ought to be estimated over a 30-second time frame by pulse palpation.
- At least two estimations in the sitting position ought to be taken.
- For subjects in whom orthostatic BP estimation is performed, HR ought to be estimated after each BP perusing.
- Results may differ as per whether HR is estimated by a specialist, a medical caretaker, or a programmed gadget.
- Patients performing self-BP estimation should likewise gather HR information.

Techniques for HR Measurement

Traditionally, HR is estimated by pulse palpation.[34] Apart from pulse palpation, different techniques to quantify HR incorporate ECG-and PPG-based wearable gadgets. A brief overview of various HR measuring techniques and their principles are given below:

Pulse palpation: The pulse rate is estimated by including the beats in a set timeframe (from 15 to 60 seconds) and multiplying that number to get the number of bpm. The pulse rate can be estimated anytime on the body where an artery is near the surface.[34] The two most regular spots to gauge HR utilizing a two-finger palpation strategy are at the wrist (using radial artery) and the neck (through the carotid artery).[36]

Electrocardiography (ECG): With the help of ECG, HR is measured more accurately and for longer periods.[34] Dynamic ECG screens show HR, yet it can likewise be determined from a printed following utilizing both of two strategies:

- When the HR is standard, count the number of large (0.2 second) boxes between 2 progressive QRS and divide 300 by this number. The number of large time boxes is divided into 300 because $300 \times 0.20 = 60$, and HR are determined in bpm or 60 seconds. For instance, if there are 3 large boxes between QRS complexes, the HR is 100 bpm because $300 \div 3 = 100$. Also, if 4 large time boxes are tallied between QRS complexes, the HR is 75 bpm (Fig. 1.5).
- If the HR is unpredictable, the principal strategy would not be precise because the stretches between QRS complexes differ from beat to beat. In most cases, the ECG chart paper is scored with marks at 3-second spans. In such cases, simply tally the number of QRS complexes every 3 or 6 seconds and multiply this number by 20 or 10, respectively.[37]

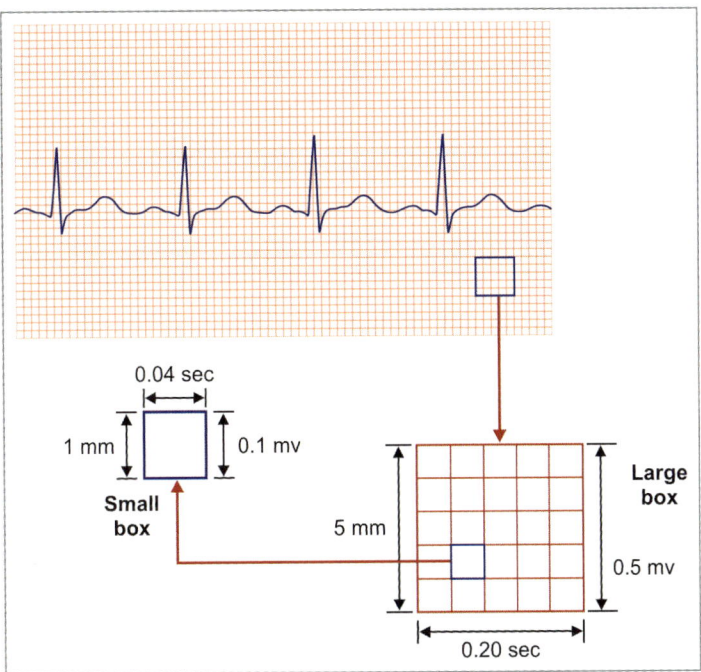

Fig. 1.5: The normal ECG tracing

- **Advantages:**[38]
    - High processing speed
    - Good reproducibility

- **Disadvantages:** An ordinary ECG is perpetually undermined by: [39]
    - Electrical impedance from encompassing hardware (for example, impacts of the electrical mains supply)
    - Measurement (or electrode contact) commotion
    - Electromyogram commotion (muscle contraction)
    - Movement heirloom
    - Instrumentation clamor (for example, an heirloom from the analog-to-digital conversion process).

Wearable devices and PPG: In the past few year's consumer wearable gadgets, include smartwatches, wristbands, wearable mobile sensors, and fitness trackers, have become exceptionally popular.[40] The ascent in the accessibility of consumer wearable devices that create well-being data gives an uncommon chance to change medical services by scientists, clinicians, and customers. These wearable gadgets depend on PPG, which is an optical method that identifies blood volume changes in the microvascular bed of tissue under the skin surface. PPG uses four segments to quantify HR: Optical producer, digital signal processor (DSP), accelerometer, and calculations (Fig. 1.6).[41,42] Wearable PPG sensors can utilize various shades of light, for example, green or red, to record these adjustments in blood volume to each having different expenses and benefits.[40]

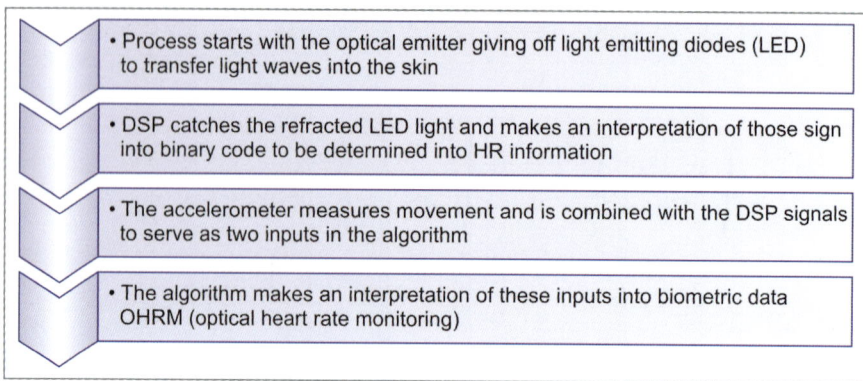

- Process starts with the optical emitter giving off light emitting diodes (LED) to transfer light waves into the skin

- DSP catches the refracted LED light and makes an interpretation of those sign into binary code to be determined into HR information

- The accelerometer measures movement and is combined with the DSP signals to serve as two inputs in the algorithm

- The algorithm makes an interpretation of these inputs into biometric data OHRM (optical heart rate monitoring)

Fig. 1.6: PPG components to measure HR

- **Advantages:**[43]
  - Non-intrusive
  - Inexpensive
  - Convenient

- **Disadvantages:** Results of PPG may differ due to: [42,44]
  - Optical commotion (a portion of the light produced, which signs as bloodstream)
  - Skin tone (more obscure skin tones and skin with tattoos)
  - Crossover issue (blunder by the algorithm mistaking other inputs as HR data because of similar continuous movement)
  - Sensor area
  - Low profusion to limits can pose challenges dependent on low bloodstream and high optical commotion.
  - Tissue modification produced by voluntary or involuntary movements can make changes of inner tissues, for example, muscle movement and dilation of tissues.

Measurement of HRV

HRV, which represents the variation of the beat-to-beat interval, is a simple and non-intrusive technique to assess ANS functions that impact CV systems.[45] Three methodologies used to screen HRV: time-domain and frequency-domain measures are linear; whereas complexity measures offer a non-linear approach.[46] Clinicians and researchers measure HRV using time-domain, frequency-domain, and non-linear indices.[47]

- **Time-domain measures:** Time-domain indices quantify the amount of HRV observed during monitoring periods that may range from <1 minute to >24 hours. The statistical metrics include the SDNN, SDANN, SDNN Index, RMSSD, SDSD, NN50, pNN50, etc.[47] Out of all these time-domain measures, the SDNN, SDANN, and SDNNi indices are obtained long-term records and represent the sympathetic and parasympathetic activity, while the rMSSD and pNN50 indexes represent the parasympathetic activity, as they are found from the analysis of adjoining RR intervals.[48] Time-domain geometric methods allow the presentation of cardiac pulse intervals (systole and diastole) and use approximations to derive the HRV measurements. The main geometric methods used are triangular index (RRtri), triangular interpolation of RR intervals (TINN), differential index, and logarithmic index.[49]

- **Frequency domain (spectral estimation of the HRV):** Frequency domain estimations gauge the distribution of absolute or relative power into four frequency bands that include ultra-low-frequency (ULF), very-low-frequency (VLF), low-frequency (LF), and high-frequency (HF).[47,50]
- **Non-linear methods:** Non-linear indices measure the unpredictability and complexity of a series of interbeat intervals (IBIs).[48] The time arrangement 1, 2, 3, 1, 2, 3 has a similar inconstancy as the time arrangement 1, 1, 2, 2, 3, 3 and 3, 1, 2, 2, 3, 1, yet different underlying patterns. The non-linear analysis enables the measurement of this additional data. Essentially, the non-linear approach methodology measures the complexity of the signal; how frequently do similar patterns reoccur? [46]

Principle Disease Linked to HRV

CVDs are one of the fundamental causes of morbidity and mortality around the world. In developing countries, CVDs are responsible for approximately 17 million deaths every year. Cardiac autonomic dysfunction is a risk factor for the progression of CVD that can be measured non-invasively using HRV. HRV has relation to a wide spectrum of ailments (Fig. 1.7). Physiologically, HRV is the result of adaptive changes in HR caused by the sympathetic nervous system (SNS) and parasympathetic nervous

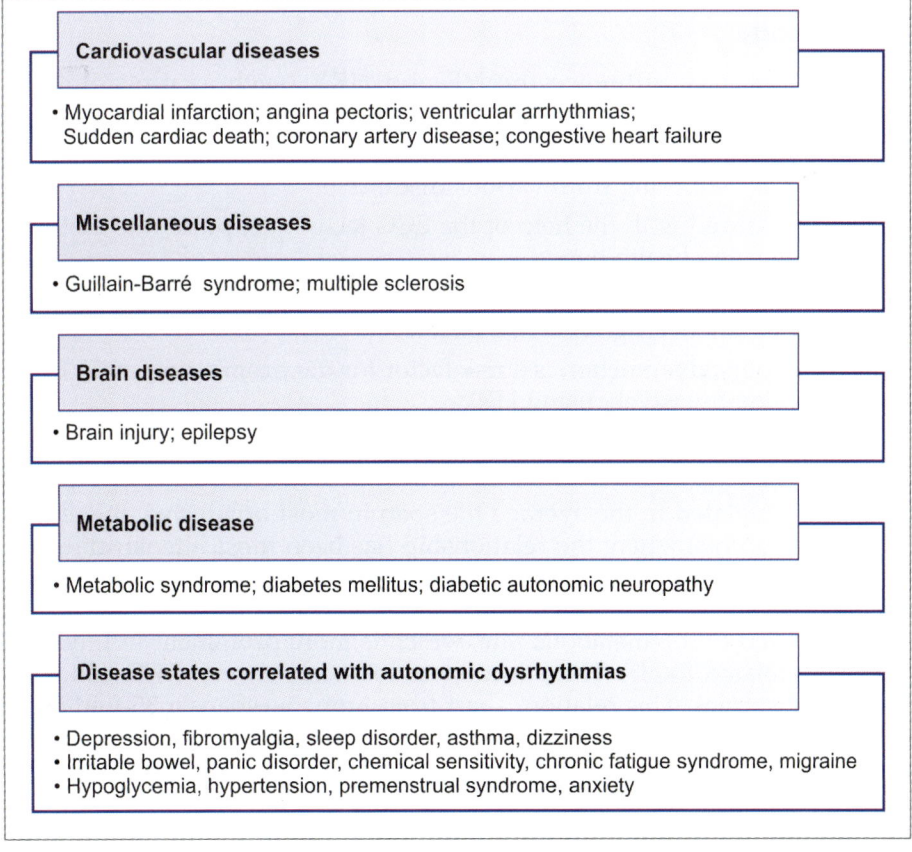

Fig. 1.7: Principal diseases related to HRV

system (PNS) with the purpose to buffer blood pressure (BP). Low HRV indicates a diminished adaptive capacity of ANS and is believed to increase morbidity. HRV has long been known to be related to morbidity and mortality after myocardial infarction (MI). Other than acute MI and cardiac death, events of congestive HF and arrhythmias have likewise been related to decreased HRV.[51,52]

When RHR should Consider Elevated?

Similar to the continuous discussion of a suitable cut-off for deciding hypertension (HTN), the limit of what ought to be viewed as an elevated HR is a discussion between the advantages and disadvantages of treatment. About 25% of the general population shows RHR above 80 bpm.[53]

In the National Health and Nutrition Examination Survey (NHANES), an RHR over 90 bpm was present in 5.2% of men and 8.4% of women. Whereas in the Cooper Clinic study, an RHR of >80 bpm was found to have a similar risk as a BP ≥140/90 mmHg. This could be utilized as a current reasonable guide. A threshold of >80 bpm ought no longer to be taken as an indication of sickness; however, a practical rule of thumb for urging people to improve the lifestyle factors identified with elevated RHR. These factors could include known CV risk factors, for example, decreasing smoking, increasing physical activity level, assessment of BP, lipids, and diabetes, and decreasing alcohol consumption and diet.[53]

Take Home Pearls

- Several factors may influence the HR and HRV (such as physiological and pathological factors, lifestyle, ecological, and neuropsychological factors).
- Monitoring and investigation of HR provide valuable information regarding health status in patients suffering from various diseases.
- HR can be measured with the help of the ECG technique, pulse rate method, PPG method, or by using health bands.
- Decreased HRV is an indicator of mortality and arrhythmic complications that is independent of other recognized risk factors.
- Cardiac autonomic dysfunction is a risk factor for the progression of CVD that can be estimated non-invasively using HRV.

GENETIC INFLUENCES ON HR AND LONGEVITY

RHR is inversely related to the average life span in most organisms. Indeed, among well-evolved creatures, where the relationship has been most intensively surveyed, there is a linear, inverse semilogarithmic relationship between average RHR and average life expectancy in all species. The association between HR and life expectancy has been attributed to the metabolic rate, which is more prominent in tiny creatures and is directly related to HR. There is a linear relation between RHR and longevity across different species. This relation, apart from humans, spans a 35-fold difference in heart rate and a 20-fold difference in the life span of other mammals. Numerous other factors influence HR, for example, genetic influences on the cell biology of electrically active atrial tissues, autonomic nervous activity, inflammatory processes, etc. Each of these factors that influence HR may likewise independently affect life expectancy.[54,55]

The average number of heartbeats per life is almost constant across species and is in the order of 10^9. Drawing from a wide allometric scale of 10^{20}-fold among living creatures, Azbel concludes that the energy utilization/body atom per HR is the equivalent in all creatures. According to his calculation, basal O_2 utilization is ~$10\ O_2$ molecules/lifetime and in those creatures with a heart ~$10^{-8}\ O_2$ molecules/heartbeat. HR is essentially hypothesized as an epiphenomenon of the rate of basal O_2 consumption and heartbeat.[55]

According to twin studies in youth- and middle-aged grown-ups, the assessments of heritability, i.e. genetic variability expressed as a portion of the total variation in HRV, ranged from 13 to 65%.[56] Whereas another twin study of time-domain HRV measures, based on 24-hour ambulatory recordings yielded noteworthy heritabilities of time-domain variables ranging from 46 to 57% and demonstrated a considerable overlap of hereditary effects on two time-domain HRV measures: Standard deviation of the R-R intervals (SDNN) and the square root of the mean squared differences between successive R-R intervals (RMSSD).[57]

Genetic Determinants of HR

RHR reflecting the balance of sympathetic and parasympathetic inputs is genetically regulated in hierarchical and yet integrative biological networks, including the autonomous nervous and hormonal frameworks. In the observational investigations, RHR was recommended to be a modifiable factor or an important treatment target for individuals with CVD. Recent observations found a positive relationship between high RHR and the risk of impaired fasting glucose, metabolic syndrome (MetS), and type-2 diabetes (T2D). Studies showed a 1.89-fold risk in developing T2D and a greater than the 4-fold risk for MetS when comparing participants in the highest quintile of RHR with those in the lowest. Guo *et al.* conducted a genome-wide association study (GWAS) to understand the genetic relationship between RHR and cardiometabolic disorders/T2D. This study analyzed the genetic relationship, causality, and shared genetic qualities among RHR and T2D utilizing low-density (LD) score regression, summed up summary data-based Mendelian randomization, and transcriptome-wide association scan (TWAS) and summary level data for T2D and 8 cardiometabolic traits. Result revealed a significant hereditary relationship between RHR and T2D ($r_g = 0.22$; 95% CI: 0.18 to 0.26; $p = 1.99 \times 10^{-22}$), and 6 cardiometabolic traits (r_g range- 0.12 to 0.24; all $p < 0.05$). RHR has a significant assessed causal impact on T2D (odds ratio: 1.12 per 10 bpm increment; $p = 7.79 \times 10^{-11}$) and weaker causal impact from T2D to RHR (0.32 bpm per doubling increment in T2D prevalence; $p = 6.14 \times 10^{-54}$). These outcomes give insights into the shared etiology for high RHR and T2D.[58]

To gain more comprehensive insights into the genetic regulation of HR, den Hoed *et al.* in 2012, performed a 2 stage meta-analysis of GWAS in data from up to 181,171 individuals. In this meta-analysis, loci associated with HR were subsequently tested for association among HR and CVD and mortality. Also, experimental studies from *Drosophila melanogaster* and *Danio rerio* models as an initial step toward recognizing the causal genes within the associated loci were included to support the meta-analysis. Den Hoed identified that 14 new loci previously unknown, to be robustly associated with HR and affirmed the relationship with all 7 previously established loci. Also, results from experiments in *Drosophila melanogaster* and *Danio rerio* models support a role in HR regulation for 20 candidate genes from 11 loci that are applicable for HR regulation, and highlight a role for genes involved in signal transmission, embryonic cardiac development, and the pathophysiology of dilated cardiomyopathy, congenital HF and/or sudden cardiac death. Also, genetic susceptibility to increased HR is related to alter cardiac conduction and diminished risk of sick sinus syndrome, and both HR- increasing and HR-decreasing variants associate with the risk of CVD. These observations provide new insights into the mechanisms that regulate or modulate HR in health and disease and provide a new perspective on the well-recognized association of HR with CVD and mortality.[59]

In several epidemiological studies, it was noticed that South Asian (SA) men and women worldwide have a high risk of CVD. Individuals of SA origin experiences a 1.5-fold increased coronary disease in contrast to the general population. SA individuals also have an increased prevalence of impaired glucose tolerance, insulin resistance, and T2D. Diabetes and dysglycemia are related to increased HR and abnormal cardiac sympathovagal balance and are indicative of increased coronary mortality. Bathula *et al.* in the study showed that on average, SA have 5 bpm higher HR-PPG than Europeans, observations that appeared to be genetically determined and were not linked with other risk factors.[60] Similarly, Neil *et al.* conducted a prospective cohort study, involving 200 SA and 200 caucasian healthy volunteers. P-wave indices, HRV, and anthropometry in SA volunteers were compared with white European healthy volunteers. SA were found to be of smaller height with lower lean body weight and smaller left atrial size. They had a higher mean HR and SA males had lower HRV, suggestive of sympathetic predominance.[61]

HR in the Indian Population

Indian population shows elevated RHR because of their increased sympathetic overactivity (SO). It relates to both systolic blood pressure (SBP) and diastolic blood pressure (DBP) as well as with BMI.[62] SO plays a significant role in the development of CVDs. It causes an elevation in HR, cardiac output, peripheral vascular resistance, and sodium reabsorption in the kidney and a consequent increase in BP. It is additionally found to be related to the prolongation of cardiac repolarization time and may plays a crucial role in increasing CVD in patients.[63] SO depends on the hormonal factors involved in the homeostatic control of the CV functions. According to a pan India, non-interventional, cross-sectional study, a noteworthy correlation has been found between SO and HR and also between SO and HTN.[63,64]

According to India Heart Study (IHS), the predominance of white coat hypertension (WCH) and masked hypertension (MH) in India is higher in comparison with worldwide data that is associated with increasing HR. In the Indian population, it was observed that the evening BP was higher than the morning SBP (127.8 ± 14.7 *vs* 129.8 ± 15.3) mmHG and DBP (81.9 ± 10.1 *vs* 82.4 ± 10.2) mmHg. The predominance of WCH was 24%, and 18% of the participants had masked HTN. More than half of the participants of IHS had an elevated RHR (79.8 ± 9.6 bpm). An elevated HR was more common in WCH.[65]

Another India Ambulatory Blood Pressure Measurement (ABPM) study was conducted between Jan 2017 to Nov 2018 to investigate sex-related differences in HR and BP patterns in 14,977 Indian subjects. The study revealed that women had higher HR both during the day and nighttime and they had a lower HR dip than men, suggesting a higher risk of all-cause mortality and CV events. During the daytime, females HR compared to men was (80.3 ± 11.2 *vs* 79.4 ± 11.5 bpm), at nighttime (71.4 ± 10.6 *vs* 68.9 ± 10.6 bpm), and over 24 hours (77.4 ± 10.6 *vs* 75.9 ± 10.6 bpm), respectively

(p <.001). For SBP, a lower daytime ABPM (131 ± 16 vs 133 ± 14 mmHg, p <.001) but higher nighttime ABPM (122 ± 18 vs 121 ± 16 mmHg, p <.001) was found in females compared to males. At nighttime in the ABPM study, it was observed that HR diminished when contrasted with daytime for both males and females, but this decrease at nighttime was larger for males than for females (−10.5 ± 8.0 vs −8.8 ± 6.8 bpm, p <0.001). Females, especially after menopause, had significant differences in ABPM limits when contrasted with males, thus indicating a less favorable CV prognosis.[66] According to the Beat survey, a cross-sectional study across India, comprising 3,743 patients with mean age 45.69 ± 6.86 years, Indian HTN patients display elevated RHR. The average RHR and BP in the Beat survey were discovered to be 82.79 ± 10.41 bpm and 146.82 ± 15.46/89.08 ± 8.8 mmHg. In this investigation, the HR was found to have relation with SBP (r = 0.247, p <0.01), DBP (r = 0.219, p <0.01); to lower extent with BMI (r = 0.041, p <0.05); yet not with age (r = 0.012, NS).[62]

Rajalakshmi et $al.$ in 2012 led a cross-sectional study, to assess HRV in obese Indian young adults (n = 150) and to build up a relationship between HRV indices and obesity indices. The results of the investigation revealed that a significant increase in the mean HR, LF (nu), and LF/HF ratio was observed in obese people compared with the normal-weight group, whereas time-domain matrices variables, total power, HF(AV), and HF (nu) were altogether lower (p <0.05). Pearson's correlation coefficient demonstrated that time-domain matrices variables negatively correspond with BMI and waist stature ratio (WSR) which was statistically significant. Furthermore, on regression analysis, BMI was found to be a major predictor for HRV variations. The study results showed reduced HRV, higher sympathetic, and lower parasympathetic nerve movement in obese subjects. HRV indices were essentially related to obesity indices, and BMI is the significant determinant for the progressions in both time and frequency domain indices.[67]

Take Home Pearls

- A linear, inverse semilogarithmic relationship is observed between RHR and average life expectancy in all species aside from humans.
- The average number of heartbeats per life is almost steady across species and is in the order of 10^9.
- RHR has been suggested to be a modifiable factor or a significant treatment target for people with CVD.
- SA men and women have a high risk of CHD. They experience a 1.5-fold increased coronary disease risk compared to the general population.
- RHR has a wide variation across the world. Asians and Indians have been found to have a higher RHR.
- Indian popultion shows increased RHR because of their increased SO.

HIGH RHR AND ITS ASSOCIATION WITH ADVERSE CLINICAL AND CV OUTCOMES

Impact of High RHR in General Population without CVD

High RHR is a risk factor for CV morbidity and mortality in normal individuals as well as in patients with cardiac disorders. Among hypertensive individuals, raised HR is a common feature.[68] The heightened sympathetic tone has a crucial role in the connection between RHR and BP on the grounds that it causes an elevation in HR, cardiac output, peripheral vascular resistance, and kidney sodium reabsorption, which thus leads to the rise of BP. High RHR is related to endothelial dysfunction, diminished artery compliance and distensibility, and thus increased arterial wall stress and raised pulsed-wave velocity, which is additionally connected with increased afterload and eventually systemic HTN.[69] Several investigations have exhibited that individuals with high HR have elevated BP readings and that this affiliation is stronger in subjects with raised sympathetic activity. The reasons may be that HTN and tachycardia having a mutual underlying factor: Increased sympathetic tone. In the Syst-Eur study (systolic hypertension in Europe); performed in elderly patients with systolic HTN, it was discovered that the patients with an HR >79 bpm had an 89% more risk of mortality than those with an HR ≤79 bpm.[70] Whereas in the Tensiopulse study, which assessed 38,145 patients, treated by 2000 general experts all over Italy, it was discovered that 30% of the hypertensive patients had an RHR ≥80 bpm.[68] On the other hand, data derived from Hypertension and Ambulatory Recording VEnetia Study (HARVEST) exhibited that baseline RHR and changes in HR in the first few months of follow-up were able to predict the development of sustained HTN in white, younger subjects assessed for stage 1 HTN.[69] The Kaliuan study furthermore indicated that around 40% of individuals without arterial HTN or cardiac arrhythmias at baseline developed HTN during the mean follow-up time of 3.5 ± 0.9 years. An increase in RHR by 10 bpm was associated with an 8% increase in new-onset of HTN.[71]

A rise in RHR is not just associated with a poorer outcome in patients with HTN but also in CAD. Among men and women without known CVD, an elevation in RHR over 10-year period was related to an elevated risk of death from IHD in patients with no known reason for mortality. Patients with RHR under 70 bpm at the first measurement yet more than 85 bpm at the subsequent assessment had a risk of death from IHD that was 90% higher, and risk of death from all causes that was 50% higher. Nauman J et al. utilized RHR as a constant variable and consolidated the squared estimation of RHR to assess nonlinear patterns. To allow visual assessment of the pattern, they presented hazard ratios for the following categories of change in RHR: (1) A decline of greater than 25 bpm; (2) a decline between 15 and 25 bpm; (3) a decline between 5 and 15 bpm; (4) a change from –5 to 5 bpm (reference); (5) an increment between 5 and 15 bpm; (6) an increment between 15 and 25 bpm; and (7) an increment of greater than 25 bpm.[72]

According to a British Regional Heart Study, during a follow-up period involving 7,735 individuals, in men with no confirmation of IHD, there was a substantial positive relationship between RHR and age-adjusted rates of all major IHD events (fatal and nonfatal), IHD-related deaths, and sudden cardiac death. After adjustment for age, SBP, cholesterol, smoking, social class, hefty drinking, and physical activity, this association was still noteworthy, though in men with prior IHD, the association was significant but less pronounced. It was observed that elevated HR ≥90 bpm is a risk factor, especially for sudden cardiac death; it is free of other built up coronary risk factors and is most obviously found in men with no past IHD at the time of the underlying examination. These findings from the study reveal that increased HR ≥90 is a risk factor for fatal IHD, especially for sudden CV death.[73]

As RHR is a non-invasive marker of cardiac function and a nice indicator of physical wellness and general well-being, raised RHR assessed at a single point is related to a higher risk of death from most causes, including cancer, independent of BP, and one of the main socio-demographic and lifestyle risk factor. According to the MCCS accomplice study, a long-term increase in RHR was related to higher mortality. It was discovered in the study that all-cause mortality risk for participants whose RHR increased from <70 bpm to 70–85 bpm was higher by 24% compared with those who kept a healthy RHR of 70 bpm or less between the benchmark and wave 2. RHR monitoring during general practitioner visits or utilizing wellness gadgets could help distinguish population subgroups at higher mortality risk.[74]

Also, it was known that the degree of relationship between RHR and the risk of all-cause and CV mortality differ across investigations. Zhang D *et al.* in 2017 conducted a meta-analysis to quantitatively assess the relationship in the general population. An aggregate of 46 investigations were included in the meta-analysis, involving 1,246,203 patients and 78,349 deaths for all-cause mortality, and 8, 48,320 patients and 25,800 deaths for CV mortality. The relative risk with 10 bpm increase of RHR was found to be 1.09 (95% CI: 1.067–1.12) for all-cause mortality and 1.08 (95% CI: 1.06–1.10) for CV mortality. Patients with an RHR of 60–80 bpm had a relative risk of 1.12 (95% CI: 1.07–1.17) for all-cause mortality and 1.08 (95% CI: 0.99–1.17) for CV mortality, and those with an RHR of more noteworthy than 80 bpm had a relative risk of 1.45 (95% CI: 1.34–1.57) for all-cause mortality and 1.33 (95% CI: 1.19–1.47) for CV mortality. When contrasted with 45 bpm, the risk of all-cause mortality increased altogether with elevated RHR in a linear relation, yet an essentially increased risk of CV mortality was seen at 90 bpm. These findings revealed that higher RHR was independently associated with increased risks of all-cause and CV mortality.[75]

As there is a substantial connection between raised RHR and increased incidence of CVDs, elevated RHR somewhere in the range of 50 and 60 years old was found to be connected with an increased risk of CVD when contrasted with individuals with stable RHR. Chen XJ *et al.* in a 25-year follow-up study, revealed that men with an RHR >75 bpm at 50 years old have twice as high-risk of all-cause death, CVD, and CHD compared with men with RHR ≤55. As per their study, participants with a baseline RHR of >75 bpm in 1993 had about a two-fold higher risk of all-cause death compared with those with <55 bpm in 1993.[76]

Impact of High RHR in Patients with CVD

High RHR adds to CVD mortality by triggering the deposition of atherosclerotic plaques by exerting mechanical stress on the walls of the arteries. Raised RHR might point to underlying arrhythmias, which increment mortality risk.[74] In patients with CAD high RHR incites CV events primarily through ventricular arrhythmias or progressive pump failure. Additionally, coronary plaque disruption is likewise related to the elevated RHR, as it represents a predictor for coronary plaque instability. Studies have demonstrated that elevated RHR was related to higher triglyceride, total cholesterol, non-HDL cholesterol, and apolipoprotein B, as well as endothelial dysfunction which could be an additional factor that associates elevated RHR and CAD. The Kailuan study demonstrated that the risk of MI was 10% higher in the most noteworthy quintile bunch contrasted and the least quintile RHR gathering (HR: 1.10; 95% CI: 1.01–1.20). Whereas Aune *et al.* in the huge meta-analysis, including 12,27,511 participants revealed that a rise of RHR above 10 bpm was related to 7% higher risk of CAD (HR 1.07; 95% CI: 1.05–1.10) and 9% for sudden cardiac death (HR: 1.09; 95% CI: 1.00–1.18).[69]

Aging of the population, worsening risk factor profile, and improved management of acute CVD have all led to increased prevalence of heart failure (HF). RHR is independently connected with outcome among patients with HF and RHR lowering has been exhibited to benefit patients with HF and reduced ejection fraction.[77] The role of RHR in HF is especially significant on account of its significance for clinical treatment in these patients. Both sympathetic and renin-angiotensin-aldosterone systems overactivity is mainly responsible for the relationship between RHR and HF. The reasons behind this association are increased oxygen consumption, decreased myocardial perfusion, and consequently decreased cardiac performance (hemodynamic changes and ultimately pro-arrhythmic effect. An additional mechanism that explains the relationship between RHR and mortality in HF is inflammation, endothelial dysfunction, and increased oxidative stress. Woodward *et al.* reported that patients with RHR >80 bpm had a 2-time higher risk of HF death than individuals with RHR <65 bpm. Whereas the Rotterdam study uncovered that every increase of 10 bpm increased the risk of development of HF for 16% in men.[69]

RHR is similarly very important for the prognosis of patients after MI. According to the meta-analysis that included around 20,000 patients from GISSI preliminaries, demonstrated the in-hospital mortality of patients after MI with HR <60 bpm was essentially lower than in patients when HR rises >100 bpm (3.3% *vs* 10.1%).[69] Whereas data from the PERFORM study, including 19,000 patients uncovered that RHR ≥70 bpm was related to 32% increased relative risk for fatal or nonfatal MI (HR 1.32; 95% CI: 1.03–1.69). Every 5-bpm RHR increment raised the relative risk for fatal and nonfatal MI by 11.3%. These findings revealed that in patients with recent non-cardio-embolic cerebral ischemia event, raised RHR ≥70 is a prognostic factor and is related to a higher risk for MI.[78]

Elevated RHR has been demonstrated to be prognostically connected with adverse events across several population studies. In the acute setting in patients with acute MI, raised HR has been additionally demonstrated to be related to poor results both in the prethrombolytic and contemporary eras. An HR >80 bpm at the time of admission was related to 3–5 times the danger of mortality compared to lower HR. Regardless of the reality that the treatment has improved fundamentally during recent years; there is still a significant relationship between increased HR at admission and increased in-hospital mortality.[4] Hjalmarson *et al.* identified in 1807 patients with acute MI, the connection between HR on hospital admittance and after discharge from the hospital and respectively total mortality from admittance to discharge and mortality at 1 year. It was observed in the study that the in-hospital mortality and post-discharge mortality increased with elevated HR on admittance. Likewise, the total mortality was found to be 15% for patients with an admittance HR in the range of 50 and 60 bpm, 41% for HR 90 bpm, and 48% for HR >110 bpm. Mortality from hospital discharge to 1 year was additionally identified with the maximal HR in the coronary care unit and to HR at discharge. In patients with moderate HF, the combined mortality for patients with an admittance HR of ≥90 bpm was more than twice that of patients with an admittance HR of 90 bpm (39% *vs* 18%). A comparative relationship was also seen in patients with mild or no HF (18% *vs* 10%).[79,80]

The prognostic implication of HR was similarly assessed in 8,915 patients with acute MI of the GISSI-2 study, treated with fibrinolytic treatment. In this examination, elevated HR on admittance was related to a progressive increment of in-hospital mortality (7.1% for HR <60 bpm to 23.4% for HR >100 bpm). A dynamic increase of 6-month mortality was noted with elevated HR (0.8% for HR <60 bpm to 14.3% for HR

>100 bpm). The multivariate assessment indicated that HR was an independent prognostic factor of mortality. Similar results were observed in the Secondary Prevention Reinfarction Israeli Nifedipine Trial (SPRINT), performed before the thrombolytic era, which demonstrated that HR on admittance in the coronary care unit was related to total mortality and the events of complications.[79]

Whereas according to a prospective, multicenter study, structured to examine the predominance of Prevalence of Peripheral Arterial Disease in Patients with Acute Coronary Syndrome (PAMISCA), an RHR ≥70 bpm in patients who have an Acute Coronary Syndrome (ACS) is an indicator of a high risk of suffering CV events during follow-up. It was discovered in the study that patients with HR ≥70 bpm had poorer prognosis, with additional hospitalizations for HF and higher CV and non-CV mortality rates, while in the multivariate analysis, HR ≥70 bpm has independently corresponded with mortality during follow-up (HR: 2.5; 95% CI: 1.26–4.97, $p = 0.009$), alongside peripheral artery disease during hospitalization, ejection fraction <40%, age, and T2D. These findings from the study revealed that the baseline HR is directly and independently related to ischemic events, sudden death, CV death, and mortality from any cause, both in patients with known ischemic events and in the normal population or patients with increased CV risk.[81]

Elevated RHR is an easily measured clinical finding in patients with stable recurring HF and sinus rhythm. But in patients with mild to severe chronic HF, raised RHR is associated with an increased risk of all-cause mortality (ACM) and CV mortality. It was known that the decrease in HR improves clinical outcomes in patients with recurring HF and in sinus rhythm, but the relationship between HR and post-discharge outcomes in patients with HHF (hospitalized for HF) is presently unclear. According to the post-hoc analysis of the Efficacy of Vasopressin Antagonism in Heart Failure: Outcome Study with Tolvaptan (EVEREST) trial study, in patients with HHF in presumed sinus rhythm, higher RHR in the early post-discharge period was independently associated with increased mortality during subsequent follow-up. It was discovered that, at HR ≥70 bpm, each 5-beat increase in 1-week post-discharge HR was independently related with increased all-cause mortality [HR: 1.13 (95% CI: 1.05 to 1.22); $p = 0.002$]. While, each 5-beat increment ≥70 bpm in 4-week post-discharge HR was foretelling all-cause mortality [HR: 1.12 (95% CI: 1.05 to 1.19); $p = 0.001$]. These findings revealed that HR at the time of discharge was found to be predictive of death within 100 days post-randomization.[82]

In the Basel Stent Kosten-Effektivitats Trial-Prospective Validation Examination (BASKETPROVE) study, including 2,029 patients who had gone through percutaneous coronary intervention (PCI) for ST-elevation myocardial infarction (STEMI) and non-ST-segment elevation acute coronary syndromes (NSTE-ACS), it was found that the mortality rises with the elevations in HR. Patients with an HR between 60 bpm and 89 bpm had a 4-fold increment in mortality contrasted with patients in the lowest HR category (<60 bpm) and those patients who were discharged with an HR above 90 bpm had a 17-fold increment in mortality contrasted with patients below 60 bpm. Conversely, none of the STEMI patients discharged with an HR below 60 bpm died during follow-up. Accordingly, it can be inferred from the investigation that elevated HR at discharge was associated with long-term all-cause mortality as well as CV deaths and nonfatal MI in "all-comer" patients going through PCI independent of ailment introduction, for example, stable angina pectoris, NSTE-ACS, and STEMI.[48,3]

The comparable outcome was found in a Dutch population of STEMI patient's as Basket prove study, an HR above 70 bpm *vs* HR below 70 bpm was related with a hazard ratio of 3.2 (1.4–7.0) for ACM, and 2.4 (1.0–5.8) for CV mortality.[4]

Take Home Pearls

- RHR is a non-invasively measured marker of cardiac function and a good indicator of physical wellness and general well-being.
- Increased RHR is related to endothelial dysfunction, reduced artery compliance, and distensibility, and consequently increased arterial wall stress and elevated pulsed-wave velocity, which are further, related to increase after burden and at last fundamental HTN.
- In acute MI, raised HR has been additionally demonstrated to be related to the poor outcomes both in the prethrombolytic and contemporary eras.
- In patients with coronary artery disease, high RHR incites CV events mainly through ventricular arrhythmias or progressive pump failure.
- In patients with mild to severe recurring HF, raised RHR is related to an increased risk of ACM and CV mortality.

Take Home Summary

RHR is an easily accessible parameter impacted by many physiological and pathological conditions. HR is mainly regulated by the sympathetic and parasympathetic input of ANS. HR varies according to age, sex, weight/BMI, and rest. Cardiac conduction system (CCS) is divided into the impulse-generating nodes (SA Node and AV Node) and the impulse-propagating His-Purkinje system. Out of all the channels, I_f plays a major role in the generation of pacemaker activity and the regulation of HR. HR and HRV both are risk markers in cardiac disease. HRV reflects beat-to-beat changes in RR intervals, which are related to the ongoing interplay between two arms of the ANS. It is also an index of the sympathovagal modulation of HR. A high HRV is a sign of a healthy heart, whereas a reduced HRV is a symptom of health problems and can affect immune functions, self-regulation, and psychological abilities. Traditionally, HR is measured by pulse palpation, but other methods can be used to measure HR, such as ECG- and PPG-based wearable devices. RHR has a wide variation across the world. Indian population shows an increased RHR because of their increased SO. RHR is strongly associated with longevity, and HRV is linked to various cardiometabolic diseases.

REFERENCES

1. Menown IB, Davies S, Gupta S, *et al*. Resting heart rate and outcomes in patients with cardiovascular disease: Where do we currently stand?. *Cardiovascular Therapeutics*. 2013 Aug; 31(4):215–23.
2. Nanchen D. Resting heart rate: What is normal? *Heart*. 2018 Jul;104(13):1048–9.
3. Avram R, Tison GH, Aschbacher K, *et al*. Real-world heart rate norms in the Health eHeart study. *npj Digital Medicine*. 2019 Jun 25;58.
4. Jensen MT. Resting heart rate and relation to disease and longevity: Past, present and future. *Scandinavian Journal of Clinical and Laboratory Investigation*. 2019;79(1–2):108–16.
5. Ghasemzadeh N, Zafari AM. A brief journey into the history of the arterial pulse. *Cardiology Research and Practice*. 2011;2011.

6. Prabhavathi K, Selvi KT, Poornima KN, *et al.* Role of biological sex in normal cardiac function and in its disease outcome—A review. *Journal of Clinical and Diagnostic Research:JCDR.* 2014 Aug;8(8):BE01–BE04.

7. Schwartz JB, Gibb WJ, Tran T. Aging effects on heart rate variation. *Journal of Gerontology.* 1991 May;46(3):M99–106.

8. Yazdanirad S, Dehghan H, Rahimi Y, *et al.* The relationship between overweight and heart rate in hot and very hot weather under controlled conditions. *Health Scope.* 2015;4(4):e30604.

9. Penzel T, Kantelhardt JW, Lo CC, *et al.* Dynamics of heart rate and sleep stages in normals and patients with sleep apnea. *Neuropsychopharmacology.* 2003 Aug;28 Suppl 1(7):S48–S53.

10. Quer G, Gouda P, Galarnyk M, *et al.* Inter- and intraindividual variability in daily resting heart rate and its associations with age, sex, sleep, BMI, and time of year: Retrospective, longitudinal cohort study of 92,457 adults. *PLoS One.* 2020 Feb 5;15(2):e0227709.

11. Gordan R, Gwathmey JK, Xie LH. Autonomic and endocrine control of cardiovascular function. *World Journal of Cardiology.* 2015 Apr 26;7(4):204–14.

12. Park DS, Fishman GI. The Cardiac Conduction System. *Circulation.* 2011 Mar 1;123(8):904–15.

13. Christoffels VM, Moorman AF. Development of the cardiac conduction system: Why are some regions of the heart more arrhythmogenic than others? *Circulation: Arrhythmia and Electrophysiology.* 2009 Apr;2(2):195–207.

14. Physiology, sinoatrial node (SA Node). Adapted from: https://www.ncbi.nlm.nih.gov/books/NBK459238/

15. Larsson HP. How is the heart rate regulated in the sinoatrial node? Another piece to the puzzle. *Journal of General Physiology.* 2010 Sep;136(3):237–41.

16. Grant AO. Cardiac ion channels. *Circulation: Arrhythmia and Electrophysiology.* 2009 Apr 1;2(2):185–94.

17. Aziz Q, Li Y, Tinker A. Potassium channels in the sinoatrial node and their role in heart rate control. *Channels (Austin).* 2018;12(1):356–66.

18. Kennedy A, Finlay DD, Guldenring D, *et al.* The cardiac conduction system: Generation and conduction of the cardiac impulse. *Critical Care Nursing Clinics of North America.* 2016 Sep;28(3):269–79.

19. Fox AA, Sharma S, Mounsey JP, *et al.* Molecular and genetic cardiovascular medicine and systemic inflammation. *Kaplan's Essentials of Cardiac Anesthesia for Cardiac Surgery.* 2017 Dec 6;94–111.

20. Klabunde R. Cardiovascular physiology concepts. *Lippincott Williams & Wilkins;* 2011 Nov 3.

21. DiFrancesco D, Borer JS. The funny current: Cellular basis for the control of heart rate. *Drugs.* 2007;67 Suppl2:15–24.

22. Scicchitano P, Carbonara S, Ricci G, *et al.* HCN channels and heart rate. *Molecules.* 2012; 17(4):4225–35.

23. Suffredini S, Mugelli A, Cerbai E. I_f channels as a therapeutic target in heart disease. *Future Cardiol.* 2007 Nov;3(6).

24. DiFrancesco D. The role of the funny current in pacemaker activity. *Circulation Research.* 2010 Feb 19;106(3):434–46.

25. Cygankiewicz I, Zareba W. Heart rate variability. *Handbook of Clinical Neurology.* 2013;117:379–93.

26. Fatisson J, Oswald V, Lalonde F. Influence diagram of physiological and environmental factors affecting heart rate variability: An extended literature overview. *Heart international.* 2016;11(1):e32.

27. van Ravenswaaij-Arts CM, Kollée LA, *et al.* Heart rate variability. *Annals of Internal Medicine.* 1993;118(6):436–47.

28. Berntson GG, Cacioppo JT, Quigley KS. Respiratory sinus arrhythmia: Autonomic origins, physiological mechanisms, and psychophysiological implications. *Psychophysiology.* 1993;30 (2):183–96.

29. Kristal-Boneh E, Raifel M, Froom P, *et al*. Heart rate variability in health and disease. *Scandinavian Journal of Work, Environment & Health*. 1995 Apr;21(2):85–95.
30. Sammito S, Böckelmann I. Factors influencing heart rate variability. *International Cardiovascular Forum Journal*. 2016 May 4; 6.
31. Dikariyanto V, Smith L, Chowienczyk PJ, *et al*. Snacking on Whole Almonds for Six Weeks Increases Heart Rate Variability during Mental Stress in Healthy Adults: A Randomized Controlled Trial. *Nutrients*. 2020 Jun;12(6):1828.
32. Kemp AH, Quintana DS, Gray MA, *et al*. Impact of depression and antidepressant treatment on heart rate variability: A review and meta-analysis. *Biological Psychiatry*. 2010 Jun;67(11):1067–74.
33. Georgiou K, Larentzakis AV, Khamis NN, *et al*. Can wearable devices accurately measure heart rate variability? A systematic review. *Folia Medica*. 2018 Mar 1;60(1):7–20.
34. Palatini P. Recommendations on how to measure resting heart rate. *Medicographia*. 2009; 31: 414–9.
35. Palatini P, Benetos A, Grassi G, *et al*. Identification and management of the hypertensive patient with elevated heart rate: statement of a European Society of Hypertension Consensus Meeting. *Journal of Hypertension*. 2006 Apr 1;24(4):603–10.
36. Biyikli T. Comparison of physical parameters of the individuals who have received NASM- OPT Model & EMS training in combination with traditional fitness training applications regularly as personal training (PT) for 20 weeks. *Journal of Education and Training Studies*. 2018 Dec;6(12):158–71.
37. Becker DE. Fundamentals of electrocardiography interpretation. *Anesthesia Progress*. 2006;53(2):53–64.
38. Li K, Rüdiger H, Ziemssen T. Spectral analysis of heart rate variability: time window matters. *Frontiers in neurology*. 2019 May 29;10:545.
39. An X, K Stylios GK. Comparison of Motion Artefact Reduction Methods and the Implementation of Adaptive Motion Artefact Reduction in Wearable Electrocardiogram Monitoring. *Sensors*. 2020 Jan;20(5):1468.
40. Nelson BW, Low CA, Jacobson N, *et al*. Guidelines for wrist-worn consumer wearable assessment of heart rate in biobehavioral research. *npj Digital Medicine*. 2020 Jun 26;3(1):90.
41. Bent B, Goldstein BA, Kibbe WA, *et al*. Investigating sources of inaccuracy in wearable optical heart rate sensors. *npj Digital Medicine*. 2020 Feb 10;3(1):18.
42. Weiler DT, Villajuan SO, Edkins L, *et al*. Wearable heart rate monitor technology accuracy in research: A comparative study between PPG and ECG technology. *Proceedings of the Human Factors and Ergonomics Society Annual Meeting*. 2017 Sep;61(1):1292–6.
43. Elgendi M. On the analysis of fingertip photoplethysmogram signals. *Current Cardiology Reviews*. 2012 Feb 1;8(1):14–25.
44. Castaneda D, Esparza A, Ghamari M, *et al*. A review on wearable photoplethysmography sensors and their potential future applications in health care. *International Journal of Biosensors and Bioelectronics*. 2018;4(4):195–202.
45. Chang YM, Huang YT, Chen IL, *et al*. Heart rate variability as an independent predictor for 8-year mortality among chronic hemodialysis patients. *Scientific Reports*. 2020 Jan 21;10(1):881.
46. Young HA, Benton D. Heart-rate variability: A biomarker to study the influence of nutrition on physiological and psychological health? *Behavioural Pharmacology*. 2018 Apr;29 (2 and 3-Special Issue):140–51.
47. Shaffer F, Ginsberg JP. An overview of heart rate variability metrics and norms. *Frontiers in Public Health*. 2017 Sep 28;5:258.
48. Vanderlei LC, Pastre CM, Hoshi RA, *et al*. Basic notions of heart rate variability and its clinical applicability. *Brazilian Journal of Cardiovascular Surgery*. 2009; 24(2):205–17.
49. Moraes JL, Rocha MX, Vasconcelos GG, *et al*. Advances in photopletysmography signal analysis for biomedical applications. *Sensors*. 2018 Jun;18(6):1894.
50. Sassi R, Cerutti S, Lombardi F, *et al*. Advances in heart rate variability signal analysis: Joint position statement by the e-Cardiology ESC Working Group and the European Heart Rhythm

Association co-endorsed by the Asia Pacific Heart Rhythm Society. *Europace*. 2015 Sep; 17(9):1341–53.

51. Hillebrand S, Gast KB, de Mutsert R, *et al*. Heart rate variability and first cardiovascular event in populations without known cardiovascular disease: Meta-analysis and dose-response meta-regression. *Europace*. 2013 May;15(5):742–9.

52. Sessa F, Anna V, Messina G, *et al*. Heart rate variability as predictive factor for sudden cardiac death. *Aging (Albany NY)*. 2018 Feb;10(2):166–77.

53. Jensen MT, Marott JL, Allin KH, *et al*. Resting heart rate is associated with cardiovascular and all-cause mortality after adjusting for inflammatory markers: The Copenhagen City Heart Study. *European Journal of Preventive Cardiology*. 2012 Feb;19(1):102–8.

54. Boudoulas KD, Borer JS, Boudoulas H. Heart rate, life expectancy and the cardiovascular system: Therapeutic considerations. *Cardiology*. 2015; 132(4): 199– 212.

55. Levine HJ. Rest heart rate and life expectancy. *Journal of the American College of Cardiology*. 1997 Oct;30(4):1104–6.

56. Uusitalo AL, Vanninen E, Levalahti E, *et al*. Role of genetic and environmental influences on heart rate variability in middle-aged men. *American Journal of Physiology-Heart and Circulatory Physiology*. 2007 Aug;293(2):H1013–H1022.

57. Golosheykin S, Grant JD, Novak OV, Heath AC, Anokhin AP. Genetic influences on heart rate variability. *International Journal of Psychophysiology*. 2017 May 1;115:65–73.

58. Guo Y, Chung W, Zhu Z, *et al*. Genome-wide assessment for resting heart rate and shared genetics with cardiometabolic traits and Type 2 Diabetes. *Journal of the American College of Cardiology*. 2019 Oct 29;74(17):2162–74.

59. den Hoed M, Eijgelsheim M, Esko T, *et al*. Identification of heart rate–associated loci and their effects on cardiac conduction and rhythm disorders. *Nature genetics*. 2013 Jun;45(6):621–31.

60. Bathula R, Francis DP, Hughes A, *et al*. Ethnic differences in heart rate: can these be explained by conventional cardiovascular risk factors? *Clinical Autonomic Research*. 2008 Apr 1;18(2):90.

61. O'Neill J, Bounford K, Anstey A, *et al*. P wave indices, heart rate variability and anthropometry in a healthy South Asian population. *PloS One*. 2019 Aug 23;14(8):e0220662.

62. Rao D, Balagopalan JP, Sharma A, *et al*. BEAT Survey: A cross-sectional study of resting heart rate in young (18–55 years) hypertensive patients. *Journal of the Association of Physicians of India*. 2015 May;63(5):14–17.

63. Padmanabhan TN, Dani S, Chopra VK, *et al*. Prevalence of sympathetic overactivity in hypertensive patients—A pan India, non-interventional, cross-sectional study. *Indian Heart Journal*. 2014;66(6):686–90.

64. Grassi G. Sympathetic overdrive and cardiovascular risk in the metabolic syndrome. *Hypertension Research*. 2006 Nov;29(11):839–47.

65. Kaul U, Verberk W, Suvarna V, *et al*. India Heart Study—IHS. *Indian Heart Journal*. 2019 Nov;71:S80– S81.

66. Upendra K, Bhagwat A, Omboni S, *et al*. Blood pressure and heart rate related to sex in untreated subjects: The India ABPM study. *Journal of Clinical Hypertension*.

67. Rajalakshmi R, VijayaVageesh Y, Nataraj SM, *et al*. Heart rate variability in Indian obese young adults. *Pakistan Journal of Physiology*. 2012;8(1):39–44.

68. Palatini P. Role of elevated heart rate in the development of cardiovascular disease in hypertension. *Hypertension*. 2011 Nov;58(5):745–50.

69. Tadic M, Cuspidi C, Grassi G. Heart rate as a predictor of cardiovascular risk. *European Journal of Clinical Investigation*. 2018 Mar;48(3):e12892.

70. Riva L, Coutsoumbas GV, Maggioni AP. Heart rate in the assessment of cardiovascular prognosis. *Medicographia*. 2012;34:414–20.

71. Wang A, Liu X, Guo X, *et al*. Resting heart rate and risk of hypertension: Results of the Kailuan cohort study. *Journal of Hypertension*. 2014;32:1600–5.

72. Nauman J, Janszky I, Vatten LJ, *et al*. Temporal changes in resting heart rate and deaths from ischemic heart disease. *Jama*. 2011 Dec 21;306(23):2579–87.

73. Shaper AG, Wannamethee G, Macfarlane PW, *et al*. Heart rate, ischaemic heart disease, and sudden cardiac death in middle-aged British men. *British Heart Journal*. 1993 Jul;70(1):49–55.

74. Seviiri M, Lynch BM, Hodge AM, *et al*. Resting heart rate, temporal changes in resting heart rate, and overall and cause-specific mortality. *Heart*. 2018 Jul;104(13):1076–85.

75. Zhang D, Wang W, Li F. Association between resting heart rate and coronary artery disease, stroke, sudden death and noncardiovascular diseases: A meta-analysis. *Canadian Medical Association Journal*. 2016 Oct 18;188(15):E384–E392.

76. Chen XJ, Barywani SB, Hansson PO, *et al*. Impact of changes in heart rate with age on all-cause death and cardiovascular events in 50-year-old men from the general population. *Open Heart*. 2019;6(1):e000856.

77. Khan H, Kunutsor S, Kalogeropoulos AP, *et al*. Resting heart rate and risk of incident heart failure: Three prospective cohort studies and a systematic meta-analysis. *Journal of the American Heart Association*. 2015 Jan 14;4(1):e001364.

78. Fox K, Bousser MG, Amarenco P, *et al*. Heart rate is a prognostic risk factor for myocardial infarction: A post hoc analysis in the PERFORM (Prevention of cerebrovascular and cardiovascular events of ischemic origin with terutroban in patients with a history of ischemic strOke or tRansient ischeMic attack) study population. *International Journal of Cardiology*. 2013 Oct 9;168(4):3500–5.

79. Fox KM. Current status: Heart rate as a treatable risk factor. *European Heart Journal Supplements*.. 2011 Sep;C30–C36.

80. Hjalmarson Å, Gilpin EA, Kjekshus J, *et al*. Influence of heart rate on mortality after acute myocardial infarction. *American Journal of Cardiology*. 1990 Mar 1;65(9):547–53.

81. Fácila L, Morillas P, Quiles J, *et al*. Prognostic significance of heart rate in hospitalized patients presenting with myocardial infarction. *World Journal of Cardiology*. 2012 Jan 26;4(1):15–19.

82. Greene SJ, Vaduganathan M, Wilcox JE, *et al*. The prognostic significance of heart rate in patients hospitalized for heart failure with reduced ejection fraction in sinus rhythm: insights from the EVEREST (Efficacy of Vasopressin Antagonism in Heart Failure: Outcome Study With Tolvaptan) trial. *JACC: Heart Failure*. 2013 Dec 1;1(6):488–96.

83. Jensen MT, Kaiser C, Sandsten KE, *et al*. Heart rate at discharge and long-term prognosis following percutaneous coronary intervention in stable and acute coronary syndromes—Results from the BASKET PROVE trial. *International Journal of Cardiology*. 2013;168(4):3802–6.

Heart Rate—a Risk Marker or a Risk Factor

Dr. CK Ponde

Learning Objectives

At the end of this chapter one should be able to:
- Resting heart rate (RHR) for cardiovascular (CV) risk evaluation
- High RHR and its association with CV risk factors
- High HR and its impact on established CVD
- Evaluation of RHR as a CV risk factor

RESTING HEART RATE (RHR) FOR CARDIOVASCULAR (CV) RISK EVALUATION

RHR is a simple parameter that can be easily obtained in all circumstances, and it allows us to provide important information on CV risk and adequate modification of lifestyle and therapy.[1] The parasympathetic nervous system (PNS) governs 80% of RHR, and the sympathetic nervous system (SNS) governs the other 20%. Both the PNS and SNS make an equal contribution up to HR of 140 bpm, after which the ratio changes quickly to a more sympathetically dominant control. Sympathetic Overactivity (SO) is the basic trigger that provokes hemodynamic changes, arrhythmias, and metabolic abnormalities, which further induces hypertension (HTN), heart failure (HF), atherosclerosis, insulin resistance, lipid abnormalities, obesity and increases CV and non-CV mortality.[2] A compelling association between RHR and all-cause and CV mortality has been found in many epidemiologic studies.[3] HR is a determinant of myocardial oxygen demand, coronary blood flow, and myocardial performance and is central to the adaptation of cardiac output (CO) to metabolic needs.[4] Thus high RHR, low RHR variability, failure to achieve the target HR during chronotropic incompetence and slow heart rate recovery (HRR) have become an established biomarker that can strongly predict CV outcomes.[5] Also, it was seen in several studies that RHR elevates with an increase in temperature, fear, immobility, and cardiometabolic risk, so physicians have considered an elevated HR to be an epiphenomenon representing 'poor conditioning'.[6]

Risk Marker *vs* Risk Factor

Risk markers help to identify the pathophysiology of diseases, improve diagnostic capabilities, and ultimately provide better risk assessment. Risk markers are most useful in identifying patients who may benefit from therapies proven to reduce risk.[7]

The goal of risk factor research is to move closer to the proximal direct causes of the disease, which includes both causal and predictive factors. Causal risk factor directly reflects the underlying biology of the disease, whereas predictor simply reflects another more proximal risk factor.[8] It plays a central part in the prediction and prevention of disease and can be used to divide a population into high-risk and low-risk subgroups.[9]

Both risk markers and risk factors are recognized from relationships between the presence of the factor and subsequent development of the disease. A risk marker becomes a risk factor if intervention to modulate these factors consequences in parallel modulation of risk provided the analysis demonstrating this risk modulation accounts for feasible confounding factors.[10]

Criteria for a Novel CV Risk Factor

For evaluating a new risk factor and to consider its routine application in patients care, the following are five characteristics that need to be considered:

- Add independent information on risk or prognosis
- Account for a clinically significant proportion of independent of other known risk factors
- Reliable or accurate
- Provide good sensitivity and predictive value
- Modification of risk factor should improve the quantum of risk

In the earliest phase of assessment, the novel risk factors should provide important independent information about the risk or prognosis. Risk is evaluated with the utilization of case-control and prospective cohort designs. These approaches produce estimates in the form of relative risks, odds ratio (OR), or hazard ratio, comparing the incidence of disease among persons who have a given risk factor with the incidence of disease among those who do not have that risk factor. Significant risk estimates, fully adjusted for other known confounders (not just age and sex), indicate that the marker adds independent information and thus has potential clinical importance.

In the second phase of assessment, the novel risk factor should account for a large proportion of the risk associated with a given disease or condition that can be determined via the frequency of risk in the population of the disease and the magnitude of its contribution to the incidence of disease.

In the third phase of the assessment of a novel risk factor, the measures should be reproducible. A low coefficient of variation (standard deviation of repeated measures divided by their mean) is an indicator of good reproducibility.

In the final definitive phase of assessment, the test for factor/marker should be available and practical to implement for widespread applications.

Careful consideration of all these factors will guide the useful transition of new markers into clinical practice and improved patient care.[8]

HR: An Emerging Risk Marker for Cardiovascular Disease (CVD)

HR is a parameter broadly utilized as a marker of health.[1] It is influenced by a various physiological process as a result of the balance of sympathetic and vagal tone. The factors and conditions that influence HR are summarized in Fig. 2.1.[11] RHR values have gained more importance with the developing proof of the relationship between elevated HR values at rest and its relation to the CV outcomes.[1] There is increasing

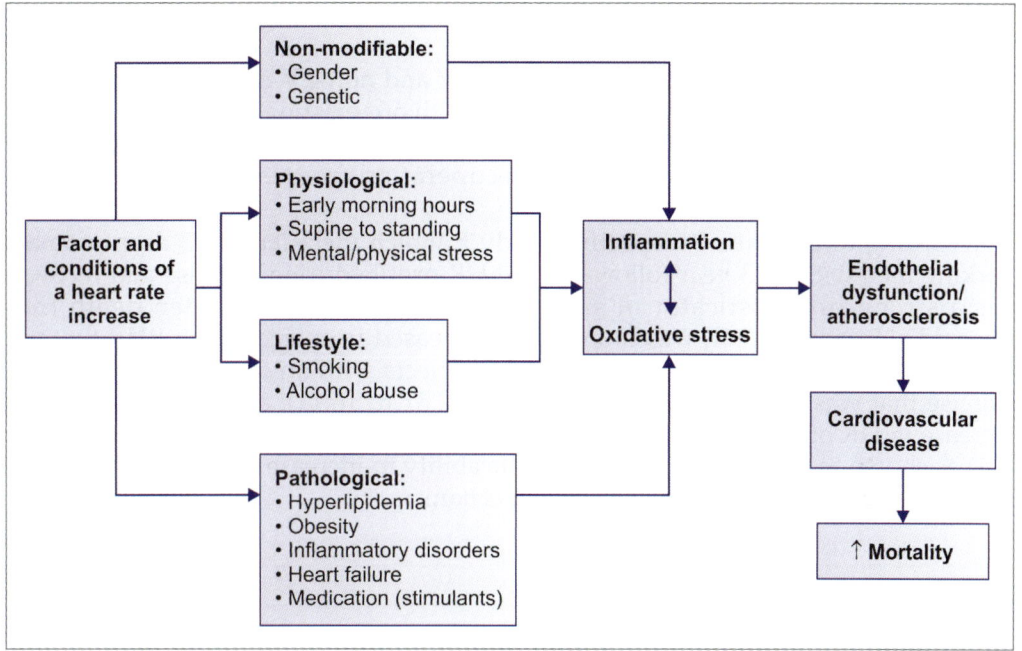

Fig. 2.1: The role of HR in the pathophysiology of CVD

epidemiological and scientific evidence suggesting that elevated RHR is associated with increased CV morbidity and mortality in populations with or without CVD. Also, statistics from trials have shown that HR is a treatable risk factor in patients with CVD and not just a prognostic marker.[12] Nonetheless, RHR is not yet foreseen in more universally known indices for assessment of global cardiac risk.[1]

According to the CORDIS trial, a follow-up of 8 years of 3,527 Israeli male industrial employees, all-cause and CVD death rates were independently associated with RHR. For all-cause mortality, workers with RHR ≥90 bpm had an adjusted relative risk (RR) of 2.23 (1.4–3.6), $p = 0.001$, whereas those with an RHR ≤79 bpm had a RR of 0.94 (0.6–1.5). A comparative outcome was achieved for CVD deaths: HR ≥90 bpm, RR: 2.02 (1.1–4.0), $p = 0.01$. Age, BMI, smoking status, and total body cholesterol, and systolic blood pressure (SBP) were all significant confounders in this relationship.[13]

Also, there is evidence of an advantageous relationship between RHR and non-CV mortality, with the specific recommendation that HR is a risk factor for cancer. Wannamethee *et al*. investigated the relation between HR, physical activity, and 9.5 years mortality from non-CVD. The study was performed on 7,735 middle-aged men. In this investigation, a strong positive affiliation was seen between the HR and all non-CV mortality, cancer mortality, and other non-CV mortality, after accounting for age, blood cholesterol, Body Mass Index (BMI), heavy alcohol drinking, physical activity, pre-existing ischemic heart disease (IHD), smoking, social class, and SBP (p <0.01). The relative risks in men with HR >90 bpm, in comparison with those with HR <60 bpm, were found to be 2.33 [95% confidence interval (CI): 1.42–3.74] for total non-CV mortality, 1.68 (95% CI: 0.92–3.10) for cancer mortality, and 3.56 (95% CI: 1.65–7.65) for mortality due to other non-CV causes. These findings suggested that in middle-aged men, RHR and physical activity are independent prognostic factors for non-CV mortality.[14]

Sudden death and unexpected death from CV and non-CV causes are a significant health burden.[15] In older subjects and patients with pre-existing disease, change in HR shows low physical fitness that is related to elevated mortality.[13] Alterations in an adjustment in HR during activity and recuperation from exercise may likewise contribute to the risk of sudden death.[15]

According to the Paris Prospective Study I, which included 5,713 asymptomatic working men with a 23-year follow-up, the HR profile during exercise and recovery was a strong prognosticator of sudden death. The risk of sudden death from myocardial infarction (MI) was found to be increased in subjects with RHR that was >75 bpm (RR: 3.92; 95% CI: 1.91 to 8.00); in subjects with an increase in HR during exercise that was <89 bpm (RR: 6.18; 95% CI: 2.37 to 16.11); and in subjects with a decrease in HR of <25 bpm after the termination of activity (RR: 2.20; 95% CI: 1.02 to 4.74) as shown in Fig. 2.2. Impairment of the ability to increase both sympathetic and vagal activity rapidly could be a possible mechanism.[15]

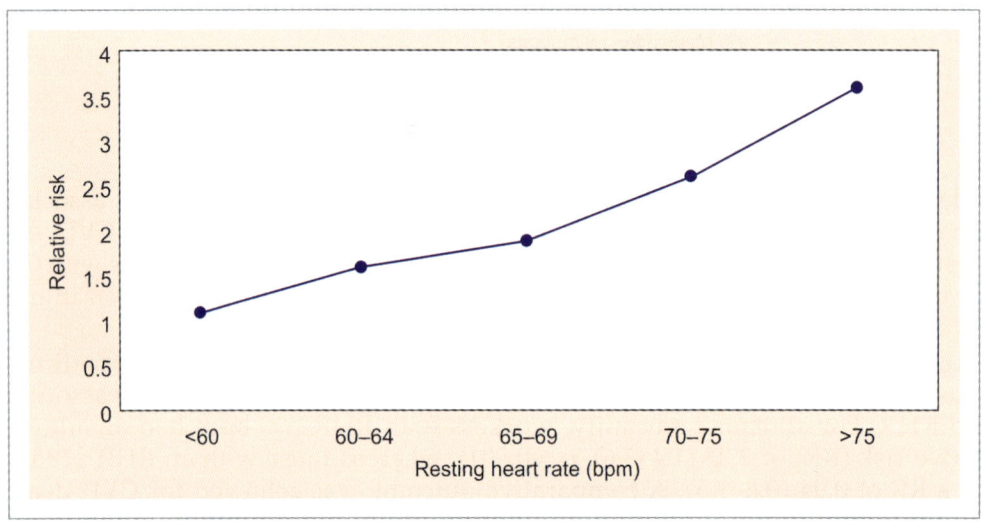

Fig. 2.2: RR of death from any cause and of non-sudden and sudden death from MI

As faster RHR is related to shorter life expectancies, several epidemiological studies have shown that elevated RHRs increase the risk of mortality from CVD. According to the National FINRISK Study, a strong, graded, independent relationship between RHR and incident CVD was seen among healthy men and women. Elevated RHR was found to be a stronger risk marker for the development of fatal as opposed to non-fatal MI. RHR >90 bpm compared to RHR <60 bpm increases the risk of CVD mortality in men by 2-fold and triples the risk in women. It was found that the RHR relationship with coronary heart disease (CHD)-specific mortality was higher and total mortality was slightly lesser, and the inclusion of non-fatal endpoints weakened this relationship.[16]

The risk for CV morbidity and mortality starts to increase in middle age and RHR changes with age. High RHR increases hemodynamic stress and abbreviates the diastolic phase that could increase the mechanical load, shear stress, and cardiac work, thereby increasing oxygen consumption. Chen XJ *et al.* conducted a prospective, population-based study to determine the effect of changes in HR with age on all- cause death and CV events in old men. During a 21-year follow-up, the study showed that men with RHR of over 75 bpm at 50 years of age have double the risk of all-cause death, CVD, and CHD compared with men with RHR of 55 bpm or below. Participants with a baseline RHR of >75 bpm in 1993 were found to have a two times higher risk of all-cause death (HR: 2.3, CI: 1.2 to 4.7, $p = 0.018$), CVD (HR: 1.8, CI: 1.1 to 3.0, $p = 0.014$), and CHD (HR: 2.2, CI: 1.1 to 4.5, $p = 0.025$) contrasted in those with <55 bpm in 1993, whereas participants with a stable RHR between 1993 and 2003 had a 44% reduced risk of CVD (HR: 0.56, CI: 0.35 to 0.87, $p = 0.011$) compared with participants with an increasing RHR. These findings suggested suggest that individuals in whom the RHR increases between 50 and 60 years of age have a worse outcome when contrasted with those with a stable RHR.[17]

Higher RHR is related to an elevated risk of all-cause and CV mortality, with certain reports demonstrating the magnitude of relationship with all-cause mortality (ACM) being stronger than that with CV mortality. It shows that the RHR relationship with mortality may not be restricted to CV death. To determine the relationship between RHR with CV and non-CV mortality, Alhalbi L *et al.* gathered the data from 6,743 participants (mean age 58.7 years, 52% females, and 48% non-Hispanic whites) from the Third National Health and Nutrition Examination Survey (NHANES-III). RHR data was acquired from a standard 12-lead electrocardiogram recorded on the NHANES participants during a physical assessment. Over a median follow-up of 13.9 years, it was observed that 906 CVDs and 1306 non-CVDs occurred. In comparison to those participants who developed non-CVD mortality and those who developed CVD death, participants were more likely to be younger, male, and with a history of chronic obstructive pulmonary disease (COPD) or cancer. Also, it was observed that those who developed CVD deaths were more likely to have dyslipidemia, prior CVD, HTN higher BMI. Higher RHR was a risk parameter in both CV mortality and non-CV mortality with a relatively similar magnitude of risk HR (95% CI): 1.19 (1.12–1.26) and 1.23 (1.17–1.29). Each 10-beat increase in RHR led to 22%, 23%, and 24% increase in all-cause, CVD, and non-CVD death, respectively ($p < 0.001$ for all). These findings suggested that RHR is probably a marker of overall well-being rather than a marker of CV health.[18]

The pathological processes known to initiate CVD include oxidative stress, endothelial dysfunction, inflammation, and vascular remodeling. These processes may prompt tissue damage characterizing atherosclerotic disease. Oxidative stress results when an increase in reactive oxygen species (ROS) generation prompts a reduction in nitric oxide (NO) activity and subsequent endothelial dysfunction. This imbalance is a known effect of established CVD risk factors such as cigarette smoking, diabetes mellitus (DM), and obesity. The latter induces pathological vascular responses, e.g. vasoconstriction, inflammation, muscle cell proliferation, and thrombosis. HR can affect all phases of the CV continuum from vascular risk factors to CV events. Experimental and clinical data suggest that sustained elevation of HR-independent of the underlying trigger-contributes to the pathogenesis of the vascular disease.[19-21] High RHR is a marker of SO, which is associated with an increased risk of CV events. SO confers an increased risk of obesity that could induce insulin resistance, higher levels of uric acid, lipid abnormalities, and HTN. These adverse events associated with SO may, therefore, account for the observed relationship between high RHR and increased risk of both CV and non-CV events.[17] The similitude of the relationship between RHR and both CV and non-CV mortality may, in part, be because of the bidirectional relationship between the autonomic nervous system (ANS) and other body systems.[18]

As high RHR is associated with high adverse CV outcomes, it can be a relevant risk marker for CVD detection. However, an essential prerequisite to meet the criteria as a risk factor, interventional studies demonstrating modulation of risk by HR reduction is still lacking. If HR reduction may reduce risk in patients with established risk factors remains an open question. Given below are the various stages of the CV continuum, which can be affected by the change in HR (Fig. 2.3).

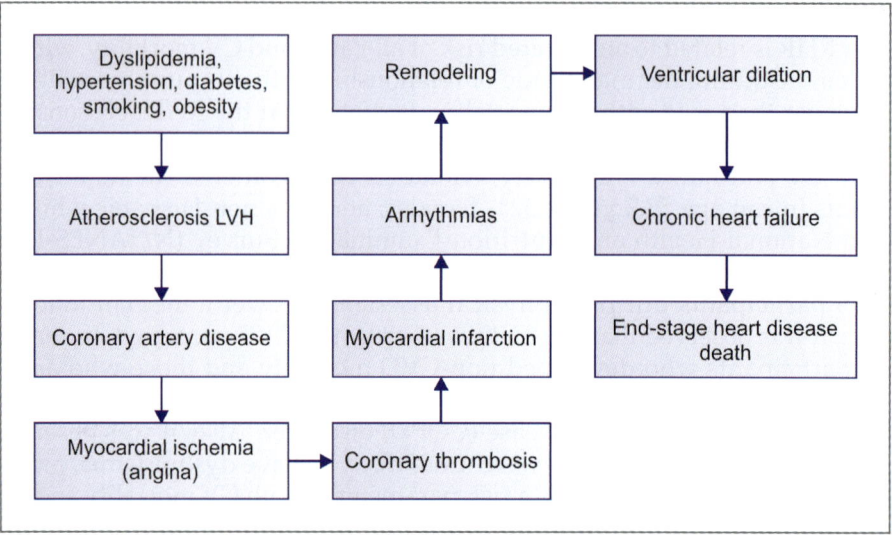

Fig. 2.3: Stages of CV continuum which can be affected by the change in HR. LVH: Left ventricular hypertrophy

Take Home Pearls

- RHR is a simple parameter that can be easily obtained in clinical practice and provides important information on CV risk.
- Risk markers help to identify people at risk and help the clinicians to apply preventive measures at the early stage of the disease, while the objective of risk factor research is to move closer to the proximal direct causes of disease.
- HR is influenced by a variety of physiological processes mainly via effects on the balance of sympathetic and vagal tone.
- SO is the basic trigger, which provokes hemodynamic changes, arrhythmias and confers an increased risk of obesity that could induce insulin resistance, high levels of uric acid, lipid abnormalities, and HTN.
- High RHR increases hemodynamic stress and shortens the diastolic phase, that could increase the mechanical load, shear stress, BP, and cardiac work, thereby increasing oxygen consumption.

HIGH RHR AND ITS ASSOCIATION WITH CV RISK FACTORS

RHR is a simple measure that reflects the integrity of the ANS.[22] In a normal person, HR varies widely and may elevate temporarily due to many different causes such as excitement, exertion, pain, ingestion of food, drinking of coffee or tea, and smoking of tobacco, etc.[23] HR elevates myocardial oxygen utilization consumption and induces fatigue and fracture of elastic fibers within the arterial wall because it may have a direct effect on the CV system.[24] Consequently, elevated RHR is related to incident CVD risk factors such as HTN, impaired glucose metabolism, dyslipidemia, and sedentary lifestyle.[25]

High RHR and its Association with HTN

Prevalent and incident HTN, both are responsible for the dysfunction of cardiac autonomic tone, including diminished vagal function and imbalance of the sympathovagal system. Therefore, it is possible that elevated RHR, as a surrogate for cardiac autonomic dysfunction, can likewise recognize individuals at risk for HTN.[26] The first evidence emphasizing the role of elevated HR as a predictor for the future development of HT was demonstrated by Levy et al. in 1945. The result of the study revealed that the frequency of transient tachycardia increased with age, up to 45. The group with transient tachycardia showed higher rates for later sustained HTN, and when both transient tachycardia and HTN were present, the incidence of later sustained HTN was more than twice as great as when either condition was present alone.[23]

Furthermore, to determine the relation between RHR and incident HTN, the Henry Ford Hospital Exercise Testing (FIT) project study was conducted. In the investigation, data from 21,873 individuals without a history of HTN was analyzed. Results showed that compared to patients with an RHR <70 bpm, those with RHR between 70–85 bpm had a 12% increased risk of HTN, and those with RHR >85 bpm had a 30% increased risk of HTN after adjustment for CHD risk factors, baseline BP, and metabolic syndrome (MetS) [Hazard Ratio (HR) = 1.15 (95% CI: 1.08–1.23)] with a p-value for trend <0.001. Also, a 10 bpm increase in RHR was found related to a 4% increase in the risk of HTN [HR (95% CI) = 1.04 (1.02–1.06)], and in age-stratified analysis, the relationship was found to remain significant only for persons younger than 60 years [HR (95% CI) = 1.20 (1.11–1.30)] for RHR >85 bpm compared to <70 bpm). It was also observed in the FIT study that older individuals have a decreased physiologic and chronotropic response to sympathetic stimulation and are more likely to develop HTN, irrespective of RHR, compared to younger individuals.[26]

RHR is a sensitive, non-invasive, and inexpensive indicator of cardiac function. Elevation in RHR increases the risk of MetS, CVD, T2DM, atrial fibrillation, and ACM.[27] A majority of the epidemiologic examinations depicts a critical connection between a high RHR and mortality (Chicago Gas Company, Chicago Heart Association Project, Framingham, British Regional Heart, Spandau, Benetos, Castel, Cordis, Reunanen, Thomas, Matiss, Ohasama, Okamura, and Jouven studies), with a global estimation of 30 to 50% mortality excess for every 20 bpm increases at rest.[28]

Furthermore, to determine the relationship of HR with the incidence of CV and non-CV disease, Gillman MW et al. analyzed evidence from a 36-years follow-up in 2,037 male subjects with HTN from the Framingham cohort. The result revealed that ACM increases progressively with RHR in HTN men. For an increment of 40 bpm in RHR, the age- and SBP-adjusted OR for ACM in men was found to be 2.18 (95% CI: 1.68 to 2.83; $p = 0.0001$), and for CV mortality 1.68 (95% CI: 1.19 to 2.37; $p = 0.0001$). These outcomes showed that HR can be an independent risk factor for CV death in persons with HTN.[29]

High RHR or autonomic imbalance is also related to subclinical inflammation represented by elevated C-reactive protein levels and leukocyte counts. Therefore, inflammation may play an important role in the relation between RHR and incident CV risk. One potential connection between RHR and HTN is leptin, an adipocytokine produced by adipose tissue that directly elevates sympathetic outflow, thereby increasing BP and HR. Elevated RHR can also be a marker of chronic stress and anxiety, that may increase the risk of HTN.[27]

High RHR and its Association with Metabolic Diseases

An increase in sympathetic tone elevates RHR and is closely related to Insulin Resistance (IR), which plays an essential part in the development of Mets. Several investigations demonstrated that a relationship between elevated RHR and diseases is characterized by a metabolic abnormality like an increase in glycemia or IR, an increase in weight and abdominal fat distribution, or an increase in lipid profile.[1,30]

High RHR or autonomic imbalance is additionally related to subclinical inflammation represented by elevated CRP level and leukocyte count, and inflammation may play a significant part in the relation of RHR and MetS. According to a dose-response meta-analysis study involving 7 cohort studies and 10 cross-sectional studies with a total of 169,786 individuals, elevation in RHR by 10 bpm increased the risk of MetS in adults by 28%. The pooled RR was observed to be 2.10 (95% CI: 1.80–2.46, $I^2 = 79.8\%$, $n = 13$) for the highest vs reference RHR category and 1.28 (95% CI: 1.23–1.34, $I^2 = 87.7\%$, $n = 15$) for each 10 bpm elevation in RHR. These outcomes showed that RHR alone might be a new target of clinical intervention like other risk factors such as hyperlipidemia and HTN.[30]

To determine the association of elevated HR to Obesity (Ob) and DM, Shigetoh Y et al. led a periodic epidemiological survey from 1979 to 1999 in the general population. The complete dataset of 614 subjects was evaluated. The outcomes showed that the ORs for the development of cardiometabolic factors in the HR ranges >80 bpm was significantly larger than 2.0, indicating a significant predictive value of higher HR ≥80 bpm for the development of Ob with an OR: 2.34 [95% CI: (1.09–5.90; $p <0.05$)], IR with OR: 2.20 [95% CI: (1.04–5.07; $p <0.05$)], and DM with OR: 5.39 [95% CI: (1.34–21.8; $p <0.01$)]. These outcomes demonstrated that an elevated HR at baseline predicts the development of Ob, IR, and DM.[31]

The HARVEST study was the principal prospective investigation, showed that persistently higher HR may incline to Ob in the early phase of HTN. As per this study, a 30% increased risk of Ob was observed for each 10-bpm elevation in baseline clinic HR (hazard ratio 1.30, CI: 1.10–1.50) and a 17% increased in risk for a 10-bpm elevation in clinic HR from baseline to study end (hazard ratio 1.17, CI: 1.06–1.28). It was also seen in the HARVEST study that sympathetic activation assumes a causative role in the development of Ob in hypertensive subjects. Besides, alterations in ANS function are believed to add to the pathogenesis of Ob and its complications.[32]

It was recently reported that high RHR is related to an increased likelihood of having diabetes. RHR is a crude index of ANS status, and diabetes may be associated with an ANS imbalance. Higher RHRs has additionally been related to increased SNS activity and may increase both chronic and acute IR, thereby inducing diabetes. The activity of SNS that are related to the elevation in HR, BP, IR, and the MetS are shown in Fig. 2.4.[33]

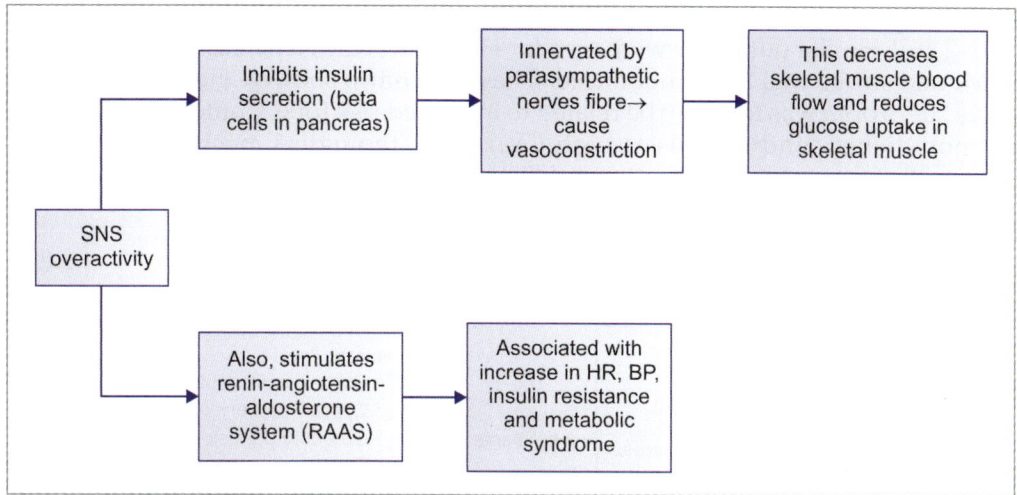

Fig. 2.4: Activity of SNS that is associated with the increases in HR, BP, insulin resistance, and the MetS. SNS: Sympathetic nervous system

As per the Korean Genome and Epidemiology Study (KoGES), an elevation in RHR is a strong risk factor for the development of DM in a dose-dependent manner and autonomous to glycometabolic parameters and baseline RHR. In participants who had more elevation in RHR at the 2-year follow-up examination, a greater cumulative incidence of diabetes was seen (either 5–10 or >10 bpm) compared to those whose elevations were <5 bpm ($p = 0.006$). The outcomes of the KoGES study also revealed that an elevation in HR >10 bpm was significantly related to the development of DM (adjusted hazard ratio: 1.31, 95% CI: 1.06–1.60), even subsequent changing for glycometabolic parameters and baseline RHR.[33]

Results from the meta-analysis study by Lee *et al.* showed that RR for the highest *vs* lowest RHR and T2D was 1.44 (95% CI: 1.20–1.74, I^2: 92.9%, 12 studies), and the summary RR per 10 bpm increase in RHR was 1.17 (95% CI: 1.09–1.26, I^2: 91.8%, 13 studies). At the point when the relationship of RHR and known risk factors with T2D risk was examined, a significant multiplicative interaction between high HR and a greater number of risk factors was seen. Men with high RHR and 3 and 4+ hazard factors, when compared with those with low RHR and ≤1 risk factor, had 7.0 and 14.8 times increased risk of T2D.[34]

To determine the association between RHR and CV risk, Bohm *et al.* examined 30,937 patients with a history of or at high risk for CVD and after MI, stroke, or with the proven peripheral vascular disease from ONTARGET/TRANSCEND trials. Data was examined by utilizing Cox regression analysis, ANOVA, and χ2 test, and the primary outcome in the study was CV death, MI, stroke, and hospitalization for HF (HHF). The outcomes showed that compared to patients without diabetes; those patients who have diabetes had a slightly higher RHR (71.8 ± 9.0 *vs* 67.9 ± 8.8,

p <0.0001). In the categories of <60 bpm, 60 <65 bpm, 65 <70 bpm, 70 <75 bpm, 75 <80 bpm, and >80 bpm, non-diabetic patients had an increased hazard of the primary outcome with a mean RHR of 75 ≤80 bpm [adjusted hazard ratio 1.17 (1.01–1.36)] compared to RHR 60 ≤65 bpm. And for patients within-trial RHR ≥80 bpm HRs were highest [diabetes: 1.96 (1.64–2.34), no diabetes: 1.73 (1.49–2.00)], for CVD hazards were also clearly increased at RHR ≥80 bpm [diabetes: 1.99 (1.53–2.58), no diabetes: 1.73 (1.38–2.16)]. Similar outcomes were seen for HHF and ACM, whereas the effect of RHR on MI and stroke was less pronounced. These outcomes showed that the mean RHR above 70–75 bpm was found to be related to increased risk for CV outcomes in diabetic and non-diabetic individuals at high CV risk. Pathological mechanisms that are responsible for causing an elevation in HR are shown in Fig. 2.5.[35]

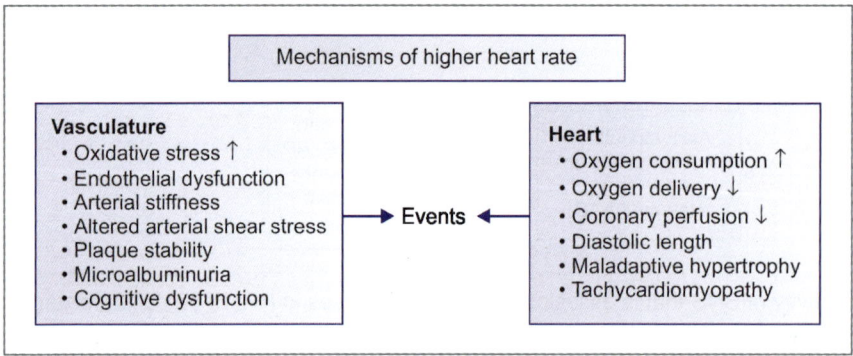

Fig. 2.5: HR as a CV outcome marker

RHR and its Association with Microalbuminuria (MAU)

MAU is a typical condition that is present in about 5–8% of apparently healthy individuals without diabetes, HTN, or other CVD, and in individuals with DM and HTN, the prevalence rises to 29% and 16%, respectively. MAU was found to be a relevant risk predictor for other CV events.[36]

As per International Survey Evaluating Microalbuminuria Routinely by Cardiologists in Patients with Hypertension (I-SEARCH) study, HR was an autonomous predictor for the prevalence of MAU in hypertensive patients with CV risk factors. The outcomes showed that with elevated HR (>80 bpm to <120 bpm), the proportion of patients with MAU increased from 63 to 69% (p <0.0001). The OR for MAU increased with elevated HR [hazard ratio (HR): 80–100 bpm compared with 60 bpm; OR: 1.47; 95% CI: 1.29–1.68; p <0.0001; and HR: 100–120 bpm compared with 60 bpm; OR: 1.56; 95% CI: 1.22–1.99; PU: 0.0004]. In summary, MAU is associated not only with high BP but also with higher HR. Consequently, the development of renal dysfunction in hypertensive individuals with high HR features another organ system that can be harmed by elevated HR in addition to the brain, the heart, and the vasculature. HR adds to the mechanical stress imposed on the kidneys by elevated BP.[36]

High RHR and its Association with Blood Lipids

Sun Ji *et al.* in a randomized study showed that patients with elevated RHR are at great risk of dyslipidemia, especially for high triglyceride (TG) and total cholesterol (TC). Multiple logistic regression analysis showed that the risk of high TG and TC was higher in subjects with RHR ≥90 bpm than in those with their RHR <70 bpm (OR: 1.42; 95% CI: 1.16–1.74 and OR: 1.33; 95% CI: 1.09–1.64, respectively). Therefore, RHR can be regarded as a powerful indicator of dyslipidemia screening and risk assessment.[37]

Whereas in the British Regional Heart Study, it was found that elevated HR was related to HTN and with an atherogenic lipoprotein profile. It was independent of factors shown an influence on HR (age, smoking, alcohol intake, physical activity, BMI, social class, and lung function). The investigation showed that HR relate essentially with the TG levels ($r = 0.15$, $p <0.0001$), and with blood cholesterol ($r = 0.07$, $p <0.0001$) and high-density lipoprotein (HDL) cholesterol levels ($r = -0.04$, $p <0.01$) and positively and significantly with blood glucose levels ($r = 0.20$, $p <0.0001$). With the elevation in HR, blood cholesterol, triglyceride, and blood glucose levels were increased significantly, whereas HDL cholesterol levels tend to decrease with elevation in HR.[14]

Around the world, CVD is the most widely recognized reason for ill-health and mortality. Therefore, understanding the novel disease marker is the key to improved disease detection and prognostication. A positive relation between RHR and mortality has been demonstrated in several investigations, and RHR has potential as an inexpensive and reliable risk marker. Therefore, to define the sex, age, and disease-specific relationship of RHR with CV and mortality outcome, Estabragh ZR *et al.* led a study involving 5,02,534 individuals from the UK BIOBANK. The main result of the study was all-cause, CV, and IHD mortality. During a 7–12 years follow-up, the study showed that in men with each 10-bpm elevation of RHR there was a 22% (HR: 1.22, CI: 1.20 to 1.24, $p = 3 \times 10^{-123}$) greater hazard of all-cause and 17% [sub-distribution hazard ratio (SHR): 1.17, CI: 1.13 to 1.21, $p = 5.6 \times 10^{-18}$] greater hazard of CV mortality; for women, corresponding figures were 19% (HR: 1.19, CI: 1.16 to 1.22, $p = 8.9 \times 10^{-45}$) and 14% (SHR: 1.14, CI: 1.07 to 1.22, $p = 0.00008$). The relationship between RHR and ischemic results were of greater magnitude among men compared to women, yet with a comparable magnitude of relationship for non-CV cancer mortality. While, the associations with all-cause, incident AMI, and cancer mortality were of greater magnitude amongst childhood than older ages. The ischemic disease appeared a more important driver of this relationship in men, and an association is more pronounced at a younger age.[38]

The possible etiological pathway by which RHR may increase CVD mortality is restricted; however, a few potential clarifications may be considered. A faster RHR is probably going to have unfavorable hemodynamic consequences prompting increased vascular shear stress, myocardial mechanical load, and tensile stress. Together, these hemodynamic changes promote adverse vascular and myocardial remodeling. Thus, increase the likelihood of endothelial injury, development of atherosclerotic disease, and acute coronary events as shown in Fig. 2.6. Also, elevated HR caused by mechanical stress may promote the weakening of the fibrous cap, which results in an increase in the risk of plaque disruption and the onset of acute CV events.[39]

Take Home Pearls

• The risk of MetS, T2DM, atrial fibrillation, CVDs, and ACM increases with elevation in RHR.
• Elevated RHR is related to raise metabolic activity and increased systemic inflammation and is present in the common final pathway of many systemic conditions, which involve inflammatory, metabolic, and neurology processes.

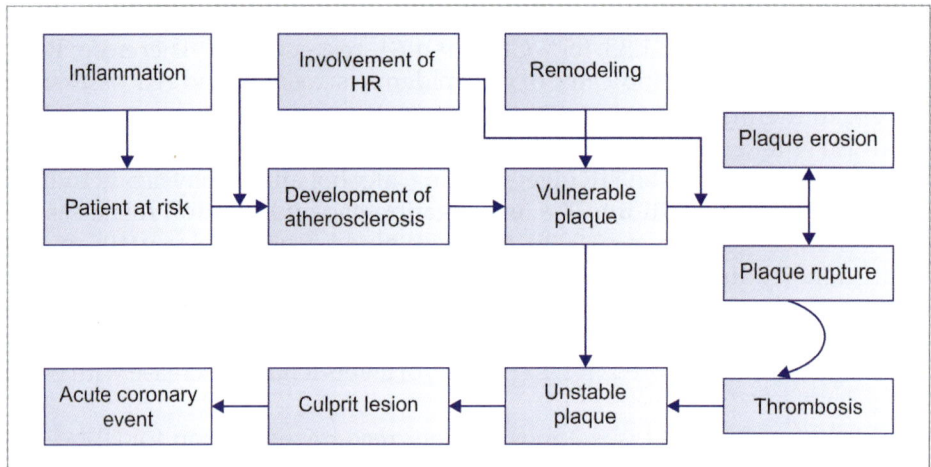

Fig. 2.6: Role of HR in the development and progression of atherosclerosis

- Both prevalent and incident hypertension has been related to the dysfunction of cardiac autonomic tone, including decreased vagal function and unevenness of the sympathovagal system.
- Elevated HR brought about by mechanical stress may promote the weakening of the fibrous cap, which eventually increases the risk of plaque disruption and the onset of acute CV events.

HIGH HR AND ITS IMPACT ON ESTABLISHED CVD

RHR is known to be a sensitive indicator of the ANS, and in several epidemiological investigations, it has been reported that elevations in RHR are related to an increased risk of CVD and total mortality because RHR is known to be a sensitive indicator of the ANS. It is plausible that an imbalance between sympathetic and parasympathetic activity may contribute to the relationship observed between elevated HR and increased chronic disease risk. Aune D et al. in 2017 led a meta-analysis study by examining the relationship between RHR and risk of CHD, SCD, HF, AF, stroke, CVD, total cancer, and ACM. The result revealed that each 10 bpm elevation in RHR is related to adverse cardiac outcomes. Also, it was observed that RR per 10 bpm elevation in RHR was 1.07 (95% CI: 1.05–1.10, I^2 = 61.9%, n = 31) for CHD, 1.09 (95% CI: 1.00–1.18, I^2 = 62.3%, n = 5) for sudden cardiac death, 1.18 (95% CI: 1.10–1.27, I^2 = 74.5%, n = 8) for HF, and (95% CI: 1.02–1.10, I^2 = 59.5%, n =16) for total stroke. The linear dose-response analysis showed an elevation in RR of 6% for total stroke, 7% for CHD, 9% for SCD, and 18% for HF for each 10-bpm elevation in RHR. These outcomes showed a positive relationship between high RHR CVD. Thus, bringing down RHR might be a potential target to decrease the risk of CVD and premature mortality.[40]

Also, according to an investigation conducted by Borer JS et al. on 19,386 white-collar employees in France followed up over 20 years, found that RHR significantly predicted non-CV mortality in both men and women. In men, the risk of CV mortality was least among those with HR <60 bpm; in correlation with this group, relative risks among men with RHR 60–80 bpm, 81–100 bpm, and 100 bpm was 1.35, 1.44, and 2.18, respectively. Coronary events were primarily and predominantly responsible for CV deaths and not because of cerebrovascular accidents. Whereas in another French cohort study involving 5,713 asymptomatic men between the age of 42 and 53 at study entry, a 23-year follow-up showed a significant relationship between RHR and both sudden and MI-related death.[10]

The CASS and BEAUTIFUL study demonstrated a positive relation between elevated RHR and CV mortality.[21] Diaz *et al.* in 2005 led an investigation to define the relationship between RHR and CV events in a large population of patients with suspected or proven CAD. The influence of HR on CV morbidity and mortality during 14.7 years in 24,913 patients with suspected or proven CAD included in the coronary artery surgery study (CASS) registry was analyzed. The outcomes revealed that ACM, CV mortality, and CV rehospitalization was increased with elevated HR (p <0.0001). Patients with RHR ≥83 bpm at baseline had a significantly higher risk for total mortality [hazard ratio (HR): 1.32, CI: 1.19–1.47, p <0.0001] and CV mortality (HR: 1.31, CI: 1.15–1.48, p <0.0001) after alteration for multiple clinical variables when compared with the reference group.[41]

Previous investigations have demonstrated a relationship between elevated RHR and the risk of CVD in the general population and individuals with stable CAD. But the threshold at which risk increases in coronary patients, and the quantitative relation between HR increase and outcome, are still less well defined. Thus, to determine the relationship between elevated HR and the risk of CV death and morbidity in individuals with CAD and left ventricular (LV) dysfunction, the BEAUTIFUL study was performed. In this investigation, the relationship of baseline RHR with CV outcomes was analyzed by utilizing Cox proportional hazard models for groups with an HR ≥70 bpm (2,693 individuals) *vs* <70 bpm (2,745 individuals). The outcomes revealed that individuals with HR ≥ 70 bpm had an increased risk for CV death (34%, p = 0.0041), admission to hospital for HF (53%, p <0.0001), admission to hospital for MI (46%, p = 0.0066), and coronary revascularization (38%, p = 0.037). Also, it was seen that with every increase of 5 bpm, there were increases in CV death (8%, p = 0.0005), admission to HHF (16%, p <0.0001), admission to hospital for MI (7%, p = 0.052), and coronary revascularization (8%, p = 0.034). These outcomes showed that in patients with LV dysfunction and CAD, elevated HR (≥70 bpm) helped to recognize those at increased risk of CV outcomes, with a higher impact on HF outcomes than coronary events.[42]

As it is known that HR is a major determinant of myocardial oxygen demand, as well as it influences coronary blood flow through diastolic filling time, but it is not defined whether simple indexes of autonomic balance such as HR may assume a role in risk stratification in AMI patients. Therefore, to determine the significance of HR as a prognostic factor in AMI patients, Zuanetti G *et al.* led an investigation (GISSI-2 trial). The results of the investigation showed that the HR values from a standard 12-lead ECG independently might predict mortality in AMI patients during the in-hospital phase and after discharge. The in-hospital mortality rate of MI patients significantly surged from 3.3 to 10.1% when patients with HR <60 bpm was compared with HR >100 bpm on admission.[43]

In investigations of patient groups with CVD, an elevation in RHR has been related to increased case fatality. Nonetheless, whether temporal changes in RHR may alter the risk of death from IHD in the general population is still not well-known. Thus, to evaluate the relation of long-term longitudinal changes in RHR with the risk of dying from IHD, Nauman J *et al.* led a prospective cohort study. A total of 13,498 men and

15,816 women without known CVD were enrolled in this cohort, and RHR was estimated at two events around 10-year apart in the Nord-Trøndelag County Health Study. Using Cox regression analyses, adjusted hazard ratios (AHRs) were assessed of death from IHD related to changes in RHR over time. During a 12 ± 2 years follow-up, the study showed that 3,038 individuals died, and 388 fatalities were caused by IHD. Compared with participants with an RHR <70 bpm at both measurements (8.2 deaths/10,000 person-years), the AHR was 1.9 (95% CI: 1.0–3.6) for participants with an RHR <70 bpm at the primary measurement but >85 bpm at the secondary measurement (17.2 deaths/10,000 person-years). For participants with RHRs between 70 and 85 bpm at the primary measurement and >85 bpm at the secondary measurement (17.4 deaths/10,000 person-years), the AHR was 1.8 (95% CI: 1.2–2.8). These findings revealed that among men and women without known CVD, elevation in RHR over 10 years was related to increased risk of death from IHD and for ACM.[44]

The studies mentioned above clearly reported a strong relationship between elevated HR and CV risk, independent of other significant risk factors. This association was seen in healthy populations among men and women, in patients with stroke, MI, IHD, CAD, or in those with LV dysfunction. Despite the substantial existent body of evidence linking elevated HR to increased CV risk, knowledge gaps remained because almost all current data are based on studies of associations between HR measured at a single point in time and subsequent CV events. However, HR may vary substantially over time. Therefore, to assess the relevance of HR in a large contemporaneous medically optimized cohort of patients with stable chronic CV disease, Lonn *et al.* evaluated the data from the ONTARGET/TRANSCEND study trials. The outcomes showed that for every 10 bpm elevation in in-trial HR, there was a 22–26% increase in the risk of major vascular events (MVE), 33–41% increase in the risk of CV death, 44–55% increase in the risk of HHF, and 33–39% increase in the risk of ACM in unadjusted, age, sex, and multivariate-adjusted models. Compared to patients who have HR <70 bpm, those with HR ≥70 bpm had a higher risk of MVE, CV death, HHF, and ACM. These findings revealed that resting and average HR were autonomously associated with significant increases in MVE, CV death, CHF, and ACM.[45]

Furthermore, to determine the relation that HR is additionally a risk factor for CV events in HF, Bohm *et al.* evaluated CV outcomes from the SHIFT placebo-controlled trial. The primary composite endpoint was CV death or HHF. The result showed that in the placebo group, patients with HR ≥87 bpm (n = 682, 286 events) were at more than twice the higher risk for the primary composite endpoint than were patients with the HR: 70 to <72 bpm [n = 461, 92 events; hazard ratio (HR) 2.34, 95% CI: 1.84–2.98, p <0.0001]. With each beat increase from baseline HR, the risk of primary composite endpoint events was increased by 3% and 16% for every 5-bpm increase. These outcomes showed that the slower the HR, the lower the CV complications.[46]

The role of RHR in HF is significant because of its importance for medical therapy in these patients. Both sympathetic and RAAS overactivity was liable for the relationship between RHR and HF. The purposes behind this affiliation are increased oxygen consumption, decreased myocardial perfusion, and consequently decreased cardiac performance, hemodynamic changes, and ultimately pro-arrhythmic effect.[2] In individuals with heart failure and reduced Ejection Fraction (HFrEF), elevated HR has been correlated with adverse results, independently of traditional risk factors.[47] Although, in a real-world setting, the effect of HR measured at the time of diagnosis and serially during follow-up and management on outcomes in HFrEF is not well-defined. Therefore, to determine the relation of HR with outcomes in HFrEF, Kurgansky *et al.* led a retrospective cohort study. In this investigation utilizing veterans affairs (VA) national electronic health records, a total of 51,194 HFrEF cases were identified. The relationship of both baseline and serially measured pulse rates (PRs) with mortality and days HHF per year and any other cause was examined by utilizing crude and multiple Cox proportional analysis. The result showed that compared to patients with PR <70 bpm, those who had a PR ≥70 bpm in the past 6-month had 36%, 25%, and 51% increased rates of mortality, all-cause hospitalization, and HHF. Additionally, it was seen that a lower PR at the time of HFrEF diagnosis and across follow-up clinical encounters was strongly associated with a lower risk of mortality and hospitalization in a real-world setting. Therefore, strategies to lower HR might be beneficial in diminishing the morbidity and mortality associated with HFrEF.[48]

Take Home Pearls

- Several epidemiological studies have suggested that elevations in RHR are related to increased risk of CVD and total mortality.
- Increased RHR is not only a significant predictor of total and CV mortality in patients with proven CAD but also in the healthy population.
- Both sympathetic and RAAS are responsible for the relationship between RHR and HF.
- In patients with HFrEF increased HR has been unfavorable outcomes, independently of traditional risk factors.

EVALUATION OF RHR AS A CV RISK FACTOR

HR is a major determinant of myocardial oxygen demand, myocardial performance, and coronary blood flow and influences nearly all stages of CVDs. Evidence that RHR may be a marker or even be a risk factor for CV morbidity and death rate has been growing since the last two decades. Recently, numerous epidemiological investigations have shown RHR to be an autonomous predictor of CV and ACM, with a global estimation of 30 to 50% death rate excess for every 20-bpm increase at rest. Studies have found a continuous elevation in risk with HR >60 bpm. Also, it was observed in the studies that RHR was an autonomous risk predictor of sudden death, even when other CV risk factors were taken into account in a multivariate analysis. This affiliation has been consistent and was seen in healthy populations among genders, various races, HTN subjects, patients with CAD or HF. This increasing evidence suggested that HR does not just foresee the outcome, but that elevated HR might be a real CV risk factor.[49,50]

HR elevation is associated with CV risk factors via SO. It is closely related to cardiometabolic abnormalities, for example, IR, glucose intolerance, HTN, dyslipidemia, and obesity. Subjects with elevated HR are likely to accumulate CV risk factors (Fig. 2.7). Also, an elevated RHR may predispose to these cardiometabolic abnormalities, proposing that an early rise in sympathetic drive may promote these metabolic changes.[51]

RHR both contributes to and reflects cardiac pathology. Due to imbalances of the ANS with increased SO or reduced vagal tone, increased HR has an impact on perfusion-contraction matching, which regulates myocardial blood supply and

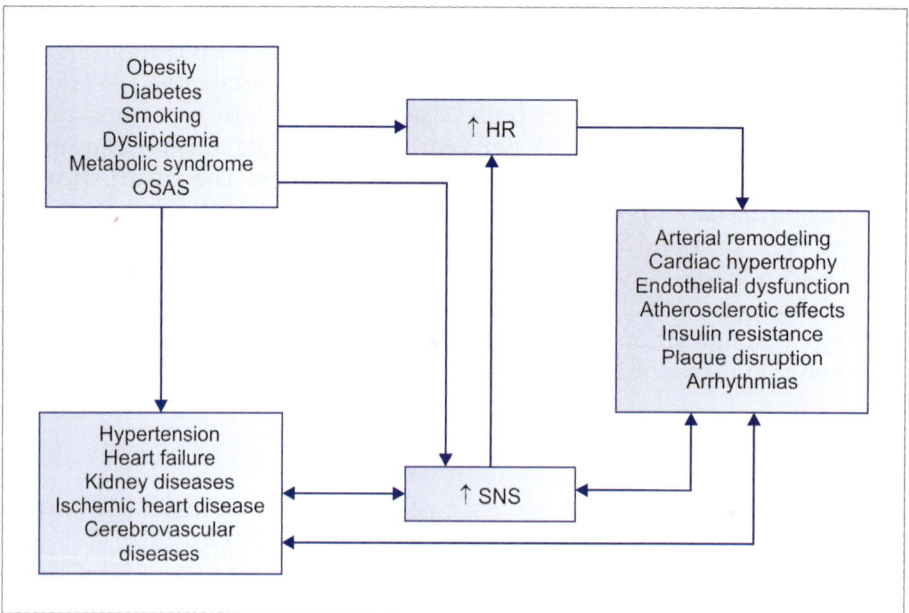

Fig. 2.7: Interplays of HR with CV risk factors and in an established CV. OSAS: Obstructive sleep apnea syndrome; SNS: Sympathetic nervous system; HR: Heart rate

function.[50] In the presence of CAD, perfusion-contraction mismatching is localized to the areas of inadequate supply. At the point when the coronary artery inflow is lacking to meet demands, contractile and diastolic functions in the affected area are correspondingly diminished. An HR elevation results not just in an elevation in myocardial oxygen demands but also in a potential impairment of supply resulting from a reduction of collateral perfusion pressure and collateral flow. This unevenness promotes arrhythmias, ischemia, and ventricular dysfunction, HF, as well as acute coronary syndromes, or SCD (Fig. 2.8).[52] The diastolic perfusion time diminishes while myocardial oxygen demand elevates with elevated HR. Peak coronary flow increases considerably during diastole, subjecting the coronary arteries to increase endothelial shear stress and pulsatile wall stress. The stressed endothelium discharges growth hormones and is related to increased platelet aggregation and a relative deficiency of NO synthesis. These factors contributed to the development of atherosclerotic lesions.[53]

Prolonged HR elevation causes cardiac noradrenaline synthesis to increase and circulate plasma noradrenaline levels to rise. This elevation in SO and myocardial oxygen requirements has a direct cytotoxic impact on myocytes and increasing apoptosis with deleterious effects on ventricular remodeling. Elevated HR reduces the flexibility of the larger arteries, resulting in a greater pulsatile arterial load on the heart; consequently, increasing the myocardial energy requirements.[46] Besides, prolonged elevated HR may also cause or exacerbate HF.[54]

Pathophysiological Effects of HR on the CVD Continuum

The CVD continuum includes risk factors initiating a process leading to tissue damage and a subsequent chain of events resulting in end-stage CVD. From vascular risk

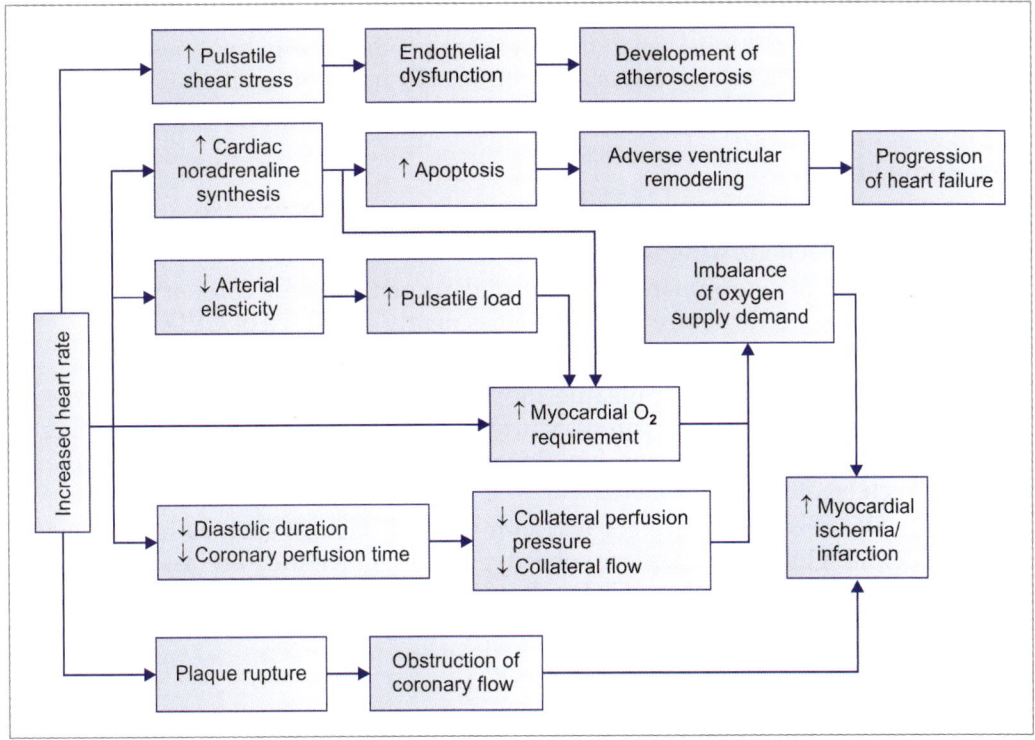

Fig. 2.8: Pathophysiological mechanisms promoted by increased HR

factors to CV events and HF, HR affects at each phase of the CV continuum and has, therefore, evolved as a relevant risk marker and goal of therapy in CV prevention and disease.[21] HR likewise firmly connected with surrogate markers, for example, inflammation, subclinical, endothelial function severity of CAD, the progression of CAD and carotid artery stenosis, and eventually plaque rupture, indicating that HR is related to every process of atherosclerosis. Moreover, high HR most of the time exists together with CV risk factors, for example, HTN, glucose metabolism abnormality, obesity, dyslipidemia, and their clustering, and related with target organ damage such as chronic kidney disease (CKD), albuminuria, atrial fibrillation, and diabetic retinopathy.[55]

RHR has developed from an ordinary clinical variable to a relevant CV risk marker based on the evidence from epidemiological and clinical investigations. Elevated RHR increases the risk and interferes at each phase of the CVD continuum, starting from endothelial dysfunction to end-stage CVD.[21] HR elevation is related to CV risk factors via SO.[55] Accelerated RHR was additionally demonstrated to be firmly connected to systemic inflammation and markers of endothelial dysfunction.[21]

Thus, it can be inferred that HR is a simple, easy, and inexpensive biomarker that can be observed without special techniques or instruments. It provides data about the patients' CV risk such as hemodynamic conditions, cardiometabolic status, autonomic nerve status, and atherosclerotic status. There is consistent evidence that RHR can predict life expectancy and is an autonomous predictor of morbidity and death rate in healthy subjects, and HR reduction can lead to a better prognosis. HR acts as a CV risk marker in the early phase of the CV continuum, where the patient does not have the CVD, whereas in the later stages when the patient has established CV disease, HR acts as a risk factor. Therefore, HR has a bidirectional relationship with CVD.

Take Home Pearls

- Evidence that RHR may be a marker or even a risk factor for CV morbidity and mortality has been growing since the last two decades.
- HR is a significant determinant of myocardial oxygen demand, coronary blood flow, and myocardial performance and influences nearly all stages of CVD.
- Elevation in HR is related to CV risk factors via SO.
- Rapid RHR intensifies the pulsatile movement of the heart and systematically changes the geometry of the coronary artery, affecting the local hemodynamics. It causes additional structural and functional changes in coronary artery endothelial cells, which leads to atherosclerosis.
- Elevated HR also frequently coexist with CV risk factors such as hypertension, dyslipidemia, glucose intolerance, obesity, and together they are associated with target organ damage such as CKD, albuminuria, atrial fibrillation, and diabetic retinopathy.

Take Home Summary

HR is a physical sign which can be easily and non-invasively estimated without special training. It is a determinant of coronary blood flow, myocardial oxygen demand, and myocardial performance and is central to the adaptation of CO to metabolic needs. HR has become an established biomarker with strong predictive of CV outcomes because it can be easily influenced by various conditions. An elevation in the RHR predisposes to cardiometabolic abnormalities and is also closely associated with them. It is also related to endothelial dysfunction, inflammation, plaque formation and progression, eventually plaque rupture, and CV death, indicating that HR is related to every process of atherosclerosis. SO is the basic trigger that causes hemodynamic changes, arrhythmias, and metabolic and elevated RHR is a surrogate of SO. Also, it was seen in a few investigations that HR is a significant risk for acute coronary events and incident HF, including CV morbidity and death rate. Therefore, the measurement of HR ought to be carried out in individuals with or without established CVD and should be viewed in the same way as other traditional risk factors. Lowering RHR might be a potential target to diminish the risk of CVD and premature mortality.

Consensus Summary

- There is a relation between high RHR and CV and ACM. However, in a healthy population, RHR can be considered a risk marker and not a risk factor.
- In individuals with stable angina, post-MI, and HFrEF, high RHR is a risk factor.
- In all other subsets of the population, one needs to be vigilant regarding RHR as a risk marker and treat the patient holistically to reduce overall CV risk.
- Lifestyle modification can be considered in individuals having high RHR without any evidence of CVD or CV risk factors.

REFERENCES

1. Seravalle G, Grassi G. Heart rate as cardiovascular risk factor. *Postgraduate Medicine.* 2020 May;132(4):358–67.

2. Tadic M, Cuspidi C, Grassi G. Heart rate as a predictor of cardiovascular risk. *European Journal of Clinical Investigation.* 2018 Jan;48(3):e12892.

3. Caetano J, Alves JD. Heart rate and cardiovascular protection. *European Journal of Internal Medicine.* 2015 May;26(4):217–22.

4. Böhm M, Schumacher HE, Teo KK, *et al.* Resting heart rate and cardiovascular outcomes in diabetic and non-diabetic individuals at high cardiovascular risk analysis from the ONTARGET/TRANSCEND trials. *European Heart Journal.* 2020 Jan;41(2):231–8.

5. Grad C, Zdrenghea D. Heart rate recovery in patients with ischemic heart disease-Risk factors. *Clujul Medical.* 2014;87(4):220–5.

6. Inoue T, Iseki K, Ohya Y. Heart rate as a possible therapeutic guide for the prevention of cardiovascular disease. *Hypertension Research.* 2013 Aug;36(10):838–44.

7. Manolio T. Novel risk markers and clinical practice. *New England Journal of Medicine.* 2003 Oct 23;349(17):1587–9.

8. Stampfer MJ, Ridker PM, Dzau VJ. Risk factor criteria. *Circulation.* 2004 Jun 29;109(25 suppl 1):IV3– 5.

9. Offord DR, Kraemer HC. Risk factors and prevention. *Evidence-Based Mental Health.* 2000;3:70–1.

10. Borer JS. Heart rate: From risk marker to risk factor. *European Heart Journal Supplements.* 2008 Aug 1;10(suppl_F):F2–F6.

11. Dominguez-Rodriguez A, Blanco-Palacios G, Abreu-Gonzalez P. Increased heart rate and atherosclerosis: Potential implications of ivabradine therapy. *World Journal of Cardiology.* 2011 Apr 26;3(4):101–4.

12. Cowie MR. Heart rate as a treatable risk factor in cardiovascular disease. *Medicographia.* 2012;34:387– 94.

13. Kristal-Boneh E, Silber H, Harari G, *et al.* The association of resting heart rate with cardiovascular, cancer and all-cause mortality. Eight year follow-up of 3527 male Israeli employees (the CORDIS Study). *European Heart Journal.* 2000 Jan;21(2):116–24.

14. Wannamethee G, Shaper AG. The association between heart rate and blood pressure, blood lipids and other cardiovascular risk factors. *Journal of Cardiovascular Risk.* 1994 Oct;1(3):223–30.

15. Jouven X, Empana JP, Schwartz PJ, *et al.* Heart-rate profile during exercise as a predictor of sudden death. *New England Journal of Medicine.* 2005 May 12;352(19):1951–8.

16. Cooney MT, Vartiainen E, Laatikainen T, *et al.* Elevated resting heart rate is an independent risk factor for cardiovascular disease in healthy men and women. *American Heart Journal.* 2010 Apr;159(4):612– 9.

17. Chen XJ, Barywani SB, Hansson PO, *et al.* Impact of changes in heart rate with age on all-cause death and cardiovascular events in 50-year-old men from the general population. *Open Heart.* 2019;6(1):e000856.

18. Alhalabi L, Singleton MJ, Oseni AO, *et al.* Relation of higher resting heart rate to risk of cardiovascular versus noncardiovascular death. *American Journal of Cardiology.* 2017 Apr 1;119(7):1003–7.

19. Dzau VJ. Tissue angiotensin and pathobiology of vascular disease: A unifying hypothesis. *Hypertension.* 2001;37:1047–52.

20. Zamorano JL. Heart rate management: A therapeutic goal throughout the cardiovascular continuum. *European Heart Journal Supplements.* 2008 Aug;10(suppl_F):F17–F21.

21. Custodis F, Reil JC, Laufs U, *et al*. Heart rate: A global target for cardiovascular disease and therapy along the cardiovascular disease continuum. *Journal of Cardiology*. 2013 Sep;62(3):183–7.

22. Farah BQ, Christofaro DG, Balagopal PB, *et al*. Association between resting heart rate and cardiovascular risk factors in adolescents. *European Journal of Pediatrics*. 2015 Dec;174(12):1621–8.

23. Levy RL, White PD, Stroud WD, *et al*. Transient tachycardia: Prognostic significance alone and in association with transient hypertension. *Journal of the American Medical Association*. 1945 Oct 27;129(9):585–8.

24. Perret-Guillaume C, Joly L, Benetos A. Heart rate as a risk factor for cardiovascular disease. *Progress in Cardiovascular Diseases*. 2009;52(1):6–10.

25. Peer N, Lombard C, Steyn K, *et al*. Elevated resting heart rate is associated with several cardiovascular disease risk factors in urban-dwelling black South Africans. *Scientific Reports*. 2020;10(1):4605.

26. Aladin AI, Al Rifai MA, Rasool SH, *et al*. The association of resting heart rate and incident hypertension: The Henry Ford Hospital Exercise Testing (FIT) Project. *American Journal of Hypertension*. 2016 Feb;29(2):251–7.

27. Shen L, Wang Y, Jiang X, *et al*. Dose-response association of resting heart rate and hypertension in adults: A systematic review and meta-analysis of cohort studies. *Medicine*. 2020 Mar; 99(10):e19401.

28. Aboyans V, Criqui MH. Can we improve cardiovascular risk prediction beyond risk equations in the physician's office?. *Journal of Clinical Epidemiology*. 2006 Jun;59(6):547–58.

29. Gillman MW, Kannel WB, Belanger A, *et al*. Influence of heart rate on mortality among persons with hypertension: The Framingham Study. *American Heart Journal*. 1993 Apr;125(4): 1148–54.

30. Liu X, Luo X, Liu Y, *et al*. Resting heart rate and risk of metabolic syndrome in adults: A dose–response meta-analysis of observational studies. *Acta Diabetologica*. 2017 Mar;54(3):223–35.

31. Shigetoh Y, Adachi H, Yamagishi SI, *et al*. Higher heart rate may predispose to obesity and diabetes mellitus: 20-year prospective study in a general population. *American Journal of Hypertension*. 2009 Feb;22(2):151–5.

32. Palatini P, Mos L, Santonastaso M, *et al*. Resting heart rate as a predictor of body weight gain in the early stage of hypertension. *Obesity*. 2011 Mar;19(3):618–23.

33. Kim G, Lee YH, Jeon JY, *et al*. Increase in resting heart rate over 2 years predicts incidence of diabetes: A 10-year prospective study. *Diabetes & Metabolism*. 2017 Feb;43(1):25–32.

34. Lee DH, de Rezende LF, Hu FB, *et al*. Resting heart rate and risk of type 2 diabetes: A prospective cohort study and meta-analysis. *Diabetes/metabolism research and reviews*. 2019 Feb;35(2):e3095.

35. Böhm M, Schumacher H, Teo KK, *et al*. Resting heart rate and cardiovascular outcomes in diabetic and non-diabetic individuals at high cardiovascular risk analysis from the ONTARGET/TRANSCEND trials. *European Heart Journal*. 2020 Jan;41(2):231–8.

36. Böhm M, Reil JC, Danchin N, *et al*. Association of heart rate with microalbuminuria in cardiovascular risk patients: Data from I-SEARCH. *Journal of Hypertension*. 2008 Jan;26(1):18–25.

37. Sun JC, Huang XL, Deng XR, *et al*. Elevated resting heart rate is associated with dyslipidemia in middle-aged and elderly Chinese. *Biomedical and Environmental Sciences*. 2014 Aug;27(8): 601–5.

38. Raisi-Estabragh Z, Cooper J, Judge R, *et al*. Age, sex and disease-specific associations between resting heart rate and cardiovascular mortality in the UK BIOBANK. *PloS ONE*. 2020 May 29;15(5):e0233898.

39. Dominguez-Rodriguez A, Blanco-Palacios G, Abreu-Gonzalez P. Increased heart rate and atherosclerosis: Potential implications of ivabradine therapy. *World Journal of Cardiology*. 2011 Apr 26;3(4):101–4.

40. Aune D, Sen A, ó'Hartaigh B, *et al*. Resting heart rate and the risk of cardiovascular disease, total cancer, and all-cause mortality—A systematic review and dose–response meta-analysis of prospective studies. *Nutrition, Metabolism, and Cardiovascular Diseases*. 2017 Jun;27(6):504–17.

41. Diaz A, Bourassa MG, Guertin MC, *et al*. Long-term prognostic value of resting heart rate in patients with suspected or proven coronary artery disease. *European Heart Journal*. 2005 May;26(10):967–74.

42. Fox K, Ford I, Steg PG, *et al*. Heart rate as a prognostic risk factor in patients with coronary artery disease and left-ventricular systolic dysfunction (BEAUTIFUL): A subgroup analysis of a randomised controlled trial. *Lancet*. 2008 Sep 6;372(9641):817–21.

43. Zuanetti G, Hernandez-Bernal F, Rossi A, *et al*. Relevance of heart rate as a prognostic factor in myocardial infarction: The GISSI experience. *European Heart Journal Supplements*. 1999;1:52–7.

44. Nauman J, Janszky I, Vatten LJ, *et al*. Temporal changes in resting heart rate and deaths from ischemic heart disease. *JAMA*. 2011 Dec 21;306(23): 2579–87.

45. Lonn EM, Rambihar S, Gao P, *et al*. Heart rate is associated with increased risk of major cardiovascular events, cardiovascular and all-cause death in patients with stable chronic cardiovascular disease: An analysis of ONTARGET/TRANSCEND. *Clinical Research in Cardiology*. 2014 Feb;103(2):149–59.

46. Böhm M, Swedberg K, Komajda M, *et al*. Heart rate as a risk factor in chronic heart failure (SHIFT): The association between heart rate and outcomes in a randomised placebo-controlled trial. *Lancet*. 2010 Sep 11;376(9744):886–94.

47. Shang X, Lu R, Liu M, *et al*. Heart rate and outcomes in patients with heart failure with preserved ejection fraction: A dose–response meta-analysis. *Medicine*. 2017 Oct;96(43):e8431.

48. Kurgansky KE, Schubert P, Parker R, *et al*. Association of pulse rate with outcomes in heart failure with reduced ejection fraction: A retrospective cohort study. *BMC Cardiovascular Disorders*. 2020 Feb;20(1).

49. Riva L, Coutsoumbas GV, Maggioni AP. Heart rate in the assessment of cardiovascular prognosis. *Medicographia*. 2012;34:414–20.

50. Arnold JM, Fitchett DH, Howlett JG, *et al*. Resting heart rate: A modifiable prognostic indicator of cardiovascular risk and outcomes? *Canadian Journal of Cardiology*. 2008 May;24(Suppl A):3A–8A.

51. Ivanoviæ BA,Tadiæ M, Dinèiæ D. Heart rate: Predictor of cardiovascular risk. *Vojnosanitetski Pregled*. 2012;69(9):799–802.

52. Heusch G, Schulz R. The role of heart rate and the benefits of heart rate reduction in acute myocardial ischaemia. *European Heart Journal Supplements*. 2007 Sep 1;9(Suppl_ F):F8–F14.

53. Kjekshus JK. Importance of heart rate in determining beta-blocker efficacy in acute and long-term acute myocardial infarction intervention trials. *American Journal of Cardiology*. 1986 Apr 25;57(12):43F–49F.

54. Khasnis A, Jongnarangsin K, Abela G, *et al*. Tachycardiainduced cardiomyopathy: A review of literature. *Pacing and Clinical Electrophysiology*. 2005 Jul;28(7):710–21.

55. Inoue T, Ohya Y. Elevated heart rate, a risk factor and risk marker of cardiovascular disease. *Current Hypertension Reviews*. 2011;7(1):29–40.

Heart Rate and Hypertension

Prof. (Dr.) JC Mohan

Learning Objectives

At the end of this chapter one should be able to:

- Hypertension (HTN) and its epidemiology
- Heart rate and its relationship with BP
- High RHR and its significance in HTN
- Management of high RHR in patients with HTN

HYPERTENSION (HTN) AND ITS EPIDEMIOLOGY

HTN is the leading preventable risk factor for cardiovascular disease (CVD) and all-cause mortality (ACM), and a major public health problem due to its high prevalence all around the globe. Around 7.5 million deaths or 12.8% of the total annual deaths worldwide occur due to high blood pressure (BP).[1,2] The prevalence of HTN and other CVD is rising globally and are strongly related to various risk factors such as aging of the populations, family history, and socioeconomic changes that favor a sedentary lifestyle, obesity, smoking, alcohol consumption, unhealthy dietary habits (i.e. high sodium and low potassium intake), stress, and lack of physical activity.[1,3]

HTN definition varies depending on the guidelines. The American College of Cardiology/American Heart Association has reduced the thresholds for diagnosis of arterial HTN to values of systolic blood pressure (SBP) of at least 130 mmHg and/or diastolic blood pressure (DBP) of at least 80 mmHg, while the 2018 European Society of Cardiology/European Society of Hypertension has left the old thresholds of 140/90 mmHg.[4] In the International Society of Hypertension (ISH) guidelines, the recommended SBP value is between 140 to 159 mmHg and for DBP 90 to 99 mmHg for stage 1 HTN.[5] While the Indian Guidelines on Hypertension IV will continue with the previous definition of 140/90 mmHg for HTN.[6] For chronic heart disease, stroke, and coronary heart disease (CHD) elevated BP is a major risk factor. Other than CHD and stroke, its complications include heart failure (HF), peripheral vascular disease, renal impairment, retinal hemorrhage, and visual impairment.[2] The latest iteration of the Global Burden of Disease (GBD) study has reported that high SBP, poor dietary intake, and tobacco use are the major risk factors for mortality and morbidity.[7] HTN-related deaths occur most commonly as a result of ischemic heart disease (IHD), hemorrhagic stroke, and ischemic stroke, which are estimated to account for 4.9, 2.0, and 1.5 million deaths, respectively. Beyond its impact on mortality, GBD has reported that in 2017, high SBP was the primary risk factor globally, accounting for 10.2 million [95% uncertainty interval (UI): 9.16–11.3 million] deaths and 208 million (UI: 188–227 million) disability-adjusted life years (DALYs) for both sexes.[4,7] Between 2007 and 2017, the number of DALYs due to hypertensive heart disease increased by 31%.[4] According to reports from the World Health Organization (WHO) and GBD study, the prevalence of HTN is increasing globally, and currently, more than 1 billion people have HTN.[7]

Global Burden of HTN

The global increase in the prevalence of HTN is consistent by sex but varied by economic development. In the past two decades, it has been observed that high-income countries (HICs) experienced a modest decrease in HTN prevalence, while low-and middle-income countries (LMICs) experienced a significant increase. These disparities in HTN prevalence suggested that the health-care systems in LMICs could be facing a rapidly increasing burden of HTN and related CVDs, in addition to a substantial load of infectious diseases. LMIC contributes to nearly two-thirds of the mortality attributable to HTN. Even though, since 1980, SBP is falling globally at the rate of 1 mmHg SBP every decade but it is growing in the case of LMICs.[8] Based on the analysis of statistics from 135 population-based studies, including 968, 419 adults from 90 countries in the year 2010, it was found that the global age-standard prevalence of HTN was 31.1% [95% confidence interval (CI): 30.0–32.2%], and the age-standardized prevalence of HTN was slightly higher in men (31.9%) than in women (30.1%) and was lower in HICs (28.5%) than in LMICs (31.5%). However, the lowest prevalence of HTN in men was observed in South Asia (26.4%), and the highest prevalence was found in Central Asia (39.0%). From 2000 to 2010, the incidence of HTN increased in LMICs and declined in HICs. LMICs experienced a sharp increase in HTN prevalence from 23.8% in 2000 to 31.5% in 2010. By contrast, HICs experienced a reduction in HTN prevalence from 31.1 to 28.5% in the same 10-year period.[8,9]

As per the American College of Cardiology (ACC), there are significant differences in BP prevalence and control rates based on race/ethnicity. In the New York City Health and Nutrition Examination Survey study, a substantially higher HTN rate for Asians (38.0%) and Hispanics (33.0%) was found when compared to non-Hispanic whites (27.5%). The prevalence was higher for South Asian (43.0%) *vs* East/Southeast Asian adults (39.9%).[10] But as per WHO estimates, HTN has become the main health concern in the Asian region affecting more than 35% of the adult population.[11] Several studies documented the incidence of HTN in South Asian countries. Cardiometabolic Risk Reduction in South Asia (CARRS) adult cohort study including a total of 16,287 individuals indicated that at baseline, HTN existed in 30.1% of men (95% CI: 28.7–31.5) and 26.8% women (25.7–27.9). Between non-hypertensive adults, average SBP increased by 2.6 mmHg (95% CI: 2.1–3.1), DBP increased by 0.7 mmHg (95% CI: 0.4–1.0, and 1 in every 6 developed HTN (82.5 per 1,000 person-years, 95% CI: 80.8–84.4). In this cohort study, the risk of incident HTN was maximum (RR = 2.95, 95% CI: 2.5–3.45) in individuals with pre-HTN compared to average BP.[8]

Similarly, Neupane *et al.* in 2014 conducted a meta-analysis study to determine the incidence of HTN in member countries of the South Asian Association for Regional Cooperation (SAARC). From the initially identified 240 articles, a total of 33 met inclusion criteria were enrolled in this study. The results indicated that the total incidence of HTN and pre-HTN was 27% and 29.6%, respectively. HTN varied between the studies ranged from 13.6 to 47.9% and was greater in the studies performed in urban areas than in rural areas. Eight out of nineteen studies with information about the incidence of HTN in both genders showed that the incidence was higher among women than men, and meta-analyzes showed that sex [men: odds ratio (OR): 1.19; 95% CI: 1.02–1.37], obesity (OR: 2.33; 95% CI: 1.87–2.78), and central obesity (OR: 2.16; 95% CI: 1.37–2.95) were associated with HTN.[11]

HTN is strongly linked to obesity and both are the main contributor to CVD, and the association between these conditions is known to vary among ethnicities. Obesity contributes to the high prevalence of HTN in Asia. In the CHPSNE Study, data has shown that overweight and obese subjects have about two-fold to five-fold risk of developing HTN compared with non-obese subjects. Waist circumference and BMI have also been linked to HTN, in which abdominal obesity may independently give rise to the risk of HTN. Similarly, Foulds *et al.* performed a trial to define the association between HTN and obesity across different ethnicities. In the study, a total of 5,084 individuals enrolled, which include: white (n = 3,566), aboriginal (n = 850), East Asian (n = 446), and South Asian (n = 222). It has been observed that the East and South Asian populations have a higher risk of emerging HTN when compared to Caucasian populations at the same level of body mass index (BMI) during a follow-up of three years.[12,13]

HTN Epidemiology in India

HTN is a big health problem in India with significant regional variations and greater urban prevalence. As per reports of the WHO, GBD Study, and Non-Communicable Disease Risk Factor Collaboration (NCD-RisC), HTN is the main reason for mortality and morbidity in India.[14] It is directly responsible for 57% of all stroke deaths and 24% of all CHD deaths in India.[15]

A study of worldwide data for the global burden of HTN in 2005 reported that 20.6% of Indian men and 20.9% of Indian women were suffering from HTN. These rates for HTN in percentage are projected to go up to 22.9 and 23.6 for Indian males and females, respectively, by 2025. While WHO in 2008, estimated that the incidence of raised BP in Indians was 32.5% (33.2% in men and 31.7% in women). An alarming rise in HTN projected by the Global Burden of Hypertension 2005 study, the GBD 2010 study, and WHO 2011 NCD India specific data portray a grim picture for the 17.8% of the world's population resided in India.[15]

Recent studies from India have shown the incidence of HTN to be 25% in urban and 10% in rural people in India.[15] The incidence of HTN was seen higher among smokers (41.3%) as compared to non-smokers (25.4%) and among obese (58%) compared to overweight (37.1%) and normal weight (25.3%). The incidence of HTN was likewise found to have increased with age among both genders, particularly after 45 years of age. Bartwal *et al.* observed in a study that the incidence of HTN was 41.7% and a relationship of HTN with an increase in age, family history of HTN, an increase in salt intake, consuming mixed diet, an increase in waist circumference, waist-hip ratio, and body mass index (BMI) is present.[3]

The Fourth National Family Health Survey (NFHS-4), which involved 749,876 eligible participants, was conducted from 2015 to 2016 in all 640 districts in India. HTN prevalence in India is high, but the proportion of adults with HTN who are aware of their diagnosis are treated and have achieved control is low. The national incidence of HTN in the sampled age range was 18.1% (95% CI: 17.8%–18.4%). It was observed that men had greater prevalence than women (19.0%, 95% CI: 18.5%–19.5%, compared to 17.2%, 95% CI: 16.9–17.4%).[5,16]

Whereas outcomes from the great India BP survey, conducted with fixed one-day BP measurement camp across 24 states and union territories of India, involving 180,335 participants (33.2% women; mean age 40.6 ± 14.9 years) revealed that the overall incidence of HTN was 30.7% (95% CI: 30.5, 30.9) and the incidence among women was 23.7% (95% CI: 23.3, 24). When the prevalence adjusted for the 2011 census population and the WHO reference population, the incidence of both females and males were found to be 29.7% and 32.8%, respectively. Both SBP and DBP were found to be higher among men than women across all age groups, except in those with age ≥65 years, where an almost equal percentage of men and women had HTN. Thus, it revealed a greater incidence of HTN in Indian adults, with nearly one in three participants having HTN.[17]

Take Home Pearls

- HTN is the leading preventable risk factor for CVD and all-cause mortality.
- HTN-related deaths occur most commonly due to ischemic heart disease, hemorrhagic stroke, and ischemic stroke.
- The global escalation in the incidence of HTN is consistent by sex but varied by economic development.
- HICs experienced a modest decrease in HTN prevalence, whereas LMICs experienced significant increases in the past two decades.
- The WHO, GBD Study, and NCD-RisC reports highlighted that HTN is the main reason for mortality and morbidity in India.

HEART RATE AND ITS RELATIONSHIP WITH BP

Heart rate (HR) and BP are two distinct measurements; however, both are related constituents of the CV system. Any disturbance in one factor may cause variations of another one. Furthermore, the existence of an uncontrolled HR or BP in common people is related to a higher risk for adverse CV effects.[18] Variability signals linked with the CV system contain relevant information about the behavior of the autonomic nervous system (ANS) that acts as a controller of many physiological parameters such as HR and BP.[19,20] In particular, BP is a complex parameter that has both physiological and neurological influences and in contrast, HR represents the cardiac cycle and determines the heart's preload and the cardiac output (CO) which positively impacts BP as the pressure on the arterial walls.[21] Both HR and BP in resting subjects are not constant but fluctuate around mean values. The short term variations in R-R interval (RRI) and BP are mainly due to respiration and to the so-called 10-second-rhythm. Respiratory sinus arrhythmia, noticeable as respiration-linked variations in HR, is a well-known phenomenon, also is the respiratory variation in BP.[22]

Changes in HR and BP are mediated through various nervous and hormonal mechanisms. The sympathetic nervous system (SNS) has an essential role in arterial BP control. The sympathetic outflow increases arterial pressure via vasoconstriction (feedforward), while elevations in BP suppress sympathetic outflow via the baroreflex (feedback) mechanism. An imbalance in the ANS, with increased sympathetic activity and/or decreased parasympathetic activity, might be implicated in the pathogenesis of higher HR and elevation in BP (Fig. 3.1).[23]

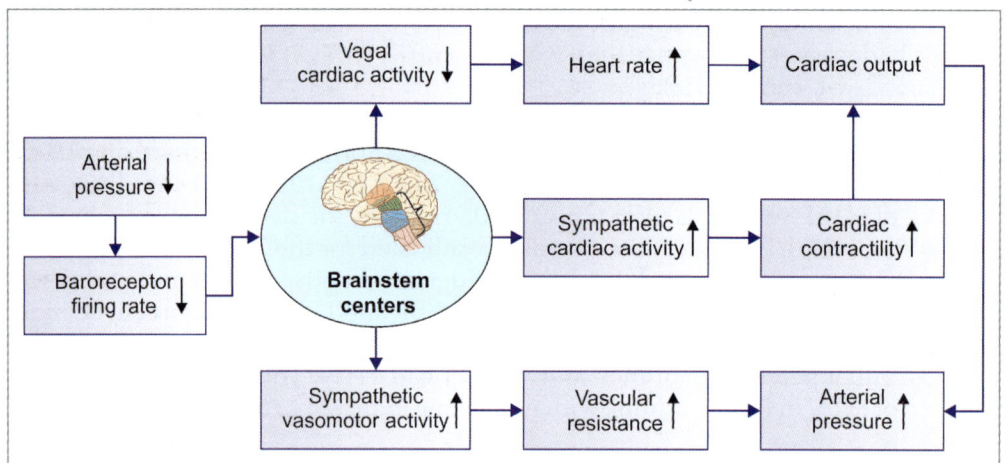

Fig. 3.1: Flow diagram showing the sequence of events after a reduction in arterial pressure results in reflex compensatory restoration of arterial pressure

HR and BP are also regulated by the ANS, which is inversely related based on baroreflex activity. Continuous recordings of SBP and interbeat intervals (IBI) revealed time sequences of spontaneously occurring consecutive beats in which BP and HR change in the opposite direction (i.e. increased SBP with increased IBI, or decreased SBP with decreased IBI). These sequences are considered to be an expression of the negative feedback mechanisms of baroreflex origin.[23] As per several epidemiological studies, higher SBP and HR are predictors of death and disability in the common people. BP-HR product or double product (DP) is a reliable surrogate measurement of myocardial oxygen consumption and an important sign of the workload of the heart. DP values are detected by using 24-hour ambulatory BP measurements, which makes it possible to retrieve accurate DP values for both daytime activity and nocturnal sleep. These values tend to change according to the circadian pattern, closely linked to changes in SBP. DP verifies whether the influence of HR depends on the level of SBP and vice versa. Due to the positive predictive value of both SBP and HR in the common people, it was expected that the DP might be useful in stratification for CV risk.[24–27]

HR Concerning Central and Peripheral BP

Changes in both peripheral and central pressures are strongly associated with HR. This relationship is quite complex, location-dependent, and differs depending on the type of BP measurement, which is to be considered. The variance between central blood pressure (CBP) and peripheral blood pressure (PBP) can be up to 20 mmHg. In particular, a direct relationship is present between elevated RHR and PBP, though an inverse relationship is present between elevated RHR and CBP. Therefore, an increase in HR is known to escalate the peripheral pressure while it reduces the central pressure.[28,22]

The association between HR and CBP is more complex than HR and PBP, mostly because of the elastic properties of the arterial network and the generation of wave reflections. In particular, the CBP is caused due to the summation of the forward pulse wave from the ventricular contraction and the reflected backward wave from the periphery to the heart. The reflected wave reaches the heart during the diastolic phase of the forward wave-enhancing diastolic aortic pressure and thereby coronary perfusion. HR variations and augmented aortic stiffness can disturb this ventricular-vascular coupling, leading to CBP alterations. Human studies have reported that HR lowering with negative chronotropic agents leads to increased CBP (as HR decreases, the reflected wave, which arrives in the heart during the systolic phase of the forward wave, leads to systolic CBP augmentation).[22,29]

HR and Arterial Stiffness

Resting HR (RHR) is a simple and useful indicator of autonomic balance and metabolic rate. Due to the greater percentage of oxygen consumption, high HR is related to oxidative stress and chronic subclinical inflammation. An elevated HR enables low, oscillatory endothelial shear stress and increased tensile stress, inducing a pro-inflammatory phenotype with elevated levels of adhesion molecules, promoting arterial stiffness.[30] Increased pulse wave velocity (PWV), a marker of arterial stiffness, has also been directly related to raised RHR. According to several trials, elevated HR promotes alterations in vascular stress results in induce endothelial dysfunction, inflammation processes, and disturbed distensibility, leading in time to atherosclerosis and increased vascular stiffness.[31] Park BJ *et al.* assessed the relationship between RHR and arterial stiffness in adults with the help of brachial-ankle pulse wave velocity (baPWV) measurement. A total of 641 adults were enrolled in the study. Odds ratios (OR) for high baPWVs were determined by multivariable logistic regression analysis after adjusting for confounding variables across HR quartiles (Q1 ≤56, Q2 = 57–62, Q3 = 63–68, Q4 ≥69 bpm). Results revealed that the age-adjusted baPWV mean values was increased progressively with HR quartile (Q1 = 1281 (17.1), Q2 = 1285 (14.8), Q3 = 1354 (14.7), and Q4 = 1416 (15.5) cm/s) (Fig. 3.2). The OR (95% CI) for high baPWVs in every HR quartile was found to be 1.00, 1.28 (0.57–2.86), 2.63 (1.20–5.79), and 3.66 (1.66–8.05), respectively. Results revealed that a higher RHR is freely related to arterial stiffness.[32]

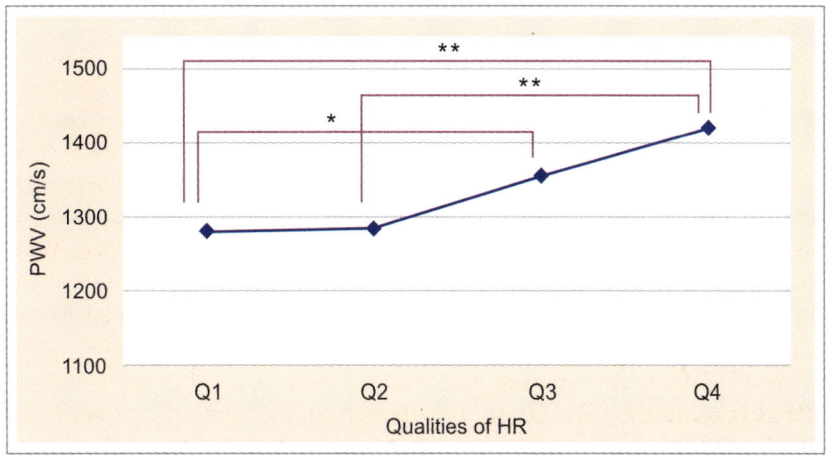

Fig. 3.2: Age-adjusted means of baPWV according to heart rate quartile. Bars represent standard errors. $^*p <0.01$, $^{**}p <0.05$

Augmentation index (AIx), an indicator of reflection waves, has also been observed to be inversely correlated with HR.[22] It is the extent of systemic arterial stiffness resulting from the ascending aortic pressure waveform. Wilkinson IB *et al.* in 2000 conducted a study including a total of 22 subjects (13 male) with a mean age of 63 years to examine the effect of HR on AIx and CBP. In this study, AIx and CBP were calculated with the help of pulse wave analysis, which further assess central arterial pressure waveforms, non-invasively throughout incremental pacing (from 60 to 110 bpm). The outcome of the trial revealed that a substantial, inverse, linear relationship was found between AIx and HR ($r = -0.76$; $p < 0.001$). With each 10-bpm increase, AIx fell by about 4%. Ejection duration and HR were inversely related ($r = -0.51$; $p < 0.001$). Peripheral systolic, diastolic, and mean arterial pressure was also increased considerably during incremental pacing because of variations in the timing of the reflected pressure wave produced by variations in the absolute duration of systole. The concern of wave reflection and aortic pressure intensification may also describe the rise in central systolic pressure throughout incremental pacing despite an increase in peripheral pressure.[33]

Take Home Pearls

- HR and BP are two separate measurements, but both are interrelated constituents of the CV system.
- HR and BP are regulated by the ANS, which is inversely related based on baroreflex activity.
- Changes in peripheral and central pressures are intensely related to HR, and its relationship is quite complex and location dependent.
- An accelerated HR enables low oscillatory endothelial shear stress and increased tensile stress, inducing a pro-inflammatory phenotype with elevated levels of adhesion molecules, thereby promoting arterial stiffness.
- AIx an indicator of arterial stiffness is inversely related to HR.

HIGH RHR AND ITS SIGNIFICANCE IN HTN

High RHR and HTN

RHR reflects autonomic control system activity and mirrors the equilibrium of sympathetic and parasympathetic nerves.[34] HR and BP are firmly connected, and hypertensive patients have higher RHR than ordinary. The increased sympathetic nervous system (SNS) tone would be the causative element in this rise in HR along with a general increment in cardiac output and the production of a hyperkinetic circulation. The elevated HR may furthermore represent a sympathetic overactivation (SO), and results in elevated BP through the four pathways (Fig. 3.3).[35]

This increased renal sympathetic activation prompts decreased renal excretory function and the progress and maintenance of HTN.[35]

Elevated RHR and HTN independently enhance the risk of mortality.[36,37] Various evidence are showing that higher RHR constitutes a powerful prognostic marker of CV events and death from cardiac and non-cardiac causes in patients with HTN. Elevated RHR is related to endothelial dysfunction, sympathetic activation, reduced artery compliance, and distensibility, and thus enlarged arterial wall stress and elevated PWV, which has been further associated with increased after burden and ultimately systemic HTN (Fig. 3.4).[38]

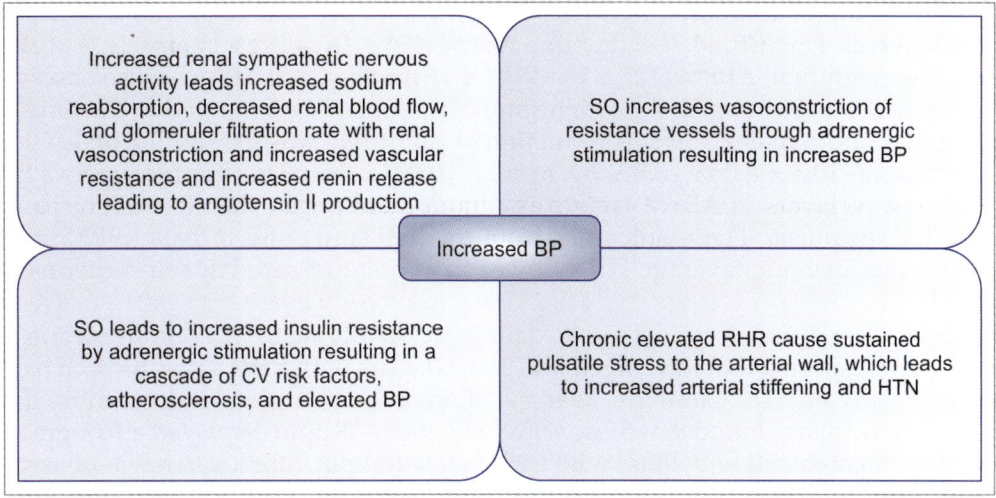

Fig. 3.3: SO pathways which contribute to the development of HTN

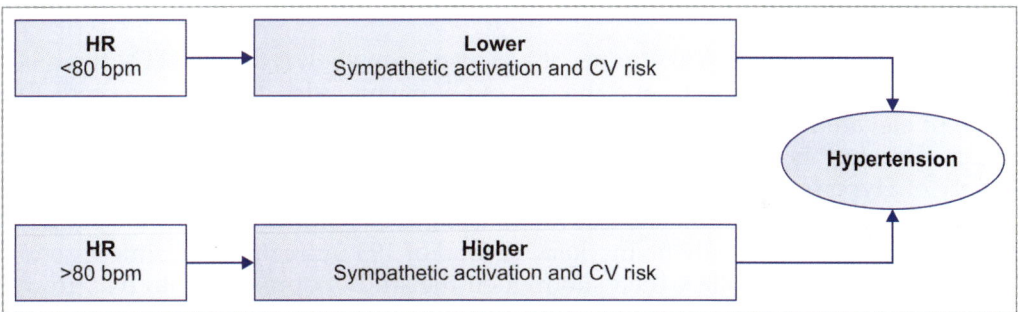

Fig. 3.4: HR value in the assessment of CV risk and sympathetic activation

According to a Pan India cross-sectional survey, involving 1,514 patients (63.58% males, 35.62% females), the prevalence of SO in newly diagnosed hypertensive patients in India was 62.42%. This statistics is consistent with statistics from Smith *et al.* study, which showed that central sympathetic activity was maximum in borderline HTN, early-stage, and complicated essential HTN, and this activity was likely to play an integral role in the growth of HTN and its complications.[39] Furthermore, according to the Indian Heart Study (IHS), incidence of white coat hypertension (WCH) and masked hypertension (MH) in India is higher in comparison with worldwide data that is associated with increasing HR. The Indian population had greater evening BP as compared to the morning SBP (127.8 ± 14.7 *vs* 129.8 ± 15.3) mmHg and DBP (81.9 ± 10.1 *vs* 82.4 ± 10.2) mmHg. The incidence of WCH was 24%, and 18% of the participants had MH. Increased RHR (79.8 ± 9.6 bpm) was present in more than half of the participants of IHS. The increased HR was more common in WCH.[40]

However, another India ambulatory blood pressure measurement (ABPM) study was performed from January 2017 to November 2018 to examine gender-related differences in BP and HR pattern. The study enrolled a total of 14,977 subjects. Outcomes revealed that women had higher HR during the daytime and nighttime and a lower HR dip as compared to men, signifying a greater risk of all-cause mortality and CV events. For SBP, a lower daytime ABPM (131 ± 16 vs 133 ± 14 mmHg, p <0.001) but higher nighttime ABPM (122 ± 18 vs 121 ± 16 mmHg, p <0.001) was also observed in females compared to males. At nighttime, HR reduced as compared to daytime for both males and females, but this reduction at nighttime was greater for males than for females (−10.5 ± 8.0 vs −8.8 ± 6.8 bpm, p <0.001). Females after menopause had significant variances in ABPM factors as compared to males, therefore, signifying a worse CV diagnosis. These outcomes from the IHS study and Indian ABPM study showed that 24 hours average HR is lower than point-of-care HR self-measured at home.[41]

Another latest study conducted by Aladin et al. involving 21,873 non-hypertensive participants reported that those aged less than 60 years with RHR above 85 bpm had a 20% more risk of HTN. Similarly, Wang et al. in an eastern population of more than 100,000 participants, found that those with RHR above 78 bpm displayed a 16% greater risk of HTN compared with those with RHR below 66 bpm. Moreover, it was observed that a higher RHR is related to several other risk factors like obesity, metabolic syndrome, and diabetes mellitus, which were also known to be associated with elevating BP as well. An imbalance in the ANS, with increased sympathetic activity and/or decreased parasympathetic activity, might be implicated in the cause of higher RHR and elevation in BP.[22]

In several epidemiological studies, it has also been shown that in HTN there is a substantial link between RHR and the risk of CV events. Also, the adverse predictive value of elevated HR is independent of the concomitant presence of other CV risk factors. Due to this evidence, the recent European Society of Cardiology/European Society of Hypertension guidelines identifies RHR values >80 bpm as interpreters of CV risk. Grassi G et al. conducted a study to test this hypothesis with the assistance of direct and indirect sympathetic markers. A total of 193 untreated moderate essential HTN patients were enrolled, then subdivided the study population into two groups as per HR< or >80 bpm (eighty-four patients displayed RHR >80 bpm). The study revealed that the clinic and ABP were similar in the two groups, whereas the left ventricular mass index (LVMI) was significantly greater in the group with HR >80 bpm. Muscle sympathetic nerve activity (MSNA) values were also significantly greater in this latter group (72.77 ± 0.9 vs 36.83 ± 1.3 bursts/min, p <0.0001); this being the case for norepinephrine (NE) level in plasma (293.0 ± 8.7 vs 254.1 ± 8.9 pg/mL, p <0.002). In the whole population, a significant direct relationship was seen between MSNA, NE, LVMI, and HR values. Also, similar results were obtained when 24-hour HR values were analyzed. Therefore, when direct adrenergic markers are used, patients with HTN showing HR >80 bpm are characterized by a noticeable sympathetic overdrive. These findings suggested that cardiac and peripheral sympathetic activation are involved in the increased CV risk identified in this group.[42]

It is well-known that high SBP is a robust CVD risk. Besides, it was reported that high HR is a risk factor for CVD and non-CVD. Although the double product (DP) is the product of SBP and HR, it has not been previously investigated whether the DP measured at rest has predictive power for the death rate in the common people. Therefore, to determine whether the DP at rest based on home BP measurement has prognostic value for mortality or not, Inoue R et al. conducted an Ohasama study. Preliminary findings in the Ohasama study suggested that the DP derived from self-measured home BP was a more precise predictor of mortality than were the constituents of the product. The respective increases in risk for total, CV and non-CV mortality were found to be 15.1%, 17.6%, and 13.9% for every 1,000 mmHg* bpm rises in the DP. Also, both SBP and HR predicted total mortality. It explains that DP at rest established on high BP measurement was considerably related to not only CVD mortality but also non-CVD mortality.[25,43]

Elevated RHR and HTN independently increase the risk of mortality. However, their combined influence on the death rate in different stages of HTN in aged people is unclear. So, to define the relation of RHR and HTN stages on all-cause and CV mortality in aged people, Ryu M *et al.* performed a Kangwha cohort study. The study enrolled a total of 6,100 residents, ages between 55- to 99-year-old. Hazard ratios were calculated for all-cause and CV mortality by RHR and HTN defined by Eighth Joint National Committee criteria using the cox proportional hazard model after adjusting for confounding factors. Hazard ratios associated with RHR >80 bpm were higher in hypertensive men compared with normotensives with HR of 61–79 bpm, with hazard ratios values of 1.43 (95% CI: 1.00–1.92) on all-cause mortality for pre-HTN, 3.01 (95% CI: 1.07–8.28) on CV mortality for pre-HTN, and 8.34 (95% CI: 2.52–28.19) for stage 2 HTN. Also, greater risk (HR: 3.54, 95% CI: 1.16–9.21) was observed among those with both an RHR ≥80 bpm and pre-HTN on CV mortality in females. Individuals with coexisting elevated RHR and HTN, even in pre-HTN have more risk for all-cause and CV mortality compared to those with elevated RHR or HTN alone. These findings proposed that elevated RHR should not be regarded as a less serious risk factor in elderly hypertensive patients.[37]

In hypertensive and normotensive patients, Li X *et al.* in 2018 examined data from two cross-sectional studies to evaluate the incidence of fast RHR and related factors. The study enrolled a total of 6,763 hypertensive patients and 2,807 normotensive subjects. Outcomes of the study revealed that the incidence of fast RHR was greater in hypertensive patients as compared with the normotensives (14.4% *vs* 7.1%, p <0.01). Fast RHR appeared as a "U-type" distribution as aging and an "inverted J type" trend as BMI increasing in both hypertensive and normotensive patients. Also, multivariate regression examination revealed that fast RHR was related with age >65 or <25 years old (OR: 1.32, 95% CI: 1.08–1.61), BMI <18.5 kg/m^2 (OR: 2.94, 95% CI: 1.47–5.87) and hypercholesterolemia (OR: 1.30, 95% CI: 1.10–1.53) in hypertensive patients. Fast RHR in the normotensives was related with a female (OR: 1.78, 95% CI: 1.27–2.48), pre-hypertensive state (OR: 2.38, 95% CI: 1.61–3.52), and rural area origin (OR: 1.50, 95% CI: 1.01–2.42). Results revealed that in patients with HTN, fast RHR might be common.[34]

The studies mentioned above clearly explain that there is a link between BP and RHR and can be used to adapt treatment. However, the variation in HR and BP levels throughout the day is common. It has been observed that a portion of the population has higher BP levels when obtained by medical personnel compared to the levels obtained by them. Once this variance is significant and established by 24-hour ABPM, it exposes the clinical conditions known as white coat syndrome, which includes: (a) White coat effect (WCE), (b) WCH, and (c) white coat normotension or MH. This phenomenon has been generally established in BP analysis and taken into account in international guidelines, though these effects have not been evaluated in HR, and there are no established values of normal RHR. Mancia *et al.* were the first to determine that HR could vary 15 bpm parallel to BP changes during a consultation with an immediate reversible effect.[42,43] Furthermore, to determine that RHR measured by the physician reflects the patient's true RHR (White-coat HR), Lequeux et al. conducted an observational, pilot study. A total of 57 ambulatory patients were enrolled and separated into three groups to look for relations with BP. Results revealed that HR was considerably greater in consultation (70.6 bpm ± 12.6 vs 68.2 bpm ± 10.1, $p = 0.034$), and was found correlated with DBP ($r = 0.45$, $p = 0.001$). In the HR subgroup analysis where patients are distributed into three groups according to the variation in HR between measurement in consultation and home self-measurement, it was observed that masked HR: [was higher at home self-measurement, 38.6% (22 patients)], white-coat-HR: [was lower at home self-measurement, 52.6% (30 patients)] and for iso HR, [no change between HR at home and consultation, 8.8% (5 patients)]. Though no difference was detected between groups in DBP measured in consultation, home DBP was found lesser in the white-coat HR group (74.3 mmHg ± 9.8 vs 77.9 mmHg ± 7.5, $p = 0.016$). The findings showed that RHR measured by the physician in the consultation does not reveal true RHR. It must be taken into account to adapt to treatment.[45]

Arterial HTN is also an essential risk factor for the worldwide burden of disease; however, its relationship with RHR has remained yet unclear. To avoid the sequelae of arterial HTN, identifying factors that may predict arterial HTN in high-risk populations would be beneficial. Therefore, for identifying the factors Wang A et al. performed a Kailuan cohort study involving 101,510 individuals. It was observed in the study that elevated RHR is related to a higher risk of the development of arterial HTN independently of other parameters such as arterial BP and diabetes mellitus in a mean follow-up of 3.5 ± 0.9 years. Likewise, it was observed that 12,565 (39.88%) individuals developed arterial HTN, and the occurrence of HTN was 104.4, 109.7, 114.2, and 124.6 per 1,000 person-years for each RHR quartile. In multivariate analysis with adjustment for BP, blood lipids, diabetes mellitus, and other parameters, hazard ratios for new-onset hypertension (NOH) increased significantly ($p < 0.0001$) with increasing RHR quartile. Furthermore, an increase in RHR by 10-bpm was related to an 8% escalation in NOH. Individuals in the highest RHR quartile revealed a 16% more risk of developing NOH when compared to participants in the lowest quartile.[46]

The Relationship between HRV and HTN

Heart rate variability (HRV), the spontaneous fluctuations around the mean HR, is a simple non-invasive measurement for investigating autonomic influence on the heart.[45] Low HRV has been identified as a robust indicator of risk related to adverse events in healthy people other than diseased patients, reflecting the vital role of the ANS in maintaining health.[46] Several trials have confirmed that decreased HRV is associated with an increased incidence of cardiac morbidity and mortality. A reduced HRV can be also used as an interpreter of HTN.[45] Huikuri et al. in 1996 conducted a research study to compare measures of HRV in subjects with HTN and normotension and to evaluate the association of HRV to lifestyle, demographic variable, systolic and diastolic pressure, and antihypertensive medication and ECG results. The study enrolled a total of 188 normotensive and 168 hypertensive males. The findings revealed that all events of HRV, except the high frequency (HF) domain, were significantly lower in subjects with HTN than in those with normotension. Subjects with HTN had significant changes in the low frequency (LF) and HF components of HRV in response to sitting compared with subjects with normotension. Multiple regression analysis showed the standard deviation of all normal to normal RR intervals (SDNN) to be predicted most strongly by BP, both in subjects with HTN and normotension. After adjustment for baseline differences in SBP and BMI between groups, no differences in HRV measures persisted. These results demonstrated that HTN results in decreased overall HRV and blunted autonomic responses during a change in body posture.[47] HRV is a non-intrusive tool to quantitatively estimate cardiac autonomic activity and has been used to document decreased cardiac autonomic activity in HTN. However, the capacity of decreased HRV to predict incident HTN has not been well-studied, and no studies are present which describe whether HTN leads to alteration in HRV. Therefore, to define the temporal sequence linking HTN, BP, and HRV in a population, Schroder et al. in 2003 investigated 11,061 individuals aged 45 to 54 years at baseline. Outcomes revealed that, among 7,099 individuals without HTN at baseline, low HRV predicted more risk of incident HTN over 9-year of follow-up. The hazard ratio (95% CI) for the lowest compared with the highest quartile of the SDNN was observed to be 1.24 (95% CI: 1.10–1.40), for the root mean square of successive differences in normal-to-normal RR intervals (RMSSD) was 1.36 (95% CI: 1.21–1.54), and for RR interval was 1.44 (95% CI: 1.27–1.63). These findings concerning HRV and incident HTN suggested that ANS dysregulation precedes the progress of clinical HTN.[50]

Another prospective cohort analysis was conducted by Singh et al. related the measures of HRV between subjects with HTN and normotension in the Framingham Heart Study and evaluated the role of HRV as an interpreter of NOH at follow-up. In the analysis, all the subjects were measured for 2 hours of ambulatory ECG recordings: 3-time domain and 5 frequency domain variables. The findings revealed that all HRV measures, except the LF/HF ratio, were considerably decreased in subjects with HTN compared with those with normotension. Among the subjects in the study (633 men and 801 women), 119 men and 125 women developed HTN at the follow-up examination 4 years later. The LF measure was associated with NOH in men. The results confirmed that HRV decreases in men and women with systemic HTN. Besides, among male subjects with normotension, lower HRV is related to a higher risk for developing HTN.[51]

High RHR as a Predictor or Precursor for HTN

It has been proved in several epidemiological studies that elevated HR can be a predictor or precursor for the development of HTN. Levy et al. in 1945 determined the first evidence highlighting the role of raised HR as a predictor/precursor for the future progress of HT. A total of 23,000 army officers with or without transient elevated HR were evaluated and screened for the future development of HT. Results revealed that the group with transient elevated HR or HTN develops HTN 2- to 3-fold more frequently than the control group.[52]

Similarly, in 1968 Paffenberg et al. cross-examined 7,500 former male college students with a consistent self-administered mail questionnaire and compared them with the college medical records 30 years earlier. They found a considerable variance in HR among the former students with self-reported HTN compared to the normotensive group (84 vs 82) and concluded that an increased HR is a risk factor for the future of HTN.[53] Whereas outcomes of the Fifth Korea National Health and Nutrition Examination Survey (KNHANES) suggested that men with RHR of 90 bpm or more were at 2.75-times increased risk of incident HTN, but the same relation was not seen in women. Higher BMI (>23 kg/m²) was also related to a greater risk of incident HTN. Further, a higher HR significantly increased the risk of diabetes and metabolic syndrome (MetS) in both genders. These outcomes suggested a significant increase in incident HTN with an increase in RHR.[28]

Inoue *et al.* in 2007 also performed a trial to decide whether a higher HR was related to the development of HTN in normotensive, screened subjects. A total of 4,300 normotensive participants with mean age 47 ± 7 were enrolled in the study, and the populations were separated into four groups depending on their HR. During a follow-up period of 3 years, the frequency of developing HTN was 4.5% in quartile 1 (HR ≤58), 6.8% in quartile 2 (HR ≤64), 6.0% in quartile 3 (65≤ HR ≤70), and 7.2% in quartile 4 (HR ≥71) ($p = 0.0424$). Subjects with greater HR have a large number of MetS components and a greater prevalence of proteinuria ($p < 0.0001$). Whereas in a logistic regression examination modified for gender, age, alcohol consumption, exercise, atherosclerotic risk factors, and lifestyle, the OR (95% CI) for the development of HTN was observed to be 1.53 (1.04–2.24) for quartile 2, 1.35 (0.90–2.02) for quartile 3 and 1.61 (1.10–2.37) for quartile 4, compared to quartile 1 as reference. These outcomes indicated that high HR was related to the development of HTN.[35]

The studies mentioned above clearly explain that a high HR is a predictor for the development of HTN, but whether HR predicts the development of sustained HTN in individuals with HTN is unclear. Therefore, to evaluate whether RHR and heart changes predict the development of sustained HTN in individuals screened for stage 1 HTN, Palatini *et al.* performed a study. A total of 1,103 patients were enrolled in the study. During a follow-up period of 6-month, it was found that clinic HR and HR changes in the first 6-month of follow-up were independent predictors of subsequent SBP and DBP regardless of initial BP and other confounders (all $p < 0.01$). Also, a significant interaction was found between sex (male) and baseline RHR on final SBP ($t = 2.4$, $p = 0.017$) and DBP ($t = 3.6$, $p < 0.001$). Patients whose HR was elevated persistently during the study had a doubled fully adjusted risk (95% CI: 1.4–2.9) of developing sustained HTN in comparison with subjects with a normal HR and transitional elevated HR. These outcomes concluded that baseline clinic HR and HR variations in the first few months of follow-up are independent predictors of the development of sustained HTN in young persons screened for stage 1 HTN.[54]

High RHR and Adverse Clinical Outcomes in Patients with HTN

HTN is the most prevalent disorder that affects a majority of adults and is an limportant risk factor for myocardial infarction and cerebrovascular disease. Among the metabolic syndrome components, HTN is the strongest predictor for CV events or carotid atherosclerosis.[35] Some evidence suggested a prognostic role for RHR in patients with CAD, heart failure, myocardial infarction, and HTN.[55] RHR is a strong predictor of total mortality and hospitalization due to CVD in HTN patients as a linear relationship was found between BP and average RHR. Also, high levels of RHR are concurrent with high BP in HTN patients. Therefore, the control of RHR is imperative for a better diagnosis of people suffering from HTN.[56] Paul *et al.* reported that among 3,364 patients with HTN, those with an RHR ranging from 81 to 90 bpm showed a greater risk of CV events and all-cause mortality. Similarly, the losartan intervention for endpoint reduction in hypertension (LIFE) study showed that in 9,190 patients with HTN with electrocardiographic signs of left ventricular hypertrophy cured with losartan- or atenolol-based regimens, the persistence of an HR 84 bpm or above, was related to an 89% and 97% increased risk of CV death and all-cause mortality, respectively. Whereas in the ABP-International study involving 7,600 untreated patients with HTN, it was found that each 10-bpm of HR increase during nighttime was related to a 13% increased risk of CV events.[22]

The usefulness of HR to assess cardiac events in treated patients with high-risk systemic HTN was further determined by evaluating the statistics from the VALUE trial, which suggested an incremental risk of cardiac events with the rise of HR. Every additional increment of 10 bpm from baseline is related to a hazard ratio (HR) of 1.16 for the composite cardiac outcomes in patients with high-risk HTN. The substantial relationship persisted in individual cardiac events like heart failure (HR: 1.24), sudden cardiac death (HR: 1.18), MI (HR: 1.10), stroke (HR: 1.09), and all-cause death (HR: 1.19). Patients in the highest quintile and the second-highest quintile had a considerably greater risk of the composite and individual cardiac events except for stroke. When the highest HR quintile as compared to the mean of the lower four quintiles, the association of the highest quintile with primary composite endpoint, heart failure, and total mortality persisted. Besides, an assessment by the controlled and the uncontrolled BP stated that the highest HR quintiles had considerably greater rates of composite endpoints in both the controlled (+53%, p <0.0001) and uncontrolled (+34%, p <0.002) BP groups. Likewise, lower four quintiles united with uncontrolled BP had a higher risk of the incident composite endpoints (p = 0.0035). These data from the VALUE trial revealed that elevated HR is a long-term predictor of CV events in patients with high-risk HTN.[57]

The investigation of the International VErapamil SR/Trandolapril STudy (INVEST) by Kolloch *et al.* also provides important information about the association between pharmacological HR reduction and outcome in patients with HTN. In the INVEST study, participants were randomly allocated to either verapamil (Ve) sustained-release or atenolol treatment. Trandolapril and/or hydrochlorothiazide were also administered to achieve BP goals. During a follow-up period of 2 years, it was observed that the HR was reduced by ≈6.5 bpm in the atenolol arm and by ≈3 bpm in the Ve arm. The mean follow-up RHR was intensely related to the risk for adverse outcomes, and a J-shaped relationship was observed. Also, it was observed in the study that the strategy reduced RHR more than Ve (at 24 months, 69.2 *vs* 72.8 bpm; p <0.001), and adverse outcomes were similar [Ve: 9.67% (rate 35/1000 patient-years) *vs* At 9.88% (rate 36/1,000 patient-years, CI: 0.90–1.06, p = 0.62)]. These findings revealed that among CAD patients with HTN, RHR predicts adverse outcomes, and on-treatment an RHR is more predictive than baseline RHR.[58]

RHR measured in the office is related to CV outcomes in the general people, HTN, and HF. But it is unclear whether in hypertensive patients, 24-hour oscillographic PR measurement is an estimation of HR resultant from ABPM associates with CV consequences or not. Bohm *et al.* in 2019 conducted a study to define the link between clinic and ambulatory HR parameters with mortality in HTN. ABPM recordings from 56,901 patients with the complete HR measures entering the final analysis from the Spanish Blood Pressure Monitoring Registry for a median follow-up time of 5.1 years were evaluated, and data were analyzed by Cox regression analysis, analysis of variance, and chi-square test. Results revealed that office HR was 3.5 bpm higher than mean 24-hour HR, office mean HR *vs* mean night was 10.4 bpm higher, and mean day *vs* mean night HR 9.3 bpm higher. It was also detected that office mean, 24-hour day and night HR more than 90 bpm were related to a higher risk for all-cause and non-CV death, whereas for CV death only mean night HR was predictive. Also, the strongest association to all-cause death was observed with mean night HR [hazard ratio (HR): 3.80 (2.87–5.03)], mean 24-hour HR [2.85 (2.30–3.54)], and mean day HR [2.22 (1.83–2.70)]. These outcomes showed that HR parameters derived from ABPM provide important information, in particular association with death by mean night HR, mean 24-hours, and reduced day-night HR dipping less than 8-bpm superior to office HR.[59]

Take Home Pearls

- RHR reflects the autonomic control system activity and mirrors the balance of sympathetic and parasympathetic nerves.
- Elevated RHR is related to diminished artery compliance, endothelial dysfunction, and distensibility, and subsequently increased arterial wall stress and increased PWV, which is further associated with increased after burden and ultimately systemic HTN.
- Increased renal sympathetic activation prompts diminished renal excretory function that leads to the progress and preservation of HT.
- Diminished HRV has been considered as a strong predictor of risk related to adverse events in healthy individuals and unhealthy patients, reflecting the vital role of the ANS in maintaining health.
- RHR is a strong predictor of total mortality and hospitalization due to CVD in HTN patients.
- RHR measured in the office has observed to be related to CV outcomes in the general people, HTN, and HF.

MANAGEMENT OF HIGH RHR IN PATIENTS WITH HTN

RHR is one of the risk factors related to the incident HTN. Treatment of an increased HR in HTN is a topic of debate because no clear proof for an ideal approach to the treatment of elevated HR in HTN is present. However, the European Society of Hypertension recommended the following methodologies in patients of HTN with increased RHR:

a. Self-measurement of HR should be done in patients who can manage at home.
b. Ambulatory HR measurements should be considered in patients with high HR in the clinic.
c. Secondary reasons for higher HR should always be considered.
d. Emphasis should always be on the improvement of lifestyle, increased physical activity, stop smoking, avoid alcohol, and reduce heavy coffee intake.
e. Dietary alteration for weight control should always be done.
f. Selective beta-blockers (BBs) should be recommended in symptomatic patients.

This consensus document signifies that no clear proof is present to recommend any specific therapy for an increased HR with HTN that is valuable and can modify the results.[28]

Non-pharmacological Management of High RHR in Patients with HTN

Non-pharmacological measures are a well-recognized mainstay in the treatment of HTN. Improvement of an unhealthy lifestyle should be particularly effective in HTN individuals with increased HR because an unfavorable lifestyle is accompanied by higher HR values. Sedentary habits, overweight, smoking, extreme alcohol consumption increase the sympathetic activity with consequent effects on RHR.

Adoption of a healthy routine could revert to mild elevations of BP and HR. Some studies proposed a possible mechanism between the SNS and dietary sodium (Na) to define the BP level.[60] As in a salt-sensitive HTN, it is observed that a high sodium intake causes plasma catecholamines to rise and pulmonary baroreceptor plasticity to fall. Piccirillo *et al.* performed a study to determine HR and BP variabilities in salt-sensitive HTN. A group of 52 subjects (37 hypertensive and 15 normotensives) was enrolled, and their ANS activity by power spectral analysis of HR and arterial pressure variabilities and baroreceptor sensitivity were determined. It has been found in the study that high sodium intake significantly enhanced the LF power of HR and arterial pressures at rest and after sympathetic stress. It also increased HR and arterial pressure variabilities. The LF/HF ratio was considerably greater in high sodium than in low sodium intake in the salt-sensitive (p <0.001) and normotensive (p <0.05) groups. In the salt-resistant hypertensive group, the LF/HF ratio stayed considerably greater than that of control subjects (p <0.001) after the low sodium regimen. These findings from the study revealed that a high sodium intake significantly improves the cardiac sympathetic activity in salt-sensitive and salt-resistant HTN.[61]

Several other studies have shown that fasting or some form of caloric restriction (CR) has considerable success in improving BP, HR, PWV, endothelial and autonomic function; this is due purely to the weight loss. CR can generally significantly improve HRV and the balance between SNS and parasympathetic nervous system (PNS) activity. A study of long-term fasters indicated that older fasters had HRV outcomes similar to those observed in a much younger cohort, or were similar to outcomes in hypertensive patients taking Atenolol, which reduces sympathetic and increases parasympathetic control of the heart. As per the study conducted by Blumenthal *et al.* CR improved carotid-femoral PWV as compared to a control group in subjects with increased BP.[62]

Aerobic exercise is also one of the most investigated and recommended lifestyle modifications for the treatment of early phases of HTN. Regular endurance exercise causes a decrease in sympathetic activity and a rise of vagal tone with beneficial effects on both BP and HR.[63] Lamina *et al.* conducted a randomized controlled trial to study the influence of training programs on RHR in patients with HTN. A total of 245 patients with mild-to-moderate essential HTN were enrolled and distributed into interval and control groups. During an 8-week follow-up interval training program of between 45 and 60 minutes, the study revealed a major influence of the exercise training programs on HR. Also, changes in VO_2 max was found negatively linked with HR ($r = -.503$) at p <0.05. These findings revealed that moderate-intensity interval training programs are effective in the non-pharmacological adjunct management of HTN and may prevent CV events through the downregulation of HR in HTN.[64]

HTN is related to higher levels of sympathetic nerve activity, decreased HRV, and delays in heart rate recovery (HRR), and the major pathophysiological mechanisms that are included in HTN autonomic dysfunction.[65] HRR is commonly defined as the decrease of HR at 1 minute after cessation of exercise.[66] Several studies have described that in hypertensive patients, a lower HRR after exercise and autonomic dysfunction is related to blunting of the nighttime BP fall. In 2019, Vicente GA *et al.* conducted a study involving 16 patients. In the study, the assumption that exercise training improves HR recovery after exercise in HTN was checked. Outcomes revealed that in hypertensive patients, the decline rate of HRR in the first and second minutes after maximal exercise testing was considerably greater in exercise-trained hypertensive patients than in untrained hypertensive patients ($p = 0.001$ and $p = 0.01$, respectively) and similar to normotensive individuals ($p = 0.52$ and $p = 0.99$, respectively. Exercise training significantly increase peak oxygen uptake in hypertensive patients (24.8 ± 1.4 vs 29.5 ± 2.3 mL/kg/min, $p = 0.01$) and normotensive individuals (29.1 ± 2.1 vs 34.1 ± 2.2 mL/kg/min, $p = 0.01$). Similarly, the preliminary variances in the HRR deterioration after exercise between hypertensive patients and normotensive individuals were no longer detected after exercise training (first minute: −34 ± 3 vs −29 ± 3 bpm, $p = 0.52$, and second minute: −49 ± 2 vs −7 ± 4 bpm, $p = 0.99$). This showed exercise training improves the HRR decline after a maximal exercise test in hypertensive HTN patients.[65]

Data from numerous observational epidemiological studies also suggest that smoking is related to a higher level of RHR. On the other hand, it was not clear by which mechanism it exerts its detrimental effect.[67] Wenyu C et al. in 2020 performed a study to define the influence of various smoking statuses on the RHR in a physical examination population with high-normal BP. A total of 210 patients were enrolled, divided into non-smoking ($n = 78$), active smoking ($n = 68$), and passive smoking ($n = 74$) groups. During a follow-up period of 2 years, it was observed that triglycerides, total cholesterol, and fasting blood glucose was considerably greater in active smoking groups than in the two other groups (all $p < 0.05$). Likewise, a considerable difference in RHR was found among the three groups (active: 76.0 ± 10.1 vs passive: 72.6 ± 5.8 vs non-smoking: 69.4 ± 4.4 bpm, $p < 0.01$. RHR was higher in subjects with high-normal BP and the passive and active smoking groups. Results revealed that strengthening smoking cessation education and avoiding exposure to secondary smoke could be beneficial to control the population with high-normal BP.[68]

Recently, a catheter-based approach to denervate the kidneys have been effectively presented into clinical practice and decrease BP and sympathetic activity in patients with resistant HTN without prominent systematic side effects. A recent study performed on 136 patients treated with renal sympathetic denervation demonstrated a marked decrease of 9 bpm in patients with a RHR >71 bpm.[69]

Pharmacological Management of High RHR in Patients with HTN

A supplementary goal of antihypertensive therapy is to decrease HR in HTN patients. Several trials retrospectively showed the beneficial effect of cardiac-slowing medications, for instance, β-adrenoceptor antagonists (β-blockers) and calcium channel antagonists on mortality, notably in patients with coronary heart disease. But no published data is present in patients with HTN free of coronary heart disease. Other antihypertensive drugs which reduce the HR are midway acting medicines and angiotensin II receptor antagonists, but their bradycardic effect is slightly weak. The f-channel antagonist Ivabradine is a selective HR-lowering agent, but it has no effect on BP. Drugs that decrease the hemodynamic burden via a decrease in sympathetic outflow or blocking peripheral effects should be useful because the sympathetic activity plays a key role in the pathogenesis of both HTN and increased HR. Though there is no proof till now that decrease in HR is useful in HTN, it is reasonable to suggest that drugs that reduce both BP and HR should be used in hypertensive patients with an increased RHR. As an alternative, drugs with a selective effect on HR can also be used along with antihypertensive drugs.[70]

In developed countries, HTN is the most important preventable cause of premature and sudden death. The benefits of antihypertensive drugs are well-recognized for the management of CV mortality and morbidity. Though the findings of an early meta-analysis of the results of 17 hypertension trials—all of which used standard diuretic or blocker therapy, or both—indicated that lowering of BP was associated with a significant fall in CHD events, the benefit noted was less than that expected from prospective observational data. Also, no individual trial had established a considerable decrease in CHD events. Dahlöf B *et al.* conducted a multicenter, prospective, randomized controlled trial in 19,257 patients with hypertension who were aged 40–79 years and had at least three other CV risk factors. Patients were prescribed either amlodipine 5–10 mg adding perindopril 4–8 mg as required (amlodipine-based regimen; n = 9639) or atenolol 50–100 mg adding bendroflumethiazide 1.25–2.5 mg and potassium as required (atenolol-based regimen; n = 9618). Non-fatal MI and fatal CHD were considered as the primary endpoint. The trial was stopped prematurely after 5.5 years median follow-up and accumulated in total 106,153 patient-years of observation. Though not significant, compared with the atenolol-based regimen, fewer individuals on the amlodipine-based regimen had a primary endpoint (429 *vs* 474; unadjusted HR: 0.90, 95% CI: 0.79–1.02, p = 0.1052), fatal and non-fatal stroke (327 *vs* 422; 0.77, 0.66–0.89, p = 0.0003), total CV events and procedures (1362 *vs* 1602; 0.84, 0.78–0.90, p <0.0001), and all-cause mortality (738 *vs* 820; 0.89, 0.81–0.99, p = 0.025). The incidence of developing diabetes was less on the amlodipine-based regimen (567 *vs* 799; 0.70, 0.63–0.78, p <0.0001). The outcomes of ASCOT-BPLA indicated that hypertensive individuals are at higher risk of developing CVD due to associated risk factors. Also, a regimen based on amlodipine and perindopril is superior to atenolol and bendroflumethiazide regimen in decreasing major CV events and all-cause mortality.[71]

Different BP-lowering medications have different effects on central aortic pressures and CV outcomes despite similar effects on brachial BP. Thus, the conduit artery function evaluation (CAFE) study, a substudy of the ASCOT, was done to examine the impact of two different BP-lowering agents (atenolol ± thiazide-based *vs* amlodipine ± perindopril-based therapy) on central aortic pressures and hemodynamics. A total of 2,199 patients in 5 ASCOT centers were enrolled in this examination. Radial artery applanation tonometry and PW analysis were utilized to determine central aortic pressures and hemodynamic indexes. Patients were given combination therapy throughout the study. In spite of comparative brachial systolic BPs between treatment groups (Δ0.7 mmHg; 95% CI: –0.4 to 1.7; p = 0.2), significant decrease was observed in central aortic pressures with the amlodipine regimen (central aortic systolic BP, Δ4.3 mmHg; 95% CI: 3.3 to 5.4; p <0.0001; central aortic pulse pressure, Δ3.0 mmHg; 95% CI: 2.1 to 3.9; p <0.0001). Cox proportional-hazards modeling shown that central pulse pressure was considerably related to a post-hoc-defined composite outcome of total CV events/procedures and development of renal impairment in the CAFE. These findings revealed that BP-lowering medications can have substantially different effects on central aortic pressures and hemodynamics despite similar influence on brachial BP. Also, central aortic pulse pressure might be a contributing factor to clinical outcomes.[72]

Beta-blockers (BBs): Cause a noticeable decrease in HR, and theoretically, should be the first-choice treatment in hypertensive patients. Recently, Xie *et al.* performed a meta-analysis to compare the efficacy of atenolol with angiotensin-converting enzyme inhibitors (ACEIs) in changing PWV, PBP, and HR among patients with essential HTN. A total of eight clinical trials were meta-analyzed, which reported atenolol to be more beneficial than ACEIs in terms of reducing peripheral diastolic pressure (WMD = −4.097 mmHg, 95% CI: −6.589 to −1.605, p = 0.001), PDBP (WMD = −6.802 mmHg, 95% CI: −8.517 to −5.087, p <0.001) and HR (WMD = −14.242 bpm, 95% CI: −16.427 to −12.058, p = 0.028) in first 3-month of treatment.[73] Another meta-analysis by Nogueira-Silva *et al.* described a decrease in BP by 10/8 mmHg, pulse pressure by 2 mmHg, and HR by 11-bpm with the usage of BB in HTN.[74]

BB decrease the HR by causing a disproportionate rise in the duration of systole that is responsible for the augmentation of central systolic pressure. The newer BBs such as carvedilol and nebivolol should be chosen as they decrease HR along with both central and peripheral pressures.[28] Shah *et al.* performed an open-label, comparative, randomized control trial to determine the brachial and central hemodynamic profile in patients taking atenolol *(n* = 22) or controlled release carvedilol *(n* = 19), a vasodilating BB, during a follow-up period of 4-week observed that carvedilol reduced AIx to a more extent than beta-selective therapy with atenolol (atenolol: 4.47% *vs* carvedilol: −0.68%; p = 0.04), also observed that at week 2, atenolol reduced HR to 61.6 bpm while carvedilol reduced HR to 64.8 bpm and at week 4, HR reduced to 60.7 bpm and 63.0 bpm in the atenolol and carvedilol groups, respectively; however, the brachial BP reductions were not considerably dissimilar between the two groups. Vasodilating BB exert their beneficial effects on the central aortic pressure by simultaneously decreasing HR and pulse wave velocity.[75] Similar results were seen in a study by comparing the usage of nebivolol, a vasodilating BB with metoprolol in 80 patients with HTN. Results after one year demonstrated no difference in brachial BP reduction but a higher decrease in central SBP (p = 0.07) and central pulse pressure (p = 0.004) in subjects treated with nebivolol.[76]

Whereas, as per data obtained from the BISO-CAD study, involved 681 hypertensive patients, bisoprolol can efficiently decrease RHR in Asian CAD patients with comorbid HTN and improve composite cardiac clinical outcome (CCCO) without affecting their BP. Bisoprolol improved CCCOs in CAD patients with comorbid HTN and RHR <65 and <70 bpm compared with RHR ≥65 and ≥75 bpm, respectively. Besides, it also decreased RHR in both intent-to-treat (ITT) and EA groups after 6, 12, and 18 months of treatment.[77]

A pharmacological reduction of HR is beneficial for patients with heart disease. However, the role of pharmacological reduction of HR using BB in preventing CV events in patients with HTN is not known. Thus, to determine the role of HR reduction with BBs on the risk of CV events in patients with hypertension, Bangalore S *et al.* conducted a meta-analysis. In this meta-analysis, randomized controlled trials were included that evaluated BBs as first-line therapy for hypertension with follow-up for at least 1-year and with data on HR. Among the 22 randomized controlled trials assessing BB for HTN, nine studies reported HR data. The 9 studies evaluated 34,096 patients who had prescribed BB against 30,139 patients who were prescribed other antihypertensive agents, and 3,987 patients taking placebo. A decrease in HR (as achieved in the BB group at study end) was related with a greater risk for the endpoints of all-cause mortality (r = −0.51; p <0.0001) CV mortality (r = −0.61; p <0.0001) MI (r = −0.85; p <0.0001), stroke (r = −0.20; p = 0.06), or HF (r = −0.56; p <0.0001). The same was true when the HR difference between the 2 treatment modalities at the end of the study was compared with the relative risk reduction for CV events. These findings revealed that in contrast to patients with MI and HF, BB-associated decrease in HR increased the risk of CV events and death for hypertensive patients.[78]

Calcium Channel Blockers (CCBs): CCBs reduce HR to a lower degree compared with BBs, and are free of adverse metabolic effects.[69] Non-dihydropyridine CCBs, such as phenylalkylamines (e.g. verapamil) and benzothiazepines (e.g. diltiazem) can be used for the treatment of elevated RHR in hypertensive patients because they exert their effect directly on sympathetic activity. These drugs act by decreasing the hemodynamic burden through a decrease in the sympathetic outflow. Besides having a peripheral action, phenylalkylamines inhibit sympathetic outflow, resulting in depletion of vascular stores, inhibition of norepinephrine (Ne) release, and attenuation of reflex tachycardia. Non-dihydropyridine calcium channel antagonists decreased the risk of cardiac events in post-MI patients with normal LV function. In the latest analysis of the first and second Danish Verapamil Infarction Trial and the multicenter Diltiazem Post-Infarction Trial evaluating the influence of HR lowering calcium channel antagonists in 1,325 hypertensive post-MI patients, a decrease in mortality rate and event rate was found in treated patients without pulmonary congestion, suggested that these drugs can be effectively used in hypertensive post-MI patients.

Dihydropyridine CCBs also exert their impact on BP and HR. Amlodipine, cilnidipine, azelnidipine, nifedipine are examples of dihydropyridine.[69] Cilnidipine is a promising 4th generation CCB with a rational pharmacological profile, i.e. dual L/N-type Ca^{2+} channel blocking action. The blockade of N-type Ca^{2+} channels effectively suppress neurohumoral regulation in the CV system, including the SNS and renin-angiotensin-aldosterone system (RAAS).[79] Studies revealed that once-daily administration of cilnidipine leads to a safe and efficient reduction of BP in essential HTN without reflex tachycardia when compared to other dihydropyridine calcium antagonists. To evaluate the effectiveness of cilnidipine on HR in patients with essential HTN, Das A *et al.* conducted a comparative study. In this study, a total of 92 patients were included and randomized into two groups (amlodipine ($n = 47$) and cilnidipine ($n = 45$)). Cilnidipine was started at 10 mg/day and then adjusted to 5–20 mg/day, and amlodipine was started at 5 mg/day and following 2.5–10 mg/day. Outcomes revealed that patients in the cilnidipine group demonstrated a significant decrease in HR from the baseline ($p = 0.00$) during a follow-up period of 24 weeks. Therefore, cilnidipine can be a favorite drug of choice in a clinical setting where HTN exists.[80]

Whereas azelnidipine showed an antihypertensive efficacy similar to that of amlodipine, but unlike amlodipine, it reduced HR, and the difference was significant in comparison with amlodipine.[70] Kuramoto *et al.* in 2003 conducted a double-blind comparison study between azelnidipine and amlodipine. In this study, azelnidipine 16 mg (23 patients) or amlodipine 5 mg (23 patients) was administered, once daily for 6-week, and BP and PR were estimated by 24-hour monitoring with a portable automatic monitor. Both drugs have shown similar effects on the office BP and PR, and during 24-hour monitoring, both drugs caused a reduction in SBP of 13 mmHg and had a similar hypotensive profile during the daytime period (07:00–21:30). The pulse rate decreased by 2-bpm in the azelnidipine group, whereas it considerably increased by 4-bpm in the amlodipine group. During the nighttime (22:00–6:30) and over 24 hours, similar trends in the BP and pulse rate were observed. These results revealed that both azelnidipine and amlodipine have a similar hypotensive effect, but pulse rate reduction was seen less in azelnidipine.[81]

Angiotensin-Converting Enzyme (ACE) Inhibitors: ACE inhibitors principally act to prevent the conversion of angiotensin I to angiotensin II in plasma and tissue and prevent the degradation of bradykinin. Clinically, during states of Na depletion, ACE inhibitors decrease peripheral vascular resistance and pulmonary capillary wedge pressure and increase cardiac output and renal blood flow. The acute response to ACE inhibitors is correlated with plasma renin activity. ACE inhibition does not increase RHR, but the postural variations in HR and BP are preserved on treatment.[82] At present, there are few statistics on the influence of antihypertensive therapy on clinic HR. Pierdomenico SD *et al.* performed a study to assess the influence of ACE inhibitors and long-acting dihydropyridine calcium antagonists on a clinic and ambulatory HR in patients with essential HTN. In the study, ACE inhibitors were prescribed to 292 hypertensive patients whereas dihydropyridine calcium antagonists were prescribed to 198 hypertensive patients. Results revealed that in patients treated with ACE inhibitors and calcium antagonists, both clinic and ambulatory BP were considerably decreased. Globally, clinic and 24-hour HR were significantly diminished in patients treated with ACE inhibitors, and remained unchanged in those treated with calcium antagonists. While patients were grouped as per baseline clinic HR (<65 bpm, 65–74 bpm, 75–84 bpm, and >85 bpm), ACE inhibitors considerably reduced clinics, 24-hour daytime and nighttime HR in those with baseline HR >75 bpm and particularly in those with baseline HR >85 bpm. However, calcium antagonists did not considerably change clinic, 24-hour daytime and nighttime HR in various subgroups. These results have showed that ACE inhibitors decrease both clinic and ambulatory HR in hypertensive patients with faster HR, they appeared to be at higher risk, and that long-acting dihydropyridine calcium antagonists do not induce significant changes in HR during chronic treatment (neither decreases nor increases).[83]

Angiotensin II Receptor Blocker (ARB): Drugs acting on the renin-angiotensin system, especially angiotensin II type 1 (AT1) receptor antagonizing agents have also shown an anti-adrenergic action since angiotensin II affects both the CNS (enhancing sympathetic outflow) and the peripheral sympathetic nerves. Selective blockade of the AT1 receptor has the additional benefit of inhibiting sympathetic activity. In elderly patients with isolated systolic HTN valsartan has been shown to reduce average daytime ambulatory HR by 3-bpm more than amlodipine.[67] ARB is usually given with a CCB for treating HTN. In an open-labeled randomized study by Daikuhara *et al.* untreated hypertensive patients were randomized to prescribe either olmesartan 20 mg/day or candesartan 8 mg/day for 12-week, and patients with BP exceeding 130/80 mmHg received add-on 16 mg/day azelnidipine to ongoing olmesartan (OL group) or 5 mg/day amlodipine to ongoing candesartan (CA group) for 24-week. Home-measured and clinic-measured BP reduced in both groups, but olmesartan and azelnidipine combination had a more determined early morning antihypertensive effect and produced more reduction in HR compared to candesartan and amlodipine.[84]

Centrally Acting Drugs: The sympathetic activity lowering action of centrally acting-adrenergic agents would appear to make them the drug of choice in hypertensive patients with increased HR, but the old centrally acting drugs such as clonidine, methyldopa, and guanfacine are rarely used because of their centrally adverse effects, which include sedation, dry mouth, and inability in men. These effects are less common with the newer anti-adrenergic drugs acting on the I1-imidazoline receptor of the rostroventrolateral medulla, such as moxonidine and rilmenidine. However, these medications had favorable metabolic effects; their influence on RHR was negligible.[71]

Take Home Pearls

- Non-pharmacological measures are a well-recognized mainstay in the management of HTN.
- Improvement of an unhealthy lifestyle should be particularly effective in HTN patients with high HR because an unfavorable lifestyle is supplemented by higher HR values.
- Regular endurance exercise causes a decrease in sympathetic activity and an increment of vagal tone with valuable effects on both BP and HR.
- Strengthening smoking cessation education and avoiding exposure to secondary smoke could be useful to control the population with high-normal BP.
- BBs, for example, carvedilol and nebivolol decrease HR as well as both central and peripheral pressures. Thus, should be favored in pharmacological management.
- Calcium antagonists are free of adverse metabolic effects and decrease HR to a lesser extent as compared to BB.

Take Home Summary

HTN is the primary preventable risk factor for CVD and all-cause mortality. In the past two decades, it has been observed that HIC experienced a modest decrease in HTN prevalence, whereas LMICs experience a remarkable increase. According to various epidemiologic and clinical studies, in patients with HTN, increased HR is a strong predictor of morbidity and mortality, underlying the importance of HR measurements. ANS dysfunction and atherosclerosis are the major contributors to the pathogenesis of untoward events. Much uncertainty is present about optimal methodologies to reduce HR in HTN and whether decreasing HR improves outcomes in uncomplicated HTN. As sympathetic activity plays important role in the pathogenesis of both HTN and high HR, drugs that reduce the hemodynamic burden through a reduction of the sympathetic outflow or blocking peripheral effects should be beneficial. The usage of selective beta-1 blockers such as carvedilol and nebivolol is recommended in pharmacological treatment because it decreases HR as well as both central and peripheral pressures. Whereas CCB reduces HR to a lesser degree compared to BBs, and they are free of adverse metabolic effects. The sympathetic activity lowering action of the new centrally acting-adrenergic agents such as moxonidine and rilmenidine would also appear the drug of choice in hypertensive patients with increased HR.

REFERENCES

1. Mills KT, Stefanescu A, He J. The global epidemiology of hypertension. *Nature Reviews Nephrology*. 2020 Apr;16(4):223–37.
2. Singh S, Shankar R, Singh GP. Prevalence and associated risk factors of hypertension: A cross-sectional study in urban Varanasi. *International Journal of Hypertension*. 2017;2017:5491838.

3. Rajkumar E, Romate J. Behavioural risk factors, hypertension knowledge, and hypertension in rural India. *International Journal of Hypertension*. 2020 Mar 9;2020:8108202.

4. Taddei S, Bruno RM, Masi S, *et al*. Epidemiology and pathophysiology of hypertension.*ESC Cardio Med*. 2018 Dec.

5. Dubey M, Rastogi S, Awasthi A. Hypertension prevalence as a function of different guidelines, India. *Bulletin of the World Health Organization*. 2019 Dec 1;97(12):799–809.

6. Shah SN, Munjal YP, Kamath SA, *et al*. Indian guidelines on hypertension-IV (2019). *Journal of Human Hypertension*. 2020 May 19.

7. Gupta R, Gaur K, Ram CV. Emerging trends in hypertension epidemiology in India. *Journal of Human Hypertension*. 2019 Aug;33(8):575–87.

8. Prabhakaran D, Jeemon P, Ghosh S, *et al*. Prevalence and incidence of hypertension: Results from a representative cohort of over 16,000 adults in three cities of South Asia. *Indian Heart Journal*. 2017 Jul-Aug 2017;69(4):434–41.

9. Mills KT, Bundy JD, Kelly TN, *et al*. Global disparities of hypertension prevalence and control: A systematic analysis of population-based studies from 90 countries. *Circulation*. 2016 Aug 9;134(6):441–50.

10. Racial disparities in hypertension prevalence and management: A crisis control?. Adapted from: https://www.acc.org/latest-in-cardiology/articles/2020/04/06/08/53/racial-disparities-in-hypertension-prevalence-and-management

11. Neupane D, McLachlan CS, Sharma R, *et al*. Prevalence of hypertension in member countries of South Asian Association for Regional Cooperation (SAARC): Systematic review and meta-analysis. *Medicine (Baltimore)*. 2014 Sep;93(13):e74.

12. Foulds HJ, Bredin SS, Warburton DE. The relationship between hypertension and obesity across different ethnicities. *Journal of Hypertension*. 2012 Feb;30(2):359–67.

13. Jin CN, Yu CM, Sun JP, *et al*. The healthcare burden of hypertension in Asia. *Heart Asia*. 2013;5(1):238–43.

14. Gupta R, Ram CV. Hypertension epidemiology in India: Emerging aspects. *Current Opinion in Cardiology*. 2019 Jul;34(4):331–41.

15. Anchala R, Kannuri NK, Pant H, *et al*. Hypertension in India: A systematic review and meta-analysis of prevalence, awareness, and control of hypertension. *Journal of Hypertension*. 2014 Jun;32(6):1170–7.

16. Prenissl J, Manne-Goehler J, Jaacks LM, *et al*. Hypertension screening, awareness, treatment, and control in India: A nationally representative cross-sectional study among individuals aged 15 to 49 years. *PLoS Medicine*. 2019 May 3;16(5):e1002801.

17. Ramakrishnan S, Zachariah G, Gupta K, *et al*. Prevalence of hypertension among Indian adults: Results from the great India blood pressure survey. *Indian Heart Journal*. 2019 Jul-Aug;71(4):309–13.

18. Yang X, Hidru TH, Wang B, *et al*. The link between elevated long-term resting heart rate and SBP variability for all-cause mortality. *Journal of Hypertension*. 2019 Jan;37(1):84–91.

19. Ernst G. Heart-rate variability—More than heart beats? *Frontiers in Public Health*. 2017;5:240.

20. Guyenet PG. The sympathetic control of blood pressure. *Nature Reviews Neuroscience*. 2006 May;7(5):335–46.

21. Sharma M, Barbosa K, Ho V, *et al*. Cuff-less and continuous blood pressure monitoring: A methodological review. *Technologies*. 2017;5(2):21.

22. Kouvas N, Tsioufis C, Vogiatzakis N, *et al*. Heart rate and blood pressure: "Connecting the dots" in epidemiology and pathophysiology. *Angiology*. 2018 Sep;69(8):660–5.

23. Sapoznikov D, Elhalel MD, Rubinger D. Heart rate response to blood pressure variations: Sympathetic activation versus baroreflex response in patients with end-stage renal disease. *PloS ONE*. 2013;8(10):e78338.

24. Rafie AH, Sungar GW, Dewey FE, *et al*. Prognostic value of double product reserve. *European Journal of Cardiovascular Prevention & Rehabilitation*. 2008 Oct;15(5):541–7.
25. Schutte R, Thijs L, Asayama K, *et al*. Double product reflects the predictive power of systolic pressure in the general population: Evidence from 9,937 participants. *American Journal of Hypertension*. 2013 May;26(5):665–72.
26. Schultz AJ, Schutte AE, Schutte R. Double product and end-organ damage in African and Caucasian men: The SABPA study. *International Journal of Cardiology*. 2013 Aug 10;167(3):792–7.
27. Wang F, Hua Y, Whelton PK, *et al*. Relationship between birth weight and the double product in childhood, adolescence, and adulthood (from the Bogalusa Heart Study). *American Journal of Cardiology*. 2017 Sep 15;120(6):1016–9.
28. Dalal J, Dasbiswas A, Sathyamurthy I, *et al*. Heart rate in hypertension: Review and expert opinion. *International Journal of Hypertension*. 2019 Feb;2019:1–6.
29. Reule S, Drawz PE. Heart rate and blood pressure: Any possible implications for management of hypertension?. *Current Hypertension Reports*. 2012 Dec;14(6):478–84.
30. Mozos I, Gug C, Mozos C, *et al*. Associations between intrinsic heart rate, P wave and QT interval durations and pulse wave analysis in patients with hypertension and high normal blood pressure. *International Journal of Environmental Research and Public Health*. 2020 Jan;17(12):4350.
31. Reed DW, McGee DA, Yano KA. Biological and social correlates of blood pressure among Japanese men in Hawaii. *Hypertension*. 1982 May;4(3):406–14.
32. Park BJ, Lee HR, Shim JY, *et al*. Association between resting heart rate and arterial stiffness in Korean adults. *Archives of Cardiovascular Diseases*. 2010 Apr 1;103(4):246–52.
33. Wilkinson IB, Mohammad NH, Tyrrell S, *et al*. Heart rate dependency of pulse pressure amplification and arterial stiffness. *American Journal of Hypertension*. 2002 Jan;15(1 Pt 1):24–30.
34. Li X, Kong T, Yao Y, *et al*. Prevalence and factors associated with fast resting heart rate in hypertensive and normotensive patients. *Clinical and Experimental Hypertension*. 2020;42(1):8–15.
35. Tjugen TB, Flaa A, Kjeldsen SE. High heart rate as predictor of essential hypertension: The hyperkinetic state, evidence of prediction of hypertension, and hemodynamic transition to full hypertension. *Progress in Cardiovascular Diseases*. 2009 Jul 1;52(1):20–5.
36. Inoue T, Iseki K, Iseki C, *et al*. Higher heart rate predicts the risk of developing hypertension in a normotensive screened cohort. *Circulation Journal*. 2007;71(11):1755–60.
37. Ryu M, Bayasgalan G, Kimm H, *et al*. Association of resting heart rate and hypertension stages on all-cause and cardiovascular mortality among elderly Koreans: The Kangwha Cohort Study. *Journal of Geriatric Cardiology*. 2016 Jul;13(7):573–9.
38. Tadic M, Cuspidi C, Grassi G. The influence of sex on left ventricular remodeling in arterial hypertension. *Heart Failure Reviews*. 2019 Nov 1;24(6):905–14.
39. Padmanabhan TN, Dani S, Chopra VK, *et al*. Prevalence of sympathetic overactivity in hypertensive patients—A pan India, non-interventional, cross sectional study. *Indian Heart Journal*. 2014 Nov- Dec;66(6):686–90.
40. Kaul U, Verberk W, Suvarna V, *et al*. India Heart Study—IHS. *Indian Heart Journal*. 2019 Nov;71:S80–S81.
41. Kaul U, Bhagwat A, Omboni S, *et al*. Blood pressure and heart rate related to sex in untreated subjects: The India ABPM Study. *Journal of Clinical Hypertension*. 2020;22(7)1154–62.
42. Grassi G, Quarti-Trevano F, Seravalle G, *et al*. Association between the European Society of Cardiology/European Society of Hypertension heart rate thresholds for cardiovascular risk and neuroadrenergic markers. *Hypertension*. 2020;76(2):577–82.
43. Inoue R, Ohkubo T, Kikuya M, *et al*. Predictive value for mortality of the double product at rest obtained by home blood pressure measurement: The Ohasama study. *American Journal of Hypertension*. 2012 May;25(5):568–75.

44. Pioli MR, Ritter AM, de Faria AP, *et al*. White coat syndrome and its variations: Differences and clinical impact. *Integrated Blood Pressure Control*. 2018;11:73–9.

45. Lequeux B, Uzan C, Rehman MB. Does resting heart rate measured by the physician reflect the patient's true resting heart rate? White-coat heart rate. *Indian Heart Journal*. 2018 Jan-Feb;70(1):93–8.

46. Wang A, Liu X, Guo X, *et al*. Resting heart rate and risk of hypertension: Results of the Kailuan cohort study. *Journal of Hypertension*. 2014 Aug;32(8):1600–5.

47. Terathongkum S, Pickler RH. Relationships among heart rate variability, hypertension, and relaxation techniques. *Journal of Vascular Nursing*. 2004 Sep;22(3):78–82.

48. Lutfi MF, Sukkar MY. Effect of blood pressure on heart rate variability. *Khartoum Medical Journal*. 2011;4(1):548–53.

49. Huikuri HV, Ylitalo A, Pikkujämsä SM, *et al*. Heart rate variability in systemic hypertension. *American Journal of Cardiology*. 1996 May 15;77(12):1073–7.

50. Schroeder EB, Liao D, Chambless LE, *et al*. Hypertension, blood pressure, and heart rate variability: The Atherosclerosis Risk in Communities (ARIC) study. *Hypertension*. 2003 Dec;42(6):1106–11.

51. Singh JP, Larson MG, Tsuji H, *et al*. Reduced heart rate variability and new-onset hypertension: Insights into pathogenesis of hypertension: The Framingham Heart Study. *Hypertension*. 1998 Aug;32(2):293–7.

52. Levy RL, White PD, Stroud WD, *et al*. Transient tachycardia: Prognostic significance alone and in association with transient hypertension. *Journal of the American Medical Association*. 1945 Oct 27;129(9):585–8.

53. Paffenbarger RS Jr, King SH, Wing AL. Chronic disease in former college students. IX. Characteristics in youth that predispose to suicide and accidental death in later life. *American Journal of Public Health and the Nation's Health*. 1969 Jun;59(6):900–8.

54. Palatini P, Dorigatti F, Zaetta V, *et al*. Heart rate as a predictor of development of sustained hypertension in subjects screened for stage 1 hypertension: The HARVEST Study. *Journal of Hypertension*. 2006 Sep;24(9):1873–80.

55. Paul L, Hastie CE, Li WS, *et al*. Resting heart rate pattern during follow-up and mortality in hypertensive patients. *Hypertension*. 2010 Feb;55(2):567–74.

56. Van de Vegte YJ, van der Harst P, Verweij N. Heart rate recovery 10 seconds after cessation of exercise predicts death. *Journal of the American Heart Association*. 2018 Apr 5;7(8):e008341.

57. Chen YD, Yang XC, Pham VN, *et al*. Resting heart rate control and prognosis in coronary artery disease patients with hypertension previously treated with bisoprolol: A sub-group analysis of the BISO-CAD study. *Chinese Medical Journal*. 2020 May 20;133(10):1155–65.

58. Julius S, Palatini P, Kjeldsen SE, *et al*. Usefulness of heart rate to predict cardiac events in treated patients with high-risk systemic hypertension. *American Journal of Cardiology*. 2012 Mar 1; 109(5):685–92.

59. Kolloch R, Legler UF, Champion A, *et al*. Impact of resting heart rate on outcomes in hypertensive patients with coronary artery disease: Findings from the INternational VErapamil-SR/trandolapril STudy (INVEST). *European Heart Journal*. 2008 May;29(10):1327–34.

60. Böhm M, Schwantke I, Mahfoud F, *et al*. Association of clinic and ambulatory heart rate parameters with mortality in hypertension. *Journal of Hypertension*. 2020 Dec;38(12):2416–26.

61. Rastenytë D, Tuomilehto J, Moltchanov V, *et al*. Association between salt intake, heart rate and blood pressure. *Journal of Human Hypertension*. 1997 Dec;11(1):57–62.

62. Piccirillo G, Bucca C, Durante M, *et al*. Heart rate and blood pressure variabilities in salt-sensitive hypertension. *Hypertension*. 1996 Dec;28(6):944–52.

63. Nicoll R, Henein MY. Caloric restriction and its effect on blood pressure, heart rate variability and arterial stiffness and dilatation: A review of the evidence. *International Journal of Molecular Sciences*. 2018 Mar 7;19(3):751.

64. Palatini P, Rosei EA, Casiglia E, *et al.* Management of the hypertensive patient with elevated heart rate: Statement of the Second Consensus Conference endorsed by the European Society of Hypertension. *Journal of Hypertension.* 2016 May;34(5):813–21.

65. Lamina S, Okaye G, Ezema C, *et al.* Effects of interval training programme on resting heart rate in subjects with hypertension: A randomized controlled trial. *Nigerian Health Journal.* 2013;13(1):26-32.

66. Amaro-Vicente G, Laterza MC, Martinez DG, *et al.* Exercise training improves heart rate recovery after exercise in hypertension. *Motriz: Revista de Educação Física.* 2019;25(1).

67. Linneberg A, Jacobsen RK, Skaaby T, *et al.* Effect of smoking on blood pressure and resting heart rate: A Mendelian randomization meta-analysis in the CARTA consortium. *Circulation: Cardiovascular Genetics.* 2015 Dec;8(6):832–41.

68. Chen w, Fang Z, Xu Y. The influence of various smoking statuses on the resting heart rate in a physical examination population with high-normal blood pressure. *Research Square.* 2020.

69. Courand PY, Lantelme P. Significance, prognostic value and management of heart rate in hypertension. *Archives of cardiovascular diseases.* 2014 Jan;107(1):48–57.

70. Palatini P, Benetos A, Julius S. Impact of increased heart rate on clinical outcomes in hypertension: Implications for antihypertensive drug therapy. *Drugs.* 2006 Feb;66(2):133–44.

71. Dahlöf B, Sever PS, Poulter NR, *et al.* Prevention of cardiovascular events with an anti-hypertensive regimen of amlodipine adding perindopril as required versus atenolol adding bendroflumethiazide as required, in the Anglo-Scandinavian Cardiac Outcomes Trial-Blood Pressure Lowering Arm (ASCOT-BPLA): A multicentre randomised controlled trial. *Lancet.* 2005;366(9489):895–906.

72. Williams B, Lacy PS, Thom SM, *et al.* Differential impact of blood pressure—Lowering drugs on central aortic pressure and clinical outcomes: Principal results of the Conduit Artery Function Evaluation (CAFE) study. *Circulation.* 2006;113(9):1213–25.

73. Xie H, Luo G, Zheng Y, *et al.* A meta-analytical comparison of atenolol with angiotensin-converting enzyme inhibitors on arterial stiffness, peripheral blood pressure and heart rate in hypertensive patients. *Clinical and Experimental Hypertension.* 2017;39(5):421–6.

74. Nogueira-Silva L, Marques PS, Lima MJ. Cochrane Corner: Antihypertensive efficacy of beta-1 selective beta blockers for primary hypertension. *Revista Portuguesa de Cardiologia.* 2017 May;36(5):385–8.

75. Shah NK, Smith SM, Nichols WW, *et al.* Carvedilol reduces aortic wave reflection and improves left ventricular/vascular coupling: A comparison with atenolol (CENTRAL Study). *Journal of Clinical Hypertension.* 2011 Dec;13(12):917–24.

76. Kampus P, Serg M, Kals J, *et al.* Differential effects of nebivolol and metoprolol on central aortic pressure and left ventricular wall thickness. *Hypertension.* 2011 Jun;57(6):1122–8.

77. Chen YD, Yang XC, Pham VN, *et al.* Resting heart rate control and prognosis in coronary artery disease patients with hypertension previously treated with bisoprolol: A sub-group analysis of the BISO-CAD study. *Chinese Medical Journal.* 2020 May 20;133(10):1155–65.

78. Bangalore S, Sawhney S, Messerli FH. Relation of beta-blocker-induced heart rate lowering and cardioprotection in hypertension. *Journal of the American College of Cardiology.* 2008 Oct 28;52(18):1482–9.

79. Chandra KS, Ramesh G. The fourth-generation calcium channel blocker: Cilnidipine.*Indian Heart Journal.* 2013 Dec;65(6):691–5.

80. Das A, Kumar P, Kumari A, *et al.* Effects of cilnidipine on heart rate and uric acid metabolism in patients with essential hypertension. *Cardiology Research.* 2016 Oct;7(5):167–72.

81. Kuramoto K, Ichikawa S, Hirai A, *et al.* Azelnidipine and amlodipine: A comparison of their pharmacokinetics and effects on ambulatory blood pressure. *Hypertension Research.* 2003; 26(3):201–8.

82. Arnett DK, Claas SA, Glasser SP. Pharmacogenetics of antihypertensive treatment. *Vascular Pharmacology*. 2006 Feb;44(2):107–18.

83. Pierdomenico SD, Bucci A, Lapenna D, *et al*. Heart rate in hypertensive patients treated with ACE inhibitors and long-acting dihydropyridine calcium antagonists. *Journal of Cardiovascular Pharmacology*. 2002 Aug;40(2):288–95.

84. Daikuhara H, Kikuchi F, Ishida T. The combination of OLmesartan and a CAlcium channel blocker (azelnidipine) or candesartan and a calcium channel blocker (amlodipine) in type 2 diabetic hypertensive patients: The OLCA study. *Diabetes and Vascular Disease Research*. 2012 Oct;9(4):280–6.

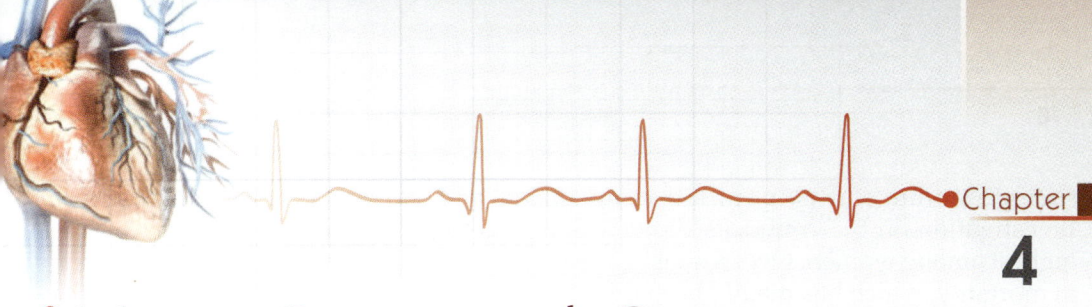

Heart Rate and Coronary Artery Disease (CAD)

Prof. (Dr.) Monotosh Panja, Dr. A Sreenivas Kumar

Learning Objectives

At the end of this chapter one should be able to:

- Epidemiology of CVD
- Clinical implications of coronary artery disease CAD and angina
- High resting heart rate and its impact on CAD and angina
- Management of high RHR—angina perspective
- Take home summary

EPIDEMIOLOGY OF CVD

Cardiovascular diseases (CVDs) consist of ischemic heart disease (IHD), stroke, heart failure (HF), peripheral arterial disease, and many other cardiac and vascular conditions. It constitutes the leading cause of global mortality and decreased quality of life (QoL). In 2017, CVD caused an estimated 17.8 million deaths worldwide, corresponding to 330 million years of life lost and another 35.6 million years lived with disability. CVD mortality is more common in middle-income countries compared with high- or low-income countries. Nearly 80% of global CVD deaths occur in low- and middle-income countries (LMIC), where CVD and risk factor burden are on the rise due to ongoing epidemiological transition.[1]

The estimated global mortality attributable to CVD was 28.2%. In 2000, the highest mortality at 5.9 million was mostly due to IHD, which accounted for 11.3% of all mortality.[2] In 2012, it was increased to approximately 7.3 million (13.2%) deaths. The second common reason for death was a stroke, responsible for 6.6 million deaths in 2012, representing 11.9% of worldwide mortality. There are three CVD categories in the top ten causes of worldwide mortality in 2012, not including diabetes mellitus (DM). Geographically, the death rate of CVD differs broadly. Generally, in 2012, Europe had the highest mortality burden because of CVD, and from 2000 onwards, a decrease in CVD burden was observed. However, CVD is the main reason for nearly half of all mortalities in the WHO European Region. In Europe itself, there is significant heterogeneity in the CVD burden across various regions. A high CVD death rate is present in Eastern Europe. These varied dissimilarities can be due to the existence of classic risk factors for CVD, like tobacco smoking, high blood pressure, and dietary risks.[2] In 2012, Russia had an estimated 1.3 million CVD mortalities, which accounted for 59.6% of all deaths. The CV death rate varies because of multiple factors, such as socioeconomic status, population specifics, and various clinical risk factors. Investigation on the Americas showed that in 2000, CVD mortality was 33.7%, the highest among women. Over the last 12 years, the Americas have seen a 20% reduction in mortality, which has mainly been driven by the high-income countries (HIC) in the region. Such large variations amongst countries in similar regions are observed and likely to be accountable for, at least in part, by access to health care and local preventative policies.[2]

Coronary heart disease (CHD) accounts for the maximum proportion of CVDs for which risk factors are hypertension, smoking, diabetes, high cholesterol, a higher level of low-density lipoprotein (LDL), obesity, and overweight causing the death of heart patients.[3]

CHD is the main cause of mortality in adults in the US, accounting for ~one-third of all deaths in patients above the age of 35.[3] Total CHD prevalence is 6.7% in US adult's ≥20 years of age. CHD prevalence is 7.4% for males and 6.2% for females.[4] From 2003 to 2013, the annual death rate causing CHD and the number of deaths dropped to 38.0% and 22.9%, respectively. In the European Union, CHD mortality decreased by 32% and 30% in men and women, respectively. Some difference was observed in Eastern Europe, where several countries had an escalation in CHD mortality in the early 1990s followed by a successive drop. From 1995 to 1998, the Russian Federation had greater CHD mortality. CHD death rate was much lesser in Japan as compared to the USA or Europe. Mortality from CHD has probably increased in developing countries from 9 million to 19 million from 1990 to 2020.[3]

As per different studies, CVDs have now become the main cause of mortality in India. One-fourth of all mortality is attributable to CVD. According to the Global Burden of Disease (GBD) study, the evaluation of age-standardized CVD death rate of 272 per 100,000 populations in India is greater than the global average of 235 per 100,000 populations. In India, some characteristics of the CVD epidemic such as early age of disease onset in the population, and high case fatality rate are reasons of concern.[5] In India, mortality increased from 1.3 million in 1990 to 2.8 million in 2016 because of CVDs, and the crude death rate increased by 34.3% from 1990 to 2016. Since 1990, the contribution to total deaths and disease burden due to CVDs has almost doubled. India reported 28·1% of total deaths and 14.1% of total Disability-Adjusted Life-Years (DALYs) in 2016 compared with 15.2% and 6.9%, respectively, in 1990.[6] The incidence of CVDs in 2016 was at a peak in Kerala, Punjab, and Tamil Nadu, followed by Maharashtra, Goa, Andhra Pradesh, West Bengal, and Himachal Pradesh.

IHD and stroke both are accountable for >80% of CVD deaths.[2] IHD cases increased from 10.2 million in 1990 to 23.8 million in 2016. The DALY rate of IHD varied 8.7 times between the states in 2016. This rate was more in the states of Tamil Nadu and Punjab, followed by Haryana, Andhra Pradesh, Karnataka, and Gujarat. High Systolic Blood Pressure (SBP), high total cholesterol, air pollution, and dietary risks are considered as the main risk factors for DALYs.[6] The study conducted by Ke C et al. reported that in 2015, CVD affected >2.1 million deaths of all ages in India. At ages 30–69 years, total CV deaths of 1.3 million included 0.9 million (68.4%) due to IHD, 0·4 million (28.0%) due to stroke 47,000 (3.5%) due to rheumatic heart diseases (RHD), and other CVD. Between 2000 and 2015, the national age-standardized death rate from IHD increased in men and women, and the pattern was similar in most states. In 2000, the age-standardized mortality rate of IHD at all ages in India was similar to HIC. But by 2015, in India, these mortality rates rose to more than double that of the UK or USA.[7]

At ages 30–69 years, the possibility of dying from IHD between 2000 and 2015 increased from 10.4 to 13.1% in men and 4.8 to 6.6% in women. Ke C *et al.* studied rural and urban dissimilarities and conducted an aging period cohort analysis. It was seen that IHD mortality at ages 30–69 years was lesser in rural areas compared with urban areas; rural rates rose rapidly, surpassing urban rates by 2015 in both the sexes.[7]

Take Home Pearls

- CVDs cause approximately one-third of deaths worldwide. Among them, IHD ranks as the most prevalent.
- CVDs are the main reason for mortality in India.
- CVDs are estimated to account for 60% of total adult deaths in India.
- The increasing prevalence of IHD is likely to continue due to population aging.

CLINICAL IMPLICATIONS OF CORONARY ARTERY DISEASE (CAD) AND ANGINA

CAD is a dynamic process of atherosclerotic plaque accumulation and functional alterations of coronary circulation that can be modified by lifestyle, pharmacological therapies, and revascularization. Due to the dynamic nature of the CAD and various clinical presentations, it can be characterized as either acute coronary syndromes (ACS) or chronic coronary syndromes (CCS).[8]

ACS covers the spectrum of clinical conditions ranging from unstable angina (UA) to non-ST-segment elevation myocardial infarction (NSTEMI) to STEMI. UA and NSTEMI have the same pathophysiologic origins and clinical presentations, however differ in severity. NSTEMI can be diagnosed when ischemia is severe to cause myocardial damage, which causes the release of a biomarker of myocardial necrosis into circulation. But in the case of UA, no such biomarker can be detected in the bloodstream hours after the initial onset of ischemic chest pain. Roughly two-thirds of patients with MI have NSTEMI, and the rest have STEMI.[8]

While CCS is a newly proposed entity by the European Society of Cardiology (ESC) that replaces stable CAD, which is known as a progressive development of plaque accumulation in coronary circulation with related functional changes.[9] The most frequently encountered clinical scenarios with suspected or established CCS are shown in Table 4.1.[10,11]

All of these scenarios are classified as CCS but involve different risks for future CV events. Progression of ACS may destabilize these clinical scenarios. The risk may decrease due to proper secondary prevention and successful revascularization. Hence, CCS is defined by the different evolutionary phases of CAD, excluding situations in

Table 4.1: CCS categories according to the ESC guidelines	
01	Patients with suspected CAD and 'stable' anginal symptoms, and/or dyspnea
02	Patients with new onset of heart failure (HF) or left ventricular (LV) dysfunction and suspected CAD
03	Asymptomatic and symptomatic patients with stabilized symptoms
04	Asymptomatic and symptomatic patients >1 year after initial diagnosis or revascularization
05	Patients with angina and suspected vasospastic or microvascular disease
06	Asymptomatic subjects in whom CAD is detected at screening

which an acute coronary artery thrombosis dominates the clinical presentation (i.e. ACS).[10,11]

Angina and its Clinical Implications

Angina pectoris (AP) is a chest discomfort of cardiac origin and a clinical manifestation of IHD.[12] Generally, angina occurs if there is an atherosclerotic narrowing of one or more epicardial coronary artery spasms with or without endothelial dysfunction.[13] In some circumstances, angina is related to coronary spasm and metabolic dysfunction. Numerous pathophysiological factors can cause myocardial ischemia. Chronic stable angina can be categorized into three main classes: stable, vasospastic, and microvascular angina (Fig. 4.1). Chronic stable angina occurs due to exercise-induced ischemia in patients with coronary flow-limiting atherosclerotic stenosis in the large coronary arteries. Stable angina occurs due to atherosclerotic narrowing of epicardial coronary arteries. In some conditions, the angina is related to coronary spasm and metabolic dysfunction. Various factors, for example, heart rate (HR), afterload, cardiac hypertrophy, and myocardial contractility can escalate myocardial oxygen demand. The numerous causes of chronic stable angina can be categorized into three broad categories: non-cardiac, cardiac ischemic, and cardiac non-ischemic causes.[14]

Vasospastic angina is seen in a minority of individuals, which is caused due to abnormal reactivity of the smooth muscles of the coronary arteries. Vasospastic angina form has specific features, for example, pain is not activated by exercise but happens at rest. Vasospasm can be induced by different triggers and requires definite analytic tests and therapies. A specific level of coronary spasm may likewise be superimposed on a non-occlusive, fixed atherosclerotic stenosis, which gets occlusive, and in this way, suggestive when the smooth muscle chokes.

In microvascular angina, myocardial ischemia is caused due to microvascular and endothelial dysfunction and by inflammation of the coronary arteries. Depending on the studies, microvascular angina presents up to 40% of patients with angina.[13,14]

Patients with stable angina have lower QoL and utilize greater healthcare resources. Many studies revealed that angina is freely linked with CV outcomes. Furthermore, large scale studies have shown that the improvement of angina symptoms by

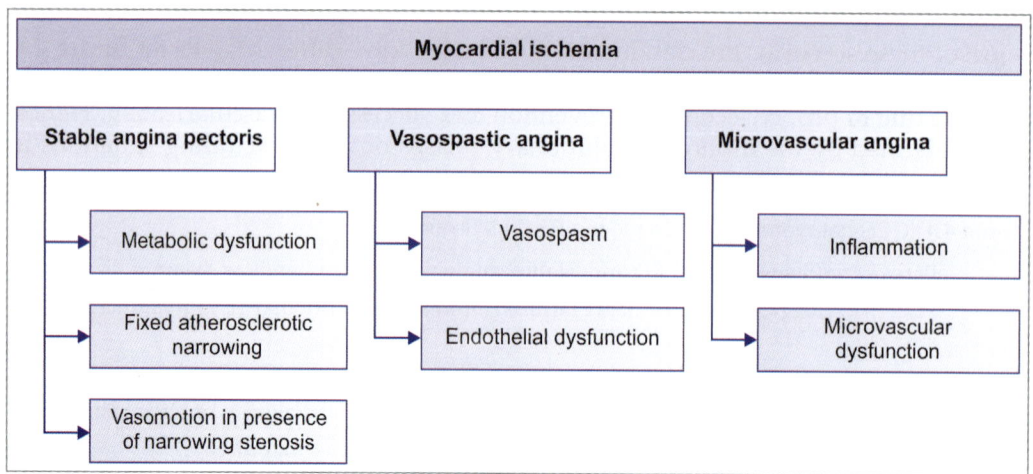

Fig. 4.1: Different manifestations of myocardial ischemia

pharmacological treatment improves QoL measures but does not decrease mortality. Also, in outpatients with stable CAD, most CV events happen in patients without prior angina. Recent studies have served as evidence that functional coronary disorders overlap and may cause angina in patients with obstructive epicardial CAD.[15]

The REduction of Atherothrombosis for Continued Health (REACH) study was conducted to determine the extent to which angina was related to CV events in patients with CAD. This study included patients with either stable symptomatic vascular disease or with multiple atherosclerotic risk factors. Patients were treated as per the best judgment practices of their primary care physicians. CV death, and myocardial infarction (MI) is the primary endpoint, whereas secondary endpoints comprised HF, CV hospitalizations, and coronary revascularization. Results showed that angina patients had higher rates of first primary endpoint event (14.2% vs 16.3%, unadjusted hazard ratio 1.19, CI: 1.11–1.27, p <0.001; adjusted hazard ratio 1.06, CI: 0.99–1.14, p = 0.11), and total primary endpoint events (adjusted risk ratio 1.08, CI: 1.01–1.16, p = 0.03) when compared with patients without angina. Patients with angina were at higher risk for coronary revascularization, HF, and CV hospitalizations. As per the REACH risk score, when patients were stratified into quartiles for recurrent CV events, it was seen that patients in higher quartiles had higher rates of the primary endpoint of CVD, MI, or stroke. Angina was linked with the primary endpoint in lower-risk patients. These findings showed that patients with stable CAD and angina had higher rates of future CV events compared with patients without angina.[15]

Also, results from several studies have shown a relation between angina and prior MI. In patients with prior MI, angina was related to a greater primary event rate. The prospective observational longitudinal registry of patients with stable coronary artery disease (CLARIFY) study was performed to define the characteristics and management of chronic coronary syndrome patients, and also the consequences and their determining factors. In this registry, a total of 32,703 chronic coronary syndrome patients (mean age of 64.2 ± 10.5 years) were enrolled (45 countries). Results revealed that interaction between angina and prior MI (p = 0.0016) was seen, and among patients with prior MI, angina was related to a higher primary event rate [11.8% (95% CI: 10.9–12.9) vs 8.2% (95% CI: 7.8–8.7). Among patients without prior MI, event rates were similar for patients with [6.3% (95% CI: 5.4–7.3)] or without angina [6.4% (95% CI: 5.9–7.0)], p >0.99. After stratification into four mutually exclusive subgroups, angina was seen related to a poorer prognosis in patients before MI history.[16]

Whereas Kaul U et al. in 2016 conducted the CLARIFY Indian cohort subgroup analysis to define the clinical characteristics, the occurrence of CAD risk factors. In this analysis, baseline data of the India cohort (n = 709) was compared with data from the rest of the World (ROW) (n = 31,994). Results showed that Indian patients were more likely to have diabetes and angina compared to ROW. Mean HR was considerably greater in Indian patients (76.1 ± 10.4 vs 68.0 ± 10.5). A significantly larger proportion of patients in India exhibited low HDL cholesterol (41.6% vs 31.2%) and HR ≥70 bpm (82.2% vs 48.5%). The risk factors control was poor in India to HR goal of ≤60 bpm achieved in 2.5%, HbA1c <7% in 9.9%, and HbA1c <6.5% in 4.6% patients. Overall, the occurrence of CV risk factors was very high in the CLARIFY India cohort compared to the ROW.[17]

Furthermore, to determine the trends in CV risk factor prevalence and pattern of use of the appropriate treatment in India compared with the ROW over 5 years, Hiremath S et al. analyzed the results from the CLARIFY registry. The analysis showed that the prevalence of angina was decreased from 27.8 to 11.2% over 5 years in India

(p <0.0001). Also, a persistent drop in mean SBP, DBP, and HR was observed over 5 years. Furthermore, a significant decrease in the percentage of patients with elevated HR (≥70 bpm) from baseline to 5 years was observed in India. Yet, the control of HR (≤60 bpm) remained poor even at 5 years in India (2.6 to 2.1%, $p = 0.43$).[18]

Take Home Pearls

- CAD is a progression of atherosclerotic plaque accumulation and functional changes of the coronary circulation.
- ACS categorized patients into STEMI, NSTEMI, or unstable angina.
- CCS is known as the altered evolutionary phases of CAD, excluding the situations in which an acute coronary artery thrombosis dominates the clinical presentation.
- Patients with stable CAD and angina had greater rates of future CV events compared with patients without angina.
- The 5-year trend of CLARIFY India registry showed variable trends in the incidence of CV risk factors such as HR >70 bpm, HbA1c >7%, higher blood pressure, and higher LDL cholesterol.

HIGH RESTING HEART RATE AND ITS IMPACT IN CAD AND ANGINA

High resting heart rate (RHR) is a simple measurement with important prognostic implications. Several epidemiologic studies demonstrated that a rise in RHR is a strong predictor for CV mortality in healthy populations and patients with various CVD, including hypertension, AMI, and HF.[19, 20] There is much evidence to suggest that elevated HR precedes many instances of myocardial ischemia during daily activities. Reduction in HR is the best way to decrease myocardial ischemia. Various studies have identified RHR as a risk factor for subsequent CV events in patients with CAD.[21]

High RHR and Outcomes in CAD

Sustained elevation of RHR plays an important role in the pathogenesis of atherosclerosis, and HR dependent acceleration of CAD development has been hypothesized as a possible pathomechanism through which elevated RHR raises CV morbidity and mortality.[22] An increase in HR leads to both greater myocardial oxygen consumption (MVO$_2$) and decreased myocardial perfusion, the latter by shortening the duration of diastole, which can induce or exacerbate myocardial ischemia. To explore the prognostic value of HR in patients with stable CAD, Diaz A *et al.* conducted a Coronary Artery Surgery Study (CASS), a multicenter research program. The study enrolled a total of 24,913 patients with suspected CAD for a median follow-up of 14.7 years. Results revealed that CV mortality and CV rehospitalizations were increased with elevated HR (p <0.0001). Patients with RHR ≥83 bpm at baseline had a higher risk for CV mortality. When patients with HR between 77–82 and ≥83 bpm compared with patients with HR ≤62 bpm, the HR values for time to first CV rehospitalization were 1.11 and 1.14, respectively (p <0.001 for both). According to subgroup analysis, the connection among HR and total mortality remained constant in all subgroups [men *vs* women, old (>65 years) *vs* young, diabetics *vs* non-diabetics, hypertensives *vs* normotensives, BMI >27 or <27, those with EF >50% or EF <50%, and patients treated with β-Blockers (BBs) *vs* those without such a treatment]. These outcomes revealed that high RHR is an indicator for CV mortality autonomous of other risk factors in patients with CAD.[19]

The patterns towards worsening outcomes related to increased baseline RHR were known to be perceptible for all-cause and CV mortality, non-fatal MI, and hospital admission for HF with a graded increase in event rate, most clearly seen for hospitalization for HF (HHF).[21] Daly CA *et al.* performed a prospective, observational, cohort study to examine RHR in a population presented with stable angina. A total of 3,779 patients with stable angina were included in the study. The mean baseline RHR was 73 bpm, and 52.3% of patients had a baseline HR >70 bpm. Results revealed that greater HR at baseline was linked with higher rates of CV mortality and hospitalization. High HRs were linked with adverse clinical outcomes in a variety of settings, including stable coronary disease.[21]

An increased HR at rest has also been found related to worse consequences in patients with hypertension, CHD, and LVD, other than those without known CVD. Though prior studies have only reported fatal outcomes, and the relationship between increased HR and non-fatal CV events are less well understood. Moreover, it is still unclear whether the influence of a rise in HR is independent of other comorbidities. Therefore, to determine the influence of the HR at rest on major CV events, Ho JE *et al.* conducted a post hoc analysis of the treating new targets (TNT) study. A total of 9,580 subjects were enrolled in the study and were followed-up for a median of 4.9 years. Results revealed that the rate of major CV events was 11.9% in those with a baseline HR of >70 bpm *vs* 8.8% in those with a baseline HR of <70 bpm. An elevated HR at rest was related to CV events, even after adjustment for differences in baseline characteristics (unadjusted hazard ratio 1.16 for each 10-bpm increase, 95% CI: 1.10 to 1.23, p <0.0001; adjusted hazard ratio 1.08 per 10-bpm increase, 95% CI: 1.02 to 1.16, p = 0.018). An HR ≥70 bpm was also found to be a significant independent predictor of all-cause mortality (hazard ratio 1.40, 95% CI: 1.14 to 1.71, p = 0.001) and HHF (hazard ratio 2.30, 95% CI: 1.80 to 2.95, p > or = 0.0001). These findings from the study revealed that each 10-bpm elevation in HR at rest was related to an 8% increase in major CV events.[23]

Whereas, depending upon comorbidities such as DM, presented statistics from several studies showed that there is a link between RHR and CV Events (CVE) in stable CAD patients with and without DM.[20] Type 2 diabetes (T2D) is the most common type of diabetes, accounting for around 90% of all diabetes worldwide. As per IDF 2019 diabetes atlas, the worldwide prevalence of diabetic patients in 2019 was 9.3% (approximate 463.0 million DM patients), and by the year 2045, the prevalence increases to 10.9% (approximate 700.2 million DM patients).[24] Moreover, this disease is more common within specific groups of patients, not the least those presenting with CAD. Thus, to determine the link between RHR and CVE in stable CAD patients with and without DM, Anselmino M *et al.* conducted a Euro Heart Survey on Diabetes. In this study, 2,608 patients were enrolled with stable CAD. Of these, 780 (30%) had known DM. Results revealed that overall, the median RHR was 70 (62–78) bpm. The RHR quartile stratification was considerably related to outcome in the overall population, whereas it was not in patients without DM. In patients with DM, the RHR quartiles correlated with survival (p = 0.032). In an adjusted regression model performed in patients without DM, RHR has been associated with neither survival nor CVE. In contrast, a 10-bpm elevation in RHR was independently related to survival, but not with CVE in patients with DM. This study demonstrated that the relationship between RHR and CVE seems to subsist in those with DM, however, not in those without DM.[20]

High RHR and High BMI both can predict severe coronary atherosclerosis burden in patients with stable AP by SYNTAX Score. Although the usefulness of RHR in determining the CHD or CVD risk of mortality in general populations has been described, the influence of RHR for coronary atherosclerosis burden in patients with stable AP, especially the combined effect of RHR and added risk factors on atherosclerosis, has not been demonstrated. Zhang M *et al.* in 2017 studied the relationship between RHR and Body Mass Index (BMI) with SYNTAX Score (SS) in patients with stable angina. The SS grades the complexity of CHD established on the lesion characteristics, and higher scores mean more complex CHD. The study enrolled a total of 312 patients and divided them into four groups as per RHR quartiles: Q1 (<65 bpm), Q2 (65–69 bpm), Q3 (70–79 bpm), and Q4 (≥80 bpm). The outcomes of the study have shown that the SS (12.0 ± 9.0, 16.0 ± 15.5, 18.0 ± 16.5, and 20.0 ± 27.5; p <0.001) was considerably greater for those in Q4 than for those in Q1, Q2, and Q3. Multivariate logistic regression analysis indicated that every 10-bpm elevation in RHR was significantly related to SS. Patients with elevated RHR and high BMI had significantly greater OR of high SS (4.03, 95% CI: 2.00–8.14), compared to participants with low RHR and low BMI. Also, it was observed that both RHR and BMI were autonomous interpreters of coronary atherosclerosis. These findings revealed that RHR, when combined with BMI highlighted the significance of the association between RHR and SS in patients with stable AP.[25]

Implications of Admission and Discharge HR in CAD

Numerous trials have confirmed that an elevation in HR during hospitalization and after discharge has been predictive of death in patients with AMI. Nevertheless, whether this relationship is mainly due to related cardiac failure is unidentified. Therefore, to define the influence of HR on mortality after AMI, Hjalmarson A *et al.* conducted a multicenter study. In this study, a total of 1,807 patients with AMI were enrolled. Results revealed that total mortality was 15% for patients with an admission HR between 50 and 60 bpm, 41% for HR >90 bpm, and 48% for HR ≥110 bpm. These outcomes reported that HR was an independent prognostic marker of 1-year mortality, and elevated HR during hospitalization for AMI is significantly and freely associated with mortality.[26]

Though admission HR foresees a higher death rate after AMI, little is identified about discharge HR. Alapati V *et al.* in 2019 conducted a study to test the assumption that greater discharge HR after AMI is related to increased long-term mortality independent of admission HR. The study also determined if BBs alter this association. The data were combined from two different prospective registries, one is PREMIER (n = 2,498), and another one is TRIUMPH (n = 4,340). Among 6,833 patients enrolled across both registries, 6,576 patients were presented for inclusion. Results revealed that discharge HR (hazard ratio = 1.14 per 10 bpm) was intensely related to the risk of death than admission HR (hazard ratio = 1.05 per 10 bpm). These outcomes stated that the higher discharge HR after AMI was more strongly associated with 3 years mortality than admission HR.[27]

Relationship of HR with Myocardial Ischemia and Plaque Stability

HR is an important determinant of oxygen utilization in patients with IHD.[28] Myocardial ischemia occurs from a mismatch between myocardial oxygen demand and supply. Both factors are influenced by HR. Analysis of several clinical studies and intervention trials indicated that HR is an important independent correlate of circadian variation in the presence of AMI and the prediction of long-term survival following AMI.[29] Most episodes of myocardial ischemia are followed by an HR rise in CAD patients. Ischemia developed is linked to both the baseline HR and the extent and period of the increase.[30] Physical exercise and mental stress are also potent triggers of myocardial ischemia. The neural mechanisms for mental stress-induced include both the PNS and SNS. Physical and mental difficulties incite transient declines in the high-frequency component of HRV. Transient variations in HRV have just been approved as a fraction of momentary changes in autonomic tone. To examine the role of autonomic changes in the start of ischemic events, Kop WM et al. examined ($n = 19$ men) whether indicators of reduced vagal tone precede ischemic events documented by ambulatory electrocardiography. He further analyzed preischemic autonomic changes during periods of high vs low physical and mental exercises during daily life. Results revealed that a significant decrease in high- and low-frequency HRV was seen in the period preceding the ischemic event ($p <0.001$). High-frequency HRV decreased in the 60- to 10-min interval before the ischemic event ($p = 0.04$). A further decrease was observed between the 4-min and 2-min intervals before the ischemic event ($p = 0.008$) and from 2-min up to the ischemic event ($p = 0.001$). Also, it was observed that ischemic events occurring at increased HR (>100 bpm; 35 episodes) were associated more with lower high-frequency HRV [3.1 ± 1.2 ln (ms^2)] than ischemic events at lesser HR [≤100 bpm; 3.9 ± 0.8 ln (ms^2); $p = 0.003$]. Low frequency HRV was also depressed during high HR events [3.8 ± 1.5 ln (ms^2) vs $5.0 \pm$ ln (ms^2); $p <0.001$], and these differences remained significant after alteration in multiple comparisons ($p <0.01$). HR gradually increased in the 60-min to the 20-min interval before the ischemic event ($p = 0.04$) after that more distinct increase was detected in the 4-min before ischemia ($p = 0.008$). A parallel time course was also detected between the HRV decreases and HR increases before the ischemic event. These results proposed that vagal withdrawal goes before transient myocardial ischemia and might help in clarifying the procedure of mental stress-induced ischemia, which ordinarily happens at low HR.[31]

Identification of whether episodes of ambulatory ischemia are caused by increases in myocardial oxygen demand or episodic coronary vasoconstriction in patients with the stable coronary disease may be important to guide the selection of optimal anti-ischemic therapy and to gain insight into mechanisms responsible for adverse cardiac events. In numerous epidemiological studies, it has been appreciated that most episodes of ambulatory ischemia are related to a preceding period of increased HR. The likelihood of emerging ischemia is anticipated by HRV and unaffected by a time of day. Thus, to define whether emerging ischemia was strongly related to HRV or not, Andrews TC et al. performed a randomized, double-blind, crossover trial. Mean minute HR activity during ambulatory ECG (AECG) monitoring was evaluated for 50 patients cured with propranolol, diltiazem, nifedipine, or placebo. Results demonstrated that 81 percent of ischemic episodes preceded a rise in HR ≥5 bpm. The possibility of ischemia related to HR increase was comparative to the extent and interval of the HR increase: likelihood ranged from 4% when the HR increased 5–9 bpm and lasted <10 minutes to 60% when the HR increased ≥20 bpm and lasted ≥40 minutes. These findings revealed that most episodes of ambulatory ischemia are related to a preceding period of increased HR.[32]

For a long time, the progression of CAD leading to ACS was due to the constant development of coronary atherosclerosis. Though, serial coronary angiography has shown that the progression of CAD happens irregularly instead of linearly with time. The rapid progression of coronary atherosclerosis leading to consecutive ACS is due to plaque disruption. Plaque disruption consists of ACS and the development of coronary atherosclerosis. Thus, to investigate the effect of hemodynamic forces in the cause of plaque disruption, Heidl and UE *et al.* conducted a study including a total of 53 patients. Patients were investigated with initially smooth stenoses that developed plaque disruption by the time of the second coronary angiogram. The investigation showed positive associations between plaque disruption, LV muscle mass >270 g, and a mean HR >80 bpm, and a negative association with BBs. These outcomes revealed that hemodynamic forces have a significant role in the pathogenesis of plaque disruption.[33]

QoL and HR in Angina

Angina is a main debilitating health condition with common chronic symptoms of intermittent, reversible chest pain, or discomfort.[34] Regardless of various efficient pharmacological medicines and the achievement of interventional cardiology; angina is always a reason for significant disability and debilitated QoL for some patients. As angina is difficult to measure objectively, clinical decisions are based on physician evaluated symptom burden.[35] Evidence showed that raised HR is an independent risk factor in patients with CAD and affect their diagnosis. Also, patients with chronic obstructive pulmonary disease (COPD) have more regular episodes of angina. Inadequate HR control is related to worse QoL in patients with CAD and COPD. The RYTHMOS study was the first prospective, a multicenter countrywide study conducted to assess the importance of HR management in the prognosis and QoL in patients with CAD and COPD.[23] In this study, 280 patients were enrolled with a mean age was 71.8 ± 9.3 years, and 76% were males. BB therapy was prescribed to 52.8% of the study patients having RHR ≤ 70 bpm (57.4% vs 42.7%, $p < 0.001$). Whereas, 16.4% of the patients were given Ivabradine, and they had a higher initial HR compared to the others (78.5 vs 71.3, $p < 0.001$). Patients with RHR >70 bpm had considerably more common angina episodes ($p < 0.001$), were less satisfied with the treatment ($p < 0.001$), and had a lower QoL ($p < 0.001$). The baseline data from the study showed that CAD and COPD patients are present with insufficient HR control and recurrent angina episodes.[36]

Impact of HR Reduction on CAD Outcomes

Raised HR induces myocardial ischemia in patients with CAD. A decrease in HR is a documented approach to avoid ischemic episodes. Moreover, a clinical trial showed that a decrease in HR decreases the symptoms of angina by improving microcirculation and coronary flow.[37] The hypothesis that the potential valuable effect of BB drugs after an AMI is quantitatively dependent on the HR reduction obtained by such treatment was examined by reviewing available data from acute and long-term intervention trials. In these trials, only patients who were given treatment within 12 hours after the start of pain were involved. It was observed that in early intervention trials, there was a close relationship between the reduction in HR and infarct size as determined by accumulated creatine kinase release ($r = 0.97$, $p < 0.001$). Similar relation was observed between the decrease in RHR and non-fatal reinfarctions ($r = 0.59$, $p < 0.05$). A joint mechanism is accountable for the decrease in death rate and non-fatal reinfarctions. This is further supported by the finding of a close link between the reductions of events in each study ($r = 0.79$, $p < 0.05$). However, in all the trials with a non-selective BB, mortality was more reduced than non-fatal reinfarctions. These findings prompted that BBs are linked to a quantifiable decrease in HR possibly indicating an anti-ischemic effect.[38]

Furthermore, to define the quantitative relationship between RHR decrease and the extent of clinical benefits in post-MI, Cucherat M conducted a meta-regression of randomized clinical trials. A total of 17 controlled randomized trials [14 with BBs and 3 with calcium channel blockers (CCBs)] met the eligibility criteria. Results revealed that a statistically significant relationship was seen between resting HR reduction and the clinical benefit including reduction in cardiac death ($p < 0.001$), all-cause death ($p = 0.008$), sudden death ($p = 0.015$), and non-fatal MI recurrence ($p = 0.024$). Each 10-bpm reduction in HR was estimated to reduce the relative risk of CV death by 30%. These consequences showed the useful effect of BBs and CCBs in post-MI patients, which proportionately linked to RHR reduction.[39]

The latest trials have demonstrated RHR to be an autonomous indicator of all-cause mortality in people with and without analyzed CVD. Comparatively, increased HR has direct harmful effects on the development of coronary atherosclerosis, myocardial ischemia, and ventricular arrhythmias. Studies have found a continuous increase in risk with HR above 60 bpm. The relationship between the mean decrease in HR and the mean change in mortality was found in different randomized, placebo-controlled trials of BBs after MI. The linear regression line ($r = 0.6$, $p < 0.05$) was fitted, excluding the smallest study (open circles). After treatment with 2 doses of 3 different CCBs, the association between the improvement in time to myocardial ischemia during bicycle exercise and the reduction in exercise HR attained in patients with stable angina.[40] Emerging data presented herein proposed that the possible role of HR and its variation should be seriously measured in future CV guidance documents.

Take Home Pearls

- Elevated RHR is an indicator of CV mortality independent of additional risk factors in patients with CAD.
- Ambulatory ischemia episodes are related to a preceding period of increased HR.
- With the help of the SYNTAX score, high RHR, and BMI, both can predict coronary atherosclerosis burden in patients with stable angina.
- Patients with HR >70 bpm had considerably poorer QoL.
- The valuable impact of BBs and CCBs in post-MI patients is relatively identified with RHR decrease.

MANAGEMENT OF HIGH RHR—ANGINA PERSPECTIVE

AP is the symptomatic sign of transitory myocardial ischemia. At the most major level, angina emerges when myocardial oxygen demand surpasses the ability of the coronary circulation to give sufficient oxygen delivery to maintain normal myocardial metabolic function.[41]

The general treatment of patients with angina must include an effort to improve prognosis. It begins with evidence-based lifestyle modification focusing on the control of CAD risk factors and patient education. Briefly, tobacco smoking, including environmental exposure, must be avoided as the benefits of smoking cessation are extensively documented. There is proof that encouragement and pharmacological aids (e.g. nicotine replacement, bupropion, and varenicline) improve success rates. Also, there is an indication that a healthy diet reduces risk. Maintaining or obtaining a healthy weight (defined as BMI <25 kg/m^2) is vital. Consumption of N-3 polyunsaturated fatty acids, mainly from oily fish rather than from supplements, is related to benefits. A 'Mediterranean diet' supplemented with extra-virgin olive oil or nuts reduce Major Adverse Cardiovascular Events (MACE) in patients at high risk. Strong evidence supports regular physical activity incorporated into the angina patient's usual daily activities. Aerobic exercise may also be suggested as part of a structured cardiac rehabilitation program, with the need for an evaluation of both exercise capacity and exercise-associated risk. Patients with stable angina may undergo moderate-intensity aerobic exercise training ≥3 times a week for 30 min per session. Sedentary patients are strongly encouraged to begin light-intensity exercise risk stratification. Exercise training offers an additional means of symptom alleviation and improves prognosis and QoL. Some psychosocial factors (e.g. depression, anxiety, and post-traumatic distress) are prevalent among CAD patients and may promote angina. Patients with angina who have symptoms of depression, anxiety, and/or hostility should be appropriately evaluated and referred for therapy. There is evidence that such an approach to management reduces symptoms and enhances QoL. Supplementary drug and physical interventions are usually applied to patients with angina. Mechanisms of action for these interventions include HR modulation, metabolic manipulation, revascularization, and others.[41]

Considerable evidence states that HR is one of the systematic contributing factors to myocardial ischemia. Therefore, reduction of and/or limiting HR increases are fundamental in the treatment of AP. Increased HR is an indicator of higher CV risk in common people and also in patients with IHD.[41] The contributors to the physiological myocardial perfusion gradient and resultant ischemia can be broken down at the patient-level into systemic, cardiac, and coronary factors (Fig. 4.2).

Benefits of HR Reduction in Angina

HR is the main factor affecting myocardial oxygen demand. The myocardium needs to work harder to complete the cardiac cycle more proficiently with higher HR. The time spent in diastole decreases with the reduced cardiac cycle. With an abbreviated cardiac cycle, the time spent in diastole diminishes. Since diastole closes prematurely, the measure of blood that typically fills the ventricles diminish, and oxygen-immersed hemoglobin is not permitted to arrive at the sub-endocardium. In ideal conditions, myocardial oxygen demand will equal myocardial oxygen supply; though, when there is structural damage from a plaque that hinders flow, there can be a mismatch between supply and demand causes ischemia.[42]

Higher HR will raise both demand and supply. It is the foremost determining factor of myocardial oxygen or energy demand or both by improving myocardial perfusion, controls oxygen supply, or energy supply or both. In humans, the heart beats an average of 100,000 times per day, which corresponds to ~36.8×10^6 times per year or 29×10^8 heartbeats in a lifetime (80 years on average). In doing so, the heart produces and immediately consumes ~30 kg of ATP every day. Decreasing the HR by 10-bpm saves ~5 kg of ATP every day.[43] Also, HR is a significant controller of oxygen consumption by mitochondrial oxidation of the myocytes, and its reduction increases

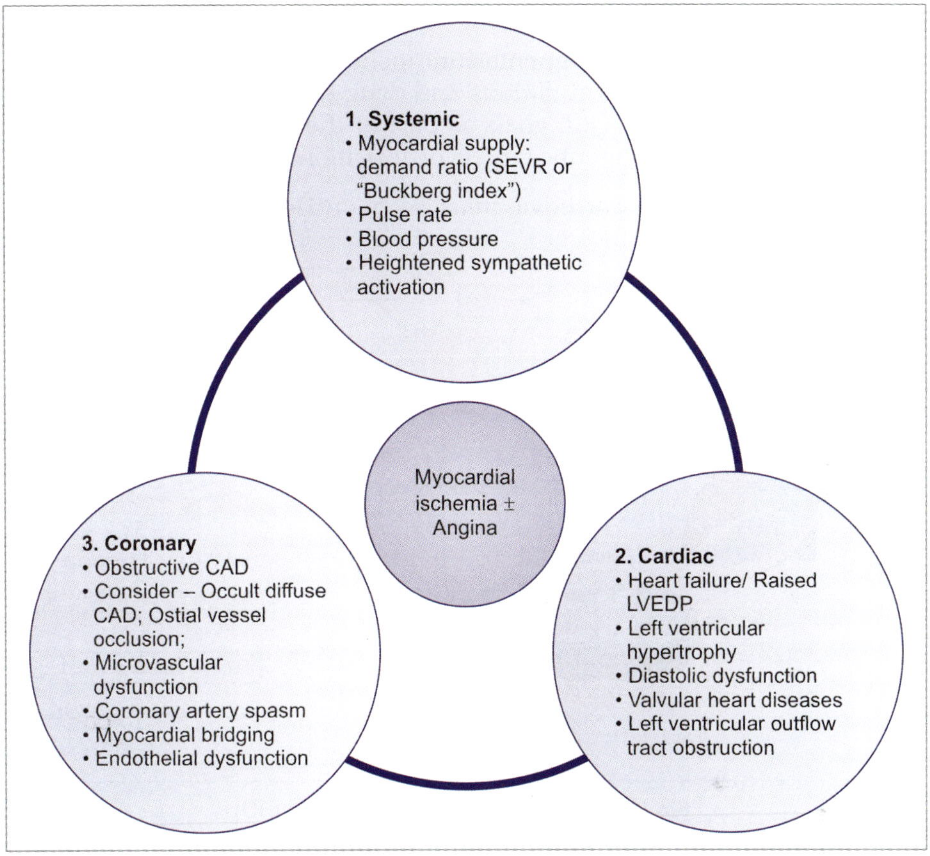

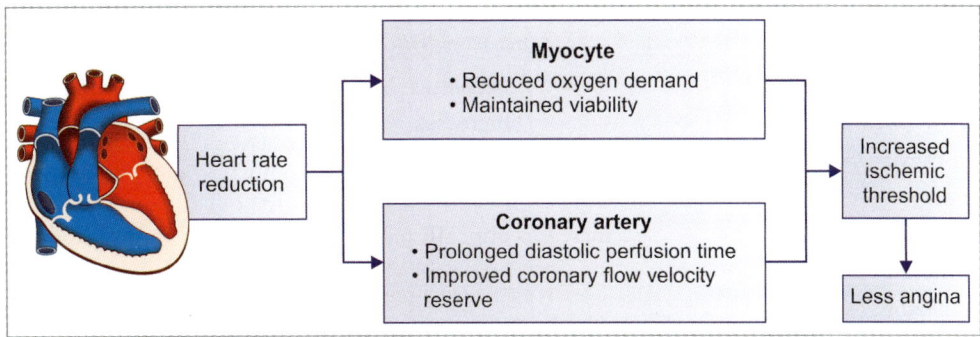

Fig. 4.2: Contributing factors to myocardial ischemia. CAD: Coronary artery disease; LVEDP: Left ventricular end-diastolic pressure; SEVR: Subendocardial viability ratio

the ischemic threshold. Also, the influence of HR reduction at the level of the coronary arteries can improve coronary flow reserve. These favorable special effects on coronary arteries could help to avoid microvascular angina and, theoretically, contribute to reducing CV events (Fig. 4.3).[44]

Fig. 4.3: Beneficial effects of HR reduction in angina

Managing Angina and High RHR

The antianginal therapeutic armamentarium includes some effective anti-ischemic agents, available in various formulations and drug delivery systems. These agents are essential in targeting the QoL goals as part of the management of stable IHD. Figure 4.4 represents the therapeutic targets of antianginal therapies.[45]

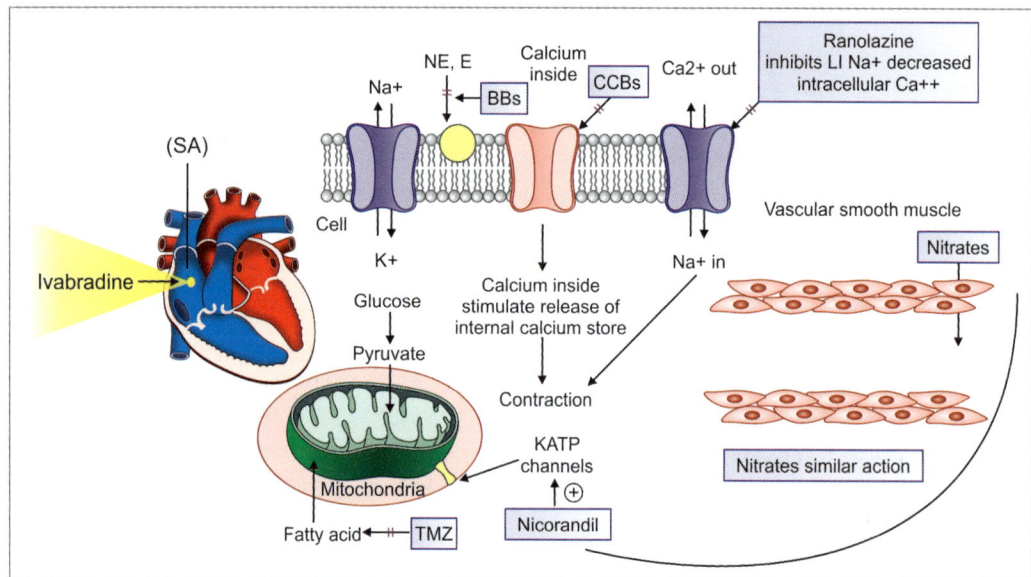

Fig. 4.4: Therapeutic target for chronic IHD

Current guidelines recommended pharmacological therapy with drugs categorized as being first-line (BBs, CCBs, short-acting nitrates) or second-line (long-acting nitrates, ivabradine, nicorandil, ranolazine, trimetazidine). Second-line drugs should be given to patients who cannot tolerate first-line agents. Pharmacological treatment has two primary objectives: initially, to reduce indications, increment angina-free strolling time, and improve QoL; furthermore, to forestall CV events. Antianginal agents improve total exercise duration along with a reduction in the daily frequency of chronic stable angina compared with placebo. In Table 4.2, first-line and second-line

Table 4.2: Antianginal therapies and their impact on HR

Antianginal drugs	Impact on HR	Line of therapy
β-Blockers	Decreases	**First-line**
Dihydropyridine CCBs	Increases	
Non-dihydropyridine CCBs	Decreases	
Nitrates	Increases	
Ivabradine	Increases pure HR reduction	**Second-line**
Nicorandil	Increases	
Ranolazine	↔	
Trimetazidine	↔	

therapy antianginal drugs mentioned with their impact on HR.[14] HR-lowering agents, for example, BBs, CCBs, and ivabradine are the chosen drugs when HR is >70 bpm (Table 4.3).[14]

Table 4.3: Properties of HR lowering antianginal agents

Property	Blood pressure	Inotropic effect	Peripheral vascular resistance	Combination therapy for further HR reduction
β-blocker	Reduced	Negative	Decreased	Synergistic effect with ivabradine
Calcium channel blockers	Reduced	Negative	Decreased	β-blockers should not be combined with verapamil, and only with caution with diltiazem due to the risk of AV block, hypotension and bradycardia
Ivabradine	No direct effect	No direct effect	No direct effect	Synergistic effect with β-blockers

Evidence that one drug is superior to another has been questioned. Between January and March 2018, Ferrari R *et al.* conducted a systematic review of articles comprising double-blind, randomized studies, including management of angina in a sample size of at least 100 patients. There is a paucity of data relating to the effectiveness of antianginal agents. Fewer studies indicated that equivalence has been shown only for three classes of drugs.[46] Similarly, a meta-analysis result of eleven trials showed that data are scarce, which compared the efficiency of antianginal agents. The classification of the antianginal drug in the first- and second-line is not established.[47] No proof is present to support the use of first- and second-line treatments for the management of angina. Rather, the medical therapy of angina should be personalized and tailored towards the individual with a consideration of the likely pathophysiological mechanisms and comorbidities.[46]

Also, angina patients have several comorbidities and symptoms due to numerous primary pathophysiologies. Several agents could be helpful based on comorbidities and the mechanisms of angina, but the guidelines do not provide recommendations on the optimal combinations of drugs. Thus, a consensus statement proposed a tailored approach, which considers the patient, their comorbidities, and the basic mechanism of ailment. As per experts, a 'diamond' approach is more suitable to choose the most suitable drug regimen, alone or in combination, for an individual patient (Figs 4.5 and 4.6).[14] "Diamond" approach is a potential framework that could assist clinicians to make the best probable therapeutic choices, independently of whether the medications are the first or second choice for angina patients.[14]

Ivabradine: Pure HR Lowering I_f Current Inhibitor

Ivabradine is a drug with a negative chronotropic influence on the Sinoatrial (SA) node. It is different from other pharmacological agents because it has an advantage in HF with reduced ejection fraction (HFrEF) in that it does not target the neurohormonal system. Ivabradine is used as a second-line medication for systolic HF and chronic stable angina.[48] As in 2005, it was first permitted by the European Medicines Agency (EMA) for use in angina patients, and the results of several trials led to its expanded indications, for instance, heart failure patients.

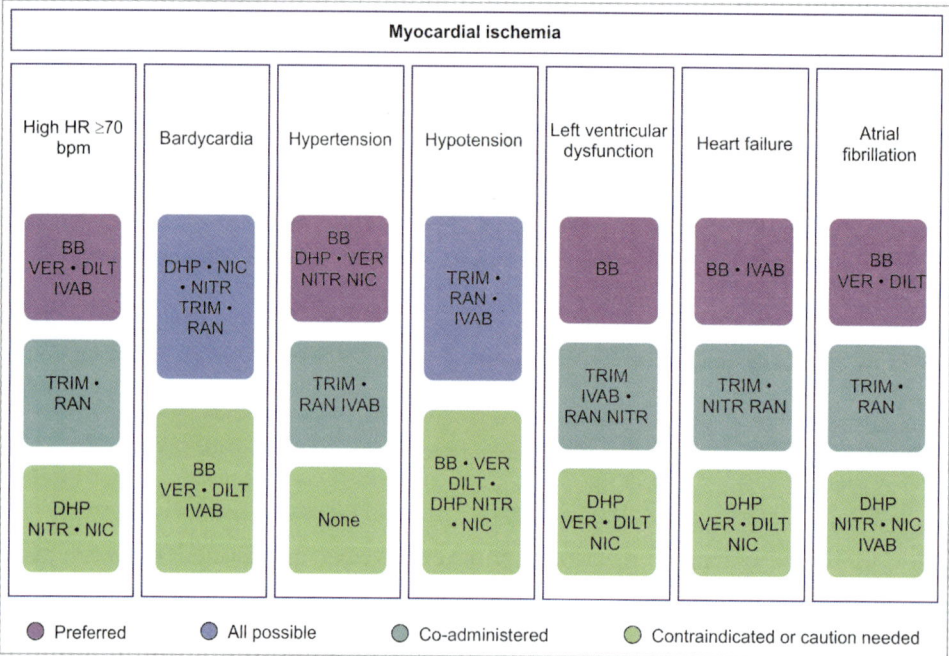

Fig. 4.5: Possible combinations of classes of antianginal drugs according to different comorbidities. BB: β-blockers; DHP: Dihydropyridine calcium channel blockers; DILT: Diltiazem; HR: Heart rate; IVAB: Ivabradine; NIC: Nicorandil; NIT/NITR: Nitrates; RAN: Ranolazine; TRIM: Trimetazidine; VER: Verapamil

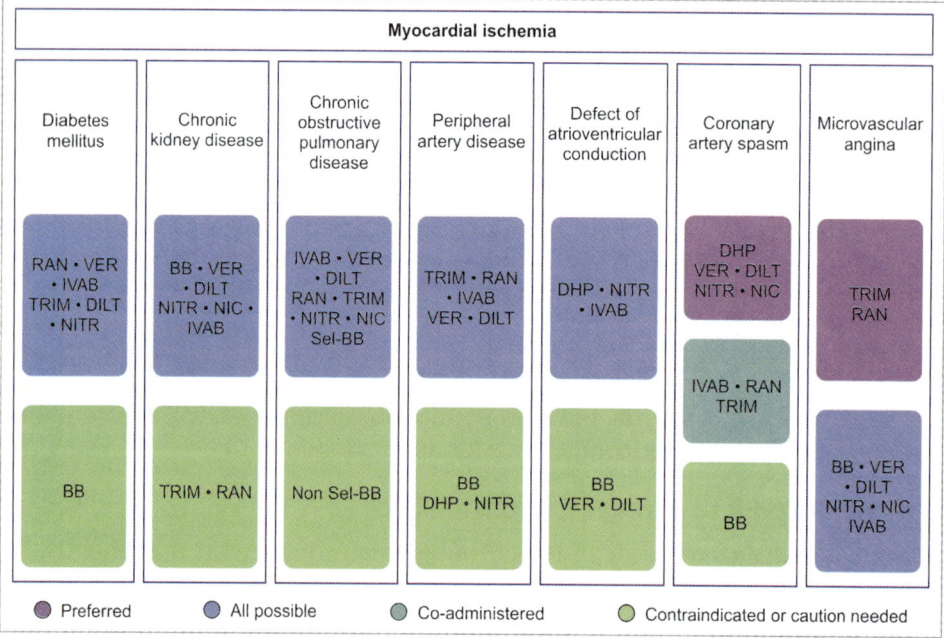

Fig. 4.6: Possible combinations of classes of other antianginal drugs according to different comorbidities. BB: β-blockers; DHP: Dihydropyridine calcium-channel blockers; DILT: Diltiazem; IVAB: Ivabradine; NIC: Nicorandil; NITR: Nitrates; Non Sel-BB: Non-selective β-blockers; RAN: Ranolazine; Sel-BB: β1-selective blockers; TRIM: Trimetazidine; VER: Verapamil

US Food and Drug Administration (FDA) has recently approved this indication (Fig. 4.7).[48] Recently in India, ivabradine has received approval from the Drugs Controller General of India (DCGI); for its once-a-day use formulation (in the form of prolonged-release tablets).[49]

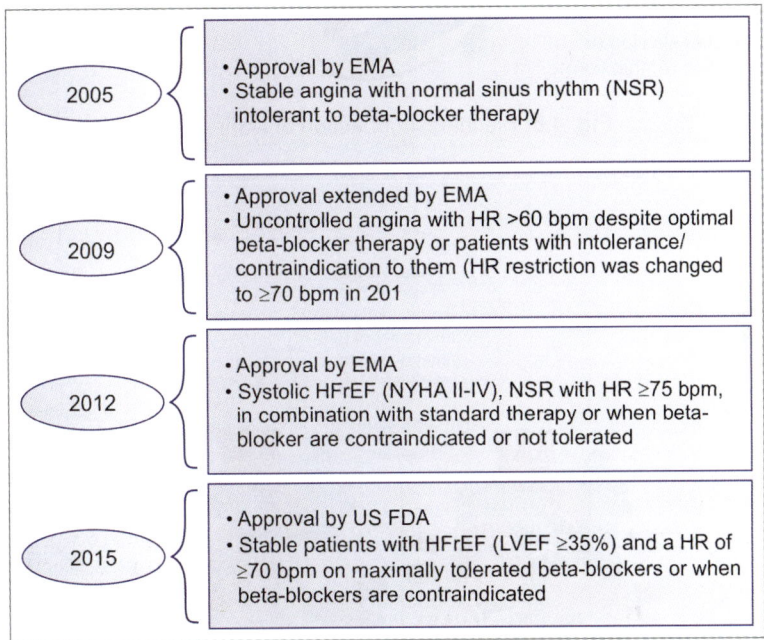

- 2005
  - Approval by EMA
  - Stable angina with normal sinus rhythm (NSR) intolerant to beta-blocker therapy

- 2009
  - Approval extended by EMA
  - Uncontrolled angina with HR >60 bpm despite optimal beta-blocker therapy or patients with intolerance/contraindication to them (HR restriction was changed to ≥70 bpm in 201

- 2012
  - Approval by EMA
  - Systolic HFrEF (NYHA II-IV), NSR with HR ≥75 bpm, in combination with standard therapy or when beta-blocker are contraindicated or not tolerated

- 2015
  - Approval by US FDA
  - Stable patients with HFrEF (LVEF ≥35%) and a HR of ≥70 bpm on maximally tolerated beta-blockers or when beta-blockers are contraindicated

Fig. 4.7: Approval timeline of Ivabradine across Europe and the United States

Ivabradine in India is indicated for the symptomatic treatment of chronic stable AP in CAD patients with normal sinus rhythm who have a contraindication or intolerance for BBs or in combination with BBs in patients inadequately controlled with an optimal BB dose and whose HR is >60 bpm. It is also indicated for the treatment of chronic HF in chronic HF New York Heart Association (NYHA) II to IV classes with systolic dysfunction, in adult patients in sinus rhythm and whose HR is >75 bpm, in combination with standard therapy including BB therapy or when BB therapy is contraindicated or not tolerated.

Ivabradine's main mechanism of action is on the SA node, which occupies mainly subepicardial location at the junction of the superior vena cava (SVC) and the right atrium (RA). Ivabradine blocks the intracellular aspect of the hyperpolarization-activated Cyclic Nucleotide-gated (HCN) trans-membrane channel in the SA node, which stops inward funny current (I_f). It causes a decrease in HR and cardioprotective effects (Figs 4.8 and 4.9).[48]

The recommended starting dosage of Ivabradine is 5 mg bid administered with food. Following fourteen days, the patient should be evaluated, and dose adjustments have to be done to attain an RHR of between 50 bpm and 60 bpm (Table 4.4). Further, additional dose adjustments have to be done based on the patient's RHR and tolerability. The maximum dosage of Ivabradine is 7.5 mg bid. No dose adjustments are required in patients with creatinine clearance values of 15 mL/min or greater.

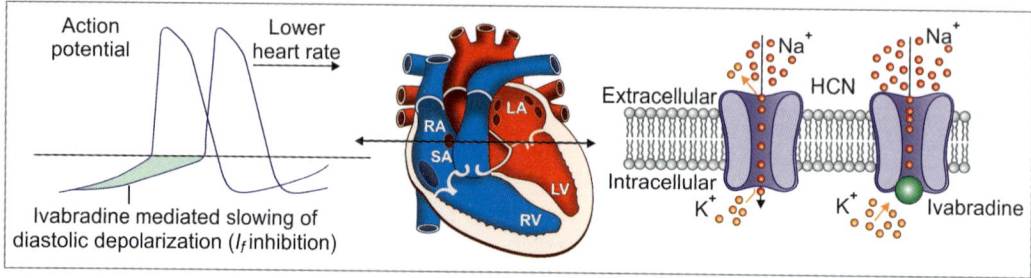

Fig. 4.8: Mechanism of action of ivabradine

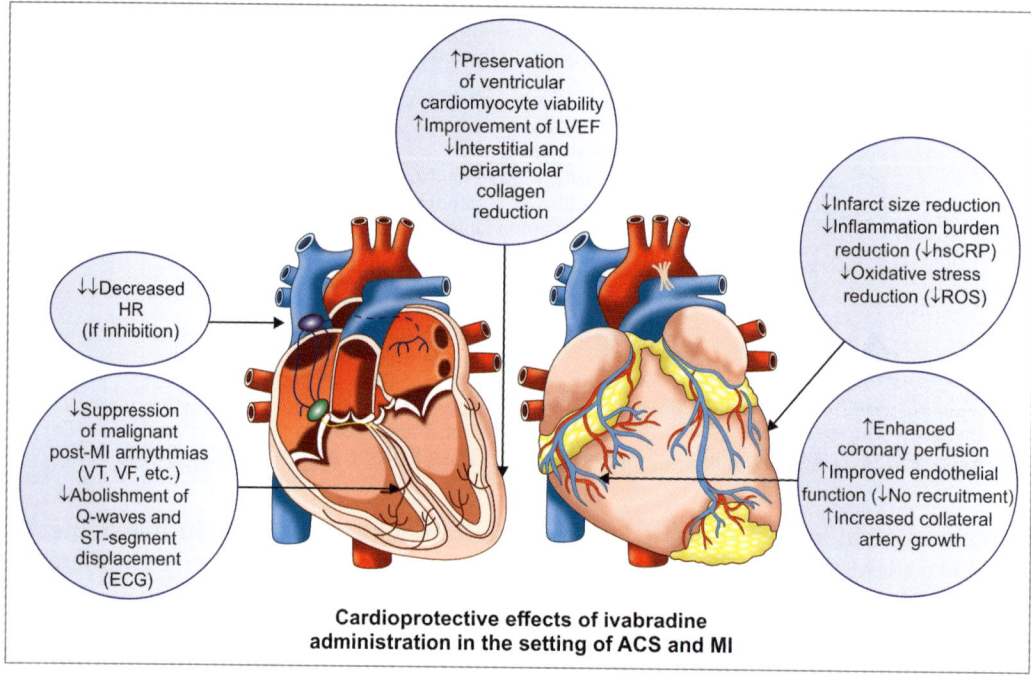

**Cardioprotective effects of ivabradine
administration in the setting of ACS and MI**

Fig. 4.9: Cardioprotective effects of ivabradine

Table 4.4: Ivabradine dosage and titration

Heart rate	Dose adjustment
Greater than 60 bpm	Increase dose by 2.5 mg twice daily up to a maximum dose of 7.5 mg twice daily
Dihydropyridine CCBs	Maintain dose
Less than 50 bpm or signs and symptoms of bradycardia	Decrease dose by 2.5 mg twice daily; I_f current dose is 2.5 mg twice daily, discontinue therapy

However, caution is advised in end-stage renal failure. The prolonged-release dosage form of ivabradine is also available for once-daily usage in 10 mg and 15 mg dosage strengths.[50]

Ivabradine should not be prescribed to patients with acute decompensated HF, severe hepatic impairment, an RHR below 60 bpm earlier to treatment, BP less than 90/50 mmHg, or pacemaker dependence. Also, Ivabradine is not prescribed to patients with sick sinus syndrome, SA block, or third-degree AV block unless a functioning demand pacemaker is present.[50]

SPECTRUM OF CLINICAL EVIDENCE WITH IVABRADINE IN CAD AND ANGINA

Increased HR by increasing myocardial oxygen demand and decreasing diastolic perfusion time causes signs of myocardial ischemia. Thus, reducing HR is an eminent approach for improving QOL and symptoms of myocardial ischemia. Ivabradine is indicated for the management of stable angina and chronic HF as it decreases myocardial oxygen consumption without disturbing myocardial contractility. Also, it is beneficial in several special populations of CAD. The spectrum of clinical evidence with ivabradine associated with CAD and angina is shown in Fig. 4.10.

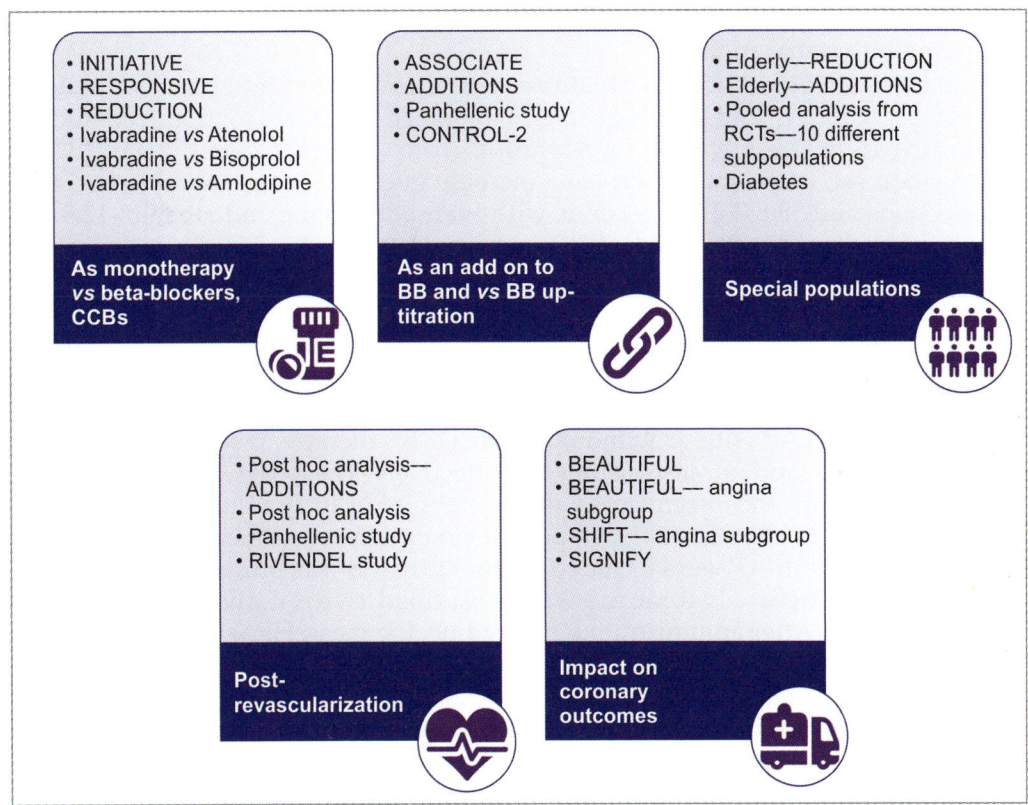

Fig. 4.10: Spectrum of clinical evidences

As Monotherapy *vs* BBs, CCBs

Angina occurs when myocardial perfusion is not enough to meet myocardial metabolic demand. Increased HR stimulates myocardial ischemia and consequent angina. Both increase myocardial oxygen demand and reduces myocardial perfusion, and finally, by shortening the period of diastole. BBs reduce angina by decreasing HR and are commonly chosen as initial therapy if contraindications are not present. Regardless of the established safety and efficacy of BBs, their use is limited by the side effects of these agents, including sexual dysfunction, tiredness, depression, cold extremities, light-headedness, intestinal disturbances, bronchospasm, and atrioventricular (AV) block.

Ivabradine is an innovative particular HR reducing agent. Tardif JC et al. conducted an INITIATIVE double-blind study to compare the antianginal and anti-ischemic properties of Ivabradine and the BB (Atenolol). A total of 939 patients with stable angina were enrolled to be given Ivabradine 5 mg BID for 4 weeks and then either 7.5 or 10 mg BID for 12 weeks or Atenolol 50 mg OD for 4 weeks and then 100 mg OD for 12 weeks. Patients underwent treadmill exercise tests at randomization (M0) and after 4 (M1) and 16 (M4) weeks of treatment. The findings of the study revealed that the rise in Total Exercise Duration (TED) at the trough at M4 was 86.8 ± 129.0 and 91.7 ± 118.8 s with Ivabradine 7.5 and 10 mg, respectively, and 78.8 ± 133.4 s with Atenolol 100 mg. Both ivabradine and atenolol reduced the anginal attacks by two-thirds. The results stated that Ivabradine and atenolol both have similar effectiveness in patients with stable angina.[51]

In another double-blind, double-dummy trial conducted by Li Y et al. patients with symptomatic AP and positive exercise tolerance tests were randomized into the Ivabradine (5 or 7.5 mg BID) or Atenolol group (12.5 or 25 mg BID). In this investigation set, in the fourth week, an increase in the TED was found to be 54.3 ± 120.1 seconds and 58.8 ± 114.7 seconds with Ivabradine 5 mg and atenolol 12.5 mg, respectively. In the 12th week, TED improved by 84.1 ± 130.5 seconds with ivabradine and 77.8 ± 126.6 seconds with atenolol (95% CI: −21.4–34.1 seconds, $p = 0.0011$ for non-inferiority). The anginal attacks and consumption of nitroglycerin both revealed a general trend of reduction ($p > 0.05$). These findings showed that Ivabradine decreases HR effectively and improving exercise capacity. It is well-tolerated and safe.[52]

In patients with AP with or without associated BB therapy, Ivabradine decreased HR, angina attacks, and nitrate consumption effectively. The RESPONSI$_f$VE study was performed, in which the effectiveness and tolerability of Ivabradine with or without BB were assessed in chronic stable AP patients in day-to-day clinical practice. A total of 1,250 patients with AP were included in the study. BB was prescribed to sixty-five percent of all patients. Ivabradine was prescribed twice daily for 4 months in patients with AP. After administrating ivabradine, the mean HR was decreased from 82.4 ± 11.8 bpm to 67.1 ± 8.4 bpm within 4 months. The average number of angina attacks/week reduced from 1.2 ± 1.9 to 0.1 ± 0.6 and the average use of short-acting nitrates/week from 1.5 ± 2.8 units to 0.2 ± 1.0 units. The response rate to ivabradine reached 87%. Results revealed that ivabradine would be the best option for better HR and symptom control in patients with chronic stable AP, regardless of simultaneous BB treatment.[53]

Similarly, one study of REDUCTION reported that the ivabradine reduces HR and is highly efficient in the management of patients with symptomatic CAD. A total of 4,954 patients with stable AP were included in the study. Patients were given Ivabradine in daily routine practice for 4 months. Results indicated that HR, AP, and consumption of short-acting nitrates were reduced during the 4 months of management with ivabradine.[54]

Coronary Flow Velocity Reserve (CFVR) was also observed to be an essential predictive marker in patients with stable CAD. BBs and Ivabradine have been shown to improve CFVR in individuals with stable CAD, but their effects were never contrasted. In a study conducted by Tagliamonte E *et al.* the outcome of bisoprolol and ivabradine was compared on CFVR in patients with stable CAD. Fifty-nine patients (38 males, 21 females; mean age 69 ± 9 years) were registered in the study. Transthoracic Doppler-derived evaluation of CFV and CFVR was effectively done in all patients. After treatment, resting peak CFV was found considerably reduced in both the ivabradine and bisoprolol groups, but without significant difference among them. However, hyperemic peak CFV significantly enlarged in both groups, but to a greater extent in the Ivabradine group. These data proved that the uses of Ivabradine treatment go beyond HR.[55]

Furthermore, in patients with stable angina, ivabradine 7.5 mg or 10 mg twice daily was presented to have similar efficacy to Amlodipine 10 mg once daily in reducing anginal symptoms. Ivabradine was observed to be superior when compared to amlodipine in decreasing myocardial oxygen consumption. To compare the antianginal and anti-ischemic effects of the novel HR-lowering agent ivabradine and the CCB (Amlodipine), Ruzyllo W *et al.* conducted 3 months randomized, double-blind, multicenter, non-inferiority trial. Patients with a ≥3-months history of chronic, stable effort induced angina were randomized to prescribe ivabradine 7.5 mg ($n = 400$) or 10 mg ($n = 391$) twice daily or amlodipine 10 mg once daily ($n = 404$) for 3 months. It was seen that at 3 months, TED was improved by 27.6 ± 91.7, 21.7 ± 94.5, and 31.2 ± 92.0 seconds with ivabradine 7.5 and 10 mg and amlodipine, respectively. HR reduced considerably by 11–13 bpm at rest and by 12–15 bpm at the peak of exercise with ivabradine but not with amlodipine. Outcomes of the study showed that ivabradine has similar efficiency and safety to amlodipine in improving exercise tolerance.[56]

As an Add on to BB and *vs* BB Up-titration

The three classifications of drugs commonly used for chronic angina include β adrenergic blocking agents, CCBs, and short- and long-acting nitrates. These drug classes reduce cardiac workload and may increase coronary blood flow—or improve its distribution—and therefore alter the difference between myocardial supply and demand. Although monotherapy is effective in some, while many patients require two or more antianginal agents to control their symptoms.[57] BBs reduce myocardial contractility and blood pressure, with both effects contributing to reducing oxygen demand.[58] Subset analyses from the BEAUTIFUL trial suggested that a decrease in HR may prevent coronary events. Despite this information showing the predictive effect of HR in CAD and the potential advantages of HR decrease, little is known concerning HRs accomplished in clinical practice, including in patients receiving HR-reducing treatments such as BBs. Likewise, there is a scarcity of data on the management of elevated HR in patients with CAD while using BBs and other HR-reducing agents.[59] To examine whether BBs may provide benefit in stable angina or not, Daly CA *et al.* in 2010 examined the outcomes from the European Heart Survey (EHS). It was seen in the analysis that slightly more than half (52%) of the patients had a mean baseline RHR >70 bpm, and even a considerable proportion of those already receiving BBs (almost 40%) had an HR >70 bpm.[60] Similarly, Steg PG *et al.* in an analysis revealed that stable CAD patients have RHR ≥70 bpm despite high usage of BBs—CLARIFY worldwide. A total of 33,177 patients were included in this study. Generally, HR ≥70 bpm was observed in 44.0% of the patients. BBs were given to 75.1% of patients. Out of 24,910 patients on BBs, 41.1% had HR ≥70 bpm. HR ≥70 bpm was freely related to wider occurrence and severity of angina, more repeated evidence of myocardial ischemia, and no use of HR-lowering agents.[59] These outcomes from the Daly and Steg analysis revealed that stable CAD patients often have RHR ≥70 bpm, which was related to worse health status, more recurrent angina, and ischemia.

Current guidelines recommended that BB doses be up-titrated to clinical trial target doses proven to improve mortality and morbidity as first-line therapy (Table 4.5). However, achieved doses of BB outside of clinical trial settings are typically lower than target; this may be in part due to side effects limiting titration of BB and clinician inertia to optimize therapies.[61] Also, when bradycardia, sinus node dysfunction, or AV block is present, β-adrenergic blockers may lead to symptomatic bradycardia or high degrees

Table 4.5: Limitations for up-titration of first-line antianginal agents

Calcium channel blockers	β-blocker	Nitrates
• Dizziness	• Fatigue	• Dizziness
• Headache	• Conduction disorders	• Flushing
• Fatigue	• Depression	• Headache
• Flushing	• Bradycardia	• Postural hypotension
• Constipation	• Hypotension	• Tachycardia
• Peripheral edema	• Bronchospasm	
• Bradycardia (rate limiting agents)	• Impairment of blood glucose	
• Hypotension	• Sexual dysfunction	

of AV block. The rate-lowering CCBs may also cause excessive bradycardia and heart block. Each class of antianginal agents has limitations described in Table 4.5. A well-known disadvantage of long-acting nitrates is their tolerance with continued use.[57]

Interestingly, a post hoc investigation of the BEAUTIFUL trial in patients with LV dysfunction whose symptom at entry was angina showed that adding ivabradine to conservative therapy, including BBs, or CCBs, further reduced HR with a benefit in terms of major cardiac events. The combination of ivabradine 7.5 mg bid and Atenolol developed extra efficacy with no untoward effect on safety or tolerability. Thus, Tardif JC et al. conducted an ASSOCIATE study to assess the antianginal and anti-ischemic efficacy of ivabradine in patients with chronic stable AP getting BB therapy. The study was a double-blinded trial that included a total of 889 patients with stable angina. The patients receiving atenolol 50 mg/day were randomized to receive ivabradine 5 mg bid for 2 months, increased to 7.5 mg bid for a further 2 months, or placebo. Results revealed that in the ivabradine group, TED at 4 months increased by 24.3 ± 65.3 compared with 7.7 ± 63.8 s with placebo (p <0.001). Ivabradine was observed to be superior to placebo for all exercise test criteria. Ivabradine and atenolol combination was well-tolerated. These findings demonstrated that the combination of ivabradine 7.5 mg bid and atenolol produced further efficacy with no untoward effect on safety or tolerability.[62]

Whereas to assess that in patients with stable AP, ivabradine combined with BB improves symptoms and QoL, ADDITIONS study was conducted. It was a non-interventional, multicenter, prospective study that enrolled a total of 2,330 patients with stable AP. Patients were prescribed ivabradine bid in addition to BB for 4 months. It was observed that after 4 months, ivabradine reduced HR by 19.4 ± 11.4 to 65.6 ± 8.2 bpm (p <0.0001). The number of anginas attacks were decreased by 1.4 ± 1.9 per week (p <0.0001), and nitrate consumption by 1.9 ± 2.9 U per week (p <0.0001). The efficiency of Ivabradine was measured by the physicians as "very good" (61%) or "good" (36%) in most patients. The study revealed that Ivabradine when combined with BB, not only decreases HR and nitrate consumption but also improves the QoL in patients.[63]

The Panhellenic study was another observational, prospective, open-label study conducted to evaluate the antianginal efficiency of 4 months of management with Ivabradine plus a BB and to record patient compliance and the effect of treatment on QOL in 2,403 patients with chronic stable angina. Patients were prescribed Ivabradine 5–7.5 mg bid in combination with BBs for 4 months. Ivabradine decreased RHR from 81.5 ± 9.7 bpm to 63.9 ± 6.0 bpm (p <–0.001), mean number of anginal attacks decreased from 2.0 ± 2.0 times/wk to 0.2 ± 0.6 times/wk (p <0.001) and nitroglycerin consumption decreased from 1.4 ± 2.0 times/wk to 0.1 ± 0.4 times/wk (p <0.001). In patients with CCS angina class I, the percentage was increased from 38% (baseline) to 84%. The mean EQ-5D visual analog scale index raised by 16.1 points (p <0.001), and compliance with management was high throughout the study (96%).[64]

Furthermore, outcomes of the CONTROL-2 study reported that Ivabradine + BB combined therapy proved better tolerability and more prominent clinical improvement, as compared to BB's up-titration. It was also observed that at week 16, Ivabradine added to BB management lead to a decrease in HR (61 ± 6 bpm vs 63 ± 8 bpm; p = 0.001), and considerably more patients were angina-free (50.6% vs 34.2%; p <0.001).[65]

Special Population

A high HR can provoke myocardial ischemia and angina in patients with CAD. Therefore, during the management of angina, HR should be decreased to 55–60 bpm. Various studies confirmed that a low RHR was linked with low CV mortality. A higher occurrence of bradycardia was found to be in patients >80 years because of age-related alteration of the sinus node, AV node, and the conduction system. Hence, the management of AP with BBs might be limited by bradycardia. The REDUCTION multicenter study assessed the viability of ivabradine in stable AP in regular practice. This subgroup examination assessed the efficacy and safety of ivabradine in octogenarians. The REDUCTION study enrolled a total of 4,954 patients with stable AP. A total of 382 octogenarians (mean age 83 ± 2.9 years) were included who were followed-up for more than 4 months. Patients had been prescribed ivabradine in flexible doses (2.5, 5, or 7.5 mg bid). HR, AP attacks, nitrate consumption, overall effectiveness, and tolerance were assessed. Results revealed that HR was reduced by 12.0 ± 12.0 bpm from 83.0 ± 15.4 to 71.0 ± 10.1 bpm (p <0.0001) after 4 months of management with ivabradine. AP occurrences were decreased from 3.0 ± 4.6 to 0.8 ± 1.8 per week (p <0.0001). Consumption of nitrates reduced from 4.2 ± 5.1 to 1.2 ± 2.7 (p <0.0001). No symptomatic bradycardia was described. The findings determined that ivabradine decreases HR effectively. Angina attacks and nitrate consumption in octogenarian patients were also reduced with ivabradine treatment. Thus, it was safe and well-tolerated without significant bradycardia.[66]

Additionally, results from a few trials have confirmed the antianginal and anti-ischemic efficacy of Ivabradine plus BBs in patients with stable AP. The subgroup analysis of the ADDITIONS study determined the efficiency of Ivabradine plus BBs and its influence on QoL in patients whose age ≥75 years in daily practice. A total of 2,330 patients were given Ivabradine twice daily, along with BBs for 4 months. HR, nitrate consumption, number of angina attacks, QoL, and tolerance were assessed. After 4 months, Ivabradine reduced HR by 19.2 ± 11.6 bpm to 65.4 ± 8.3 bpm. The angina attacks per week were reduced by 1.6 ± 1.8 to 0.4 ± 1.3, and the average consumption of short-acting nitrates per week was decreased by 2.2 ± 3.2 to 0.6 ± 1.8 units (both p <0.0001). Thus, adding Ivabradine plus BBs combination was successful in lessening HR, angina attacks, and nitrate consumption in older patients (≥75 years) with stable AP.[67]

The antianginal and anti-ischemic efficacy of ivabradine have been further verified in large-scale trials. Data on the existence of angina attacks, HR, and short-acting nitrate consumption were pooled from 5 randomized studies. Patients were prescribed 5, 7.5, or 10 mg of ivabradine bid for 3 or 4 months. Efficacy data were present for 2,425 patients in whom ivabradine decrease the level of recurrence of diary-based angina attacks by 59.4% and nitrate consumption by 53.7%. All subpopulations experienced 51–70% reductions in the angina attacks, with similar reductions for the other parameters studied. Ivabradine decreased HR by 14.5% in the safety set. In all the subpopulations, ivabradine had a good safety and tolerability profile with constant antianginal efficacy.[68]

Ivabradine was also seen to be effective in preventing angina in patients with DM and was not related to specific safety concerns on glucose metabolism. In 2010, Borer JS *et al.* examined pharmacokinetics, effectiveness, safety, and effects on glucose metabolism of ivabradine in DM patients. Maximum of the studies comprised data from 535 patients with DM. Outcomes revealed no difference in the pharmacokinetics of ivabradine in patients with DM *vs* without DM. A decrease in the HR at rest with ivabradine was similar in those with (15.2%) and without (15.7%) DM. Also, ivabradine was not related to adverse effects on glucose metabolism. These outcomes revealed that ivabradine is an attractive substitute to BBs in patients with stable AP and DM.[69]

Post-Revascularization

The antianginal effectiveness of ivabradine is well-recognized. In patients who had undergone coronary revascularization, ivabradine was found to be effective. In a post hoc analysis from ADDITIONS, ivabradine 5.0 mg or 7.5 mg bid was used in the management of 1,193 patients with angina and a history of PCI for 4 months. Angina attacks were decreased from 1.9 ± 2.4 per week to 0.5 ± 1.5 per week, and the frequency of nitrate consumption demolish from 2.7 ± 3.7 per week to 1.0 ± 1.9 per week (p <0.0001).[70] Moreover, results from a post hoc analysis conducted by Zarifis *et al.* including a total of 926 stable angina patients with a history of coronary revascularization were prescribed ivabradine for 4 months. Outcomes showed that ivabradine decreased the number of anginal attacks from 2.2 ± per week to 0.3 ± 0.6 per week (p <0.001), nitroglycerin consumption from 1.5 ± 2.2 per week to 0.1 ± 0.4 per week (p <0.001), and improved QoL, compared with baseline (p <0.001).[71]

As it was known that ivabradine reduces HR without affecting blood pressure, but whether ivabradine may exert benefits on endothelial function in humans is still unclear. Therefore, to examine the influence of decrease HR obtained with Ivabradine on endothelial function of patients with CAD treated with Percutaneous Coronary

Intervention (PCI). Mangiacapra F *et al.* conducted HR reduction by IVabradine for improvement of ENDothELial function in patients with CAD (RIVENDEL) study. It was a relatively small size prospective, randomized, controlled open-label study, involves 70 patients who underwent successful PCI. It determined the influence of ivabradine on brachial artery reactivity, as assessed by Flow-Mediated Dilatation (FMD) and Nitroglycerin-Mediated Dilatation (NMD). A substantial decrease was detected in the Ivabradine group at both 4 weeks and 8 weeks, respectively, in HR (65.2 ± 5.9 bpm and 62.2 ± 5.7 bpm; p <0.001), related to the development of FMD (12.2% ± 6.2% and 15.0% ± 7.7%; p <0.001) and enhancement of NMD (16.6% ± 10.4% and 17.7 ± 10.8; p <0.001) compared with standard therapy. Data obtained from post hoc analysis, or using surrogate endpoints, although reflecting important findings in real-life medical practice, must be interpreted with caution.[72]

Impact on Coronary Outcomes

Ivabradine is a unique HR-lowering drug in patients with sinus rhythm. BP, myocardial contractility, intracardiac conduction, or ventricular repolarization is not affected by ivabradine. Treatment with ivabradine, in this way, allows assessing the impacts of bringing down HR without legitimately adjusting different aspects of cardiac function. Ivabradine is beneficial for patients with stable CAD and Left-Ventricular Systolic Dysfunction (LVSD). BEAUTIFUL is a randomized, double-blind, placebo-controlled study conducted to determine whether decreasing the HR with ivabradine decreases CV death and morbidity in patients with CAD and LVSD. The study enrolled 10,917 eligible patients who had CAD and an LVSD. Results revealed that ivabradine decreased HR by 6 bpm at 12 months, corrected for placebo. Ivabradine treatment was also related to a reduction in coronary revascularization (HR: 0.70, 95% CI: 0.52–0·93, p = 0.016). The results of the study stated that the reduction in HR with ivabradine was used to decrease the incidence of CAD outcomes in a subgroup of patients who have HR of 70 bpm or greater.[73]

Similarly, post hoc analysis of BEAUTIFUL reported that ivabradine is beneficial in decreasing CV events in patients with stable CAD and LVSD who were presented with limiting angina. Also, it was found related to a 24% reduction in the primary endpoint (CV mortality or HHF and non-fatal MI or HF) (HR: 0.76; 95% CI: 0.58–1.00) and a 42% reduction in hospitalization for MI (HR: 0.58, 95% CI: 0.37–0.92). Whereas in patients with HR 70 bpm, there was a 73% reduction in hospitalization for MI (HR: 0.27, 95% CI: 0.11–0.66) and a 59% reduction in coronary revascularization (HR: 0.41, 95% CI: 0.17–0.99). Ivabradine was safe and well-tolerated.[74]

Pharmacologically, decreasing the HR improves consequences in patients with systolic CHF, demonstrated by trials with BBs and, most recently, with ivabradine, in the systolic heart failure treatment with the I_f inhibitor ivabradine trial (SHIFT). In 6,558 patients with symptomatic CHF, LVSD (LVEF ≤35%), and HR of 70 bpm or higher, SHIFT was carried out to evaluate the outcome of ivabradine on clinical consequences in this patient population. As reported by Swedberg *et al.* SHIFT was a randomized, double-blind, parallel-group, multicenter, placebo-controlled study that examined the influence of ivabradine when added to current guideline-based therapy. Ivabradine considerably decreased the risk of CV death and hospitalization because of HF by 18% (29% *vs* 24%; HR: 0.82; 95% CI: 0.75 to 0.90; p <0.0001), compared with placebo. Ivabradine also decreased the composite endpoint of CV death and HHF by 15%, 20%, and 18% in the respective subgroups (p for interaction = 0.52).[75]

Whereas SIGNIFY (Study Assess ING the morbidity-mortality benefits of the *If* inhibitor Ivabradine in patients with CoronarY artery disease) trial assessed whether HR reduction with Ivabradine would improve clinical outcomes in patients with stable CAD. It was a randomized, double-blind, placebo-controlled trial of ivabradine given on top of standard antianginal therapy, involving 19,102 patients without clinically apparent HF and a baseline HR ≥70 bpm. The study also included 12,049 patients with effort-limiting angina (CCS class ≥II)). Patients were randomized to placebo or Ivabradine. Results have shown that the mean (±SD) HR in the Ivabradine group was 60.7 ± 9.0 bpm *vs* 70.6 ± 10.1 bpm in the placebo group at 3 months. There was no interaction between the usage of Ivabradine and adverse events in other pre-specified sub-groups, defined according to age, BB use at randomization, gender, baseline HR, history of DM, previous MI, or previous coronary revascularization. Ivabradine treatment, contrasted with placebo, was linked with considerably higher rates of symptomatic (7.9% *vs* 1.2%, *p* <0.001) and asymptomatic (11.0% *vs* 1.3%, *p* <0.001)) bradycardia, atrial fibrillation (5.3% *vs* 3.8%, *p* <0.001) and phosphenes (5.4% *vs* 0.5%, *p* <0.001). Interestingly, QT interval prolongation was prominent more repeatedly in patients treated with ivabradine. These results indicated that adding ivabradine to standard therapy to reduce the HR did not improve clinical outcomes in patients with stable CAD.[76]

The outcomes of SIGNIFY were perplexing—patients with symptomatic angina who were treated with ivabradine therapy were at greater risk of increased adverse events. In the pre-specified chronic stable angina subgroup, an increase appeared to take place in the primary composite endpoint of CV death and non-fatal MI. Anyhow, the clarification of these outcomes could be the higher dosage used and/or the concomitant use of diltiazem or verapamil; or there may be potentially significant pro-arrhythmic effects of ivabradine treatment; or the possibility of statistical error.[77]

QoL

To further discover the influence of ivabradine on angina-related QoL, Tendera M *et al.* analyzed SIGNIFY QoL substudy data. Data were presented for 4,187 patients (2,084 ivabradine and 2,103 placebos). Results revealed that QoL was improved in both treatment groups. At 12 months, the primary result of the change in physical limitation score was 4.56 points for ivabradine *vs* 3.40 points for placebo (E: 0.96; 95% CI: –0.14 to 2.05; *p* = 0.085). Patients with the worst QoL at baseline had the best improvement in QoL for 12 months, with improvement in physical limitation and a substantial decrease in angina frequency (*p* = 0.034).[61] The ivabradine group had greater values for angina frequency score, which was considerably better with ivabradine at 12, 24, and 36 months. The outcomes of the study revealed that at 12 months, ivabradine treatment did not affect the primary outcome of change in physical limitation score.[78]

Take Home Pearls

- Angina occurs when there is inadequate oxygen supply to maintain normal myocardial metabolic function.
- The reduction of HR is considered important in the treatment of AP.
- Ivabradine decreases HR and is extremely effective and well-tolerated in the treatment of patients with symptomatic CAD.

- Ivabradine's main mechanism of action on cardiac tissue is on the SA node, present at a subepicardial position at the junction of the SVC and the right atrium.
- Ivabradine + BB combination has good tolerability and safety compared to BB up-titration in patients with stable angina.
- Adding ivabradine to regular therapy creates a substantial perfection in endothelial function in CAD patients undergoing revascularization with PCI.

TAKE HOME SUMMARY

CVDs constitute the primary reason for worldwide mortality and reduced QoL. The estimated global death rate due to CVD was 28.2%. In India, one-fourth of all death rates are due to CVD. IHD and stroke are mainly responsible for >80% of CVD deaths. Higher rates of future CV events were present in patients with stable CAD and angina when contrasted with patients without angina. RHR has important predictive consequences. There is much evidence to propose that elevated HR precedes many instances of myocardial ischemia during everyday activities. An increase in HR at rest was found to be linked with worse consequences in patients with hypertension, CHD, and LVD, and in those without known CV disease. As high RHR is a significant determinant of angina and adverse CV outcomes, it can be effectively managed with the help of HR decreasing antianginal agents. Current guidelines suggested pharmacological treatment with drugs classified as being first-line (BBs, CCBs, short-acting nitrates) or second-line (long-acting nitrates, ivabradine, nicorandil, ranolazine, trimetazidine). Nevertheless, despite the established safety and efficiency of first-line medications, their use is limited by the side effects of these agents. However, ivabradine is a unique precise HR lowering agent. Results from numerous epidemiological trials reported that among the HR lowering antianginal agents, ivabradine is a favorable efficiency and tolerability as a monotherapy and as a combination with improvement in QoL and coronary outcomes.

REFERENCES

1. Mensah GA, Roth GA, Fuster V. The global burden of cardiovascular diseases and risk factors: 2020 and beyond. *Journal of the American College of Cardiology*. 2019 Nov 19;74(20): 2529–32.

2. McAloon CJ, Osman F, Glennon P, *et al*. Chapter 4—Global epidemiology and incidence of cardiovascular disease. 2016;57–96.

3. Sanchis-Gomar F, Perez-Quilis C, Leischik R, *et al*. Epidemiology of coronary heart disease and acute coronary syndrome. *Annals of Translational Medicine*. 2016 Jul;4(13):256.

4. Benjamin EJ, Muntner P, Alonso A, *et al*. Heart disease and stroke statistics-2019 update: A report from the American Heart Association. *Circulation*. 2019;139(10):e56–e528.

5. Prabhakaran D, Jeemon P, Roy A. Cardiovascular diseases in India: Current epidemiology and future directions. *Circulation*. 2016 Apr 19;133(16):1605–20.

6. Prabhakaran D, Jeemon P, Sharma M, *et al*. The changing patterns of cardiovascular diseases and their risk factors in the states of India: The Global Burden of Disease Study 1990–2016. *The Lancet Global Health*. 2018 Dec 1;6(12):E1339–E1351.

7. Ke C, Gupta R, Xavier D, *et al*. Divergent trends in ischaemic heart disease and stroke mortality in India from 2000 to 2015: A nationally representative mortality study. *The Lancet Global Health*. 2018 Aug;6(8):E914–E923.

8. Kumar A, Cannon CP. Acute coronary syndromes: Diagnosis and management, part I. *Mayo Clin Proc*. 2009;84(10):917–38.

9. Hussain S, AlRashed M, Rajan R, *et al*. Chronic coronary syndrome: A review of the literature. *Annals of Clinical Cardiology*. 2020 Sep.

10. Knuuti J, Wijns W, Saraste A, *et al*. 2019 ESC guidelines for the diagnosis and management of chronic coronary syndromes. *European Heart Journal*. 2020 Jan 14;41(3):407–77.

11. Thygesen K, Alpert JS, Jaffe AS, *et al*. Fourth universal definition of myocardial infarction (2018). *Journal of the American College of Cardiology*. 2018 Oct 30;72(18):2231–64.

12. Ford TJ, Berry C. Angina: Contemporary diagnosis and management. *Heart*. 2020 Mar;106(5): 387–98.

13. Ferrari R, Pavasini R, Balla C. The multifaceted angina. *European Heart Journal Supplements*. 2019 Apr;21(Supplement_C):C1–C5.

14. Ferrari R, Camici PG, Crea F, *et al*. Expert consensus document: A 'diamond' approach to personalized treatment of angina. *Nature Reviews Cardiology*. 2018 Feb;15(2):120–32.

15. Eisen A, Bhatt DL, Steg PG, *et al*. Angina and future cardiovascular events in stable patients with coronary artery disease: Insights from the Reduction of Atherothrombosis for Continued Health (REACH) registry. *Journal of the American Heart Association*. 2016 Sep 28;5(10):e004080.

16. Sorbets E, Fox KM, Elbez Y, *et al*. Long-term outcomes of chronic coronary syndrome worldwide: Insights from the international CLARIFY registry. *European Heart Journal*. 2020 Jan 14;41(3):347–56.

17. KauL U, Natrajan S, Dalal J, *et al*. Prevalence and control of cardiovascular risk factors in stable coronary artery outpatients in India compared with the rest of the world: An analysis from international CLARIFY registry. *Indian Heart Journal*. 2017 Jul-Aug;69(4):447–52.

18. Hiremath S, Vala DR, Roy T, *et al*. Changing patterns in the prevalence and management of cardiovascular risk factors in India and their comparison with the rest of the world along with clinical outcomes at 5-year: An analysis of stable coronary artery disease patients from The Prospective Observational Longitudinal Registry of patients with stable coronary artery disease (CLARIFY) registry. *Indian Heart Journal*. 2018 Dec;70(Suppl 3):S36–S42.

19. Diaz A, Bourassa MG, Guertin MC, *et al*. Long-term prognostic value of resting heart rate in patients with suspected or proven coronary artery disease. *European Heart Journal*. 2005 May;26(10):967–74.

20. Anselmino M, Öhrvik J, Ryden L, *et al*. Resting heart rate in patients with stable coronary artery disease and diabetes: A report from the euro heart survey on diabetes and the heart. European Heart Journal. 2010 Dec;31(24):3040–5.

21. Daly CA, Clemens F, Sendon JL, *et al*. Inadequate control of heart rate in patients with stable angina: Results from the European heart survey. *Postgraduate Medical Journal*. 2010 Apr;86 (1014):212–7.

22. Kohler A, Muzzarelli S, Leibundgut G, *et al*. Relationship between the resting heart rate and the extent of coronary artery disease as assessed by myocardial perfusion SPECT. *Swiss Medical Weekly*. 2012 Aug 13;142:w13660.

23. Ho JE, Bittner V, DeMicco DA, *et al*. Usefulness of heart rate at rest as a predictor of mortality, hospitalization for heart failure, myocardial infarction, and stroke in patients with stable coronary heart disease (Data from the Treating to New Targets [TNT] trial). *American Journal of Cardiology*. 2010 Apr 1:105(7):905–11.

24. IDF DIABETES ATLAS: Ninth edition 2019. Adapted from: https://www.diabetesatlas.org/upload/resources/2019/IDF_Atlas_9th_Edition_2019.pdf

25. Zhang B, Pei C, Zhang Y, *et al*. High resting heart rate and high BMI predicted severe coronary atherosclerosis burden in patients with stable angina pectoris by SYNTAX Score. *Angiology*. 2018 May;69(5):380–6.

26. Hjalmarson Å, Gilpin EA, Kjekshus J, *et al.* Influence of heart rate on mortality after acute myocardial infarction. *American Journal of Cardiology.* 1990 Mar 1;65(9):547–53

27. Alapati V, Tang F, Charlap E, *et al.* Discharge heart rate after hospitalization for myocardial infarction and long-term mortality in 2 US registries. *Journal of the American Heart Association.* 2019 Feb 5;8(3):e010855.

28. Singh BN. Increased heart rate as a risk factor for cardiovascular disease. *European Heart Journal Supplements.* 2003 Sep 1;5(Suppl_G):G3–G9.

29. Indolfi C, Ross J. The role of heart rate in myocardial ischemia and infarction: Implications of myocardial perfusion-contraction matching. *Progress in Cardiovascular Diseases.* 1993 Jul-Aug;36(1):61–74.

30. Rosano GM, Vitale C, Volterrani M. Heart rate in ischemic heart disease. The innovation of ivabradine: More than pure heart rate reduction. *Advances in Therapy.* 2010 Apr;27(4):202–10.

31. Kop WJ, Verdino RJ, Gottdiener JS, *et al.* Changes in heart rate and heart rate variability before ambulatory ischemic events. *Journal of the American College of Cardiology.* 2001 Aug;38(3):742–9.

32. Andrews TC, Fenton T, Toyosaki N, *et al.* Subsets of ambulatory myocardial ischemia based on heart rate activity. Circadian distribution and response to anti-ischemic medication. The Angina and Silent Ischemia Study Group (ASIS). *Circulation.* 1993 Jul;88(1):92–100.

33. Heidland UE, Strauer BE. Left ventricular muscle mass and elevated heart rate are associated with coronary plaque disruption. *Circulation.* 2001 Sep 25;104(13):1477–82.

34. Wu J, Han Y, Xu J, *et al.* Chronic stable angina is associated with lower health-related quality of life: Evidence from Chinese patients. *PLoS One.* 2014 May 19;9(5):e97294.

35. Manolis AJ, Ambrosio G, Collins P, *et al.* Impact of stable angina on health status and quality of life perception of currently treated patients. The BRIDGE 2 survey. *European Journal of Internal Medicine.* 2019 Dec;70:60–7.

36. Andrikopoulos G, Pastromas S, Kartalis A, *et al.* Inadequate heart rate control is associated with worse quality of life in patients with coronary artery disease and chronic obstructive pulmonary disease. The RYTHMOS study. *Hellenic Journal of Cardiology.* 2012 Mar;53(2):118–26.

37. Ferrari R, Fox K. Heart rate reduction in coronary artery disease and heart failure. *Nature Reviews Cardiology.* 2016 Aug;13(8):493–501.

38. Kjekshus JK. Importance of heart rate in determining beta-blocker efficacy in acute and long-term acute myocardial infarction intervention trials. *American Journal of Cardiology.* 1986 Apr 25;57(12):43F–49F.

39. Cucherat M. Quantitative relationship between resting heart rate reduction and magnitude of clinical benefits in post-myocardial infarction: A meta-regression of randomized clinical trials. *European Heart Journal.* 2007 Dec;28(24):3012–9.

40. Fox K, Borer JS, Camm AJ, *et al.* Resting heart rate in cardiovascular disease. *Journal of the American College of Cardiology.* 2007 Aug 28;50(9):823–30.

41. Winchester DE, Pepine CJ. Angina treatments and prevention of cardiac events: An appraisal of the evidence. *European Heart Journal Supplements.* 2015 Dec;17(Suppl G):G10–G18.

42. Boyette LC, Manna B. Physiology, Myocardial Oxygen Demand. In: StatPearls [Internet]. *Treasure Island (FL): StatPearls Publishing.* 2020 Jan. Available from: https://www.ncbi.nlm.nih.gov/books/NBK499897/

43. Ferrari R, Ceconi C, Guardigli G. Pathophysiological role of heart rate: From ischaemia to left ventricular dysfunction. *European Heart Journal Supplements.* 2008 Aug;10(Suppl_F):F7–F10.

44. Ferrari R, Fox K. Heart rate reduction in coronary artery disease and heart failure. *Nature Reviews Cardiology.* 2016 Aug;13(8):493–501.

45. Padala SK, Lavelle MP, Sidhu MS, *et al.* Antianginal therapy for stable ischemic heart disease: A contemporary review. *Journal of Cardiovascular Pharmacology and Therapeutics.* 2017 Nov;22(6):499–510.

46. Ferrari R, Pavasini R, Camici PG, *et al.* Anti-anginal drugs–beliefs and evidence: Systematic review covering 50 years of medical treatment. *European Heart Journal.* 2019 Jan 7;40(2):190–4

47. Pavasini R, Camici PG, Crea F, *et al.* Anti-anginal drugs: Systematic review and clinical implications. *International Journal of Cardiology.* 2019 May 15;283:55–63.

48. Kaski JC, Gloekler S, Ferrari R, Fox K, *et al.* Role of ivabradine in management of stable angina in patients with different clinical profiles. *Open Heart.* 2018 Mar 9;5(1):e000725.

49. DCGI green flag to Abbott heart failure, angina treatment drug ivabradine. Available from:https://www.medicaldialogues.in/news/industry/pharma/dcgi-green-flag-to-abbott-heart- failure-angina-treatment-drug-ivabradine-69213

50. Tse S, Mazzola N. Ivabradine (Corlanor) for heart failure: The first selective and specific *If* inhibitor. *Pharmacy and Therapeutics.* 2015 Dec;40(12):810–4.

51. Tardif JC, Ford I, Tendera M, *et al.* Efficacy of ivabradine, a new selective I(f) inhibitor, compared with atenolol in patients with chronic stable angina. *European Heart Journal.* 2005 Dec;26 (23):2529–36.

52. Li Y, Jing L, Li Y, *et al.* The efficacy and safety of ivabradine hydrochloride versus atenolol in Chinese patients with chronic stable angina pectoris. *Pharmacoepidemiology and Drug Safety.* 2014 Nov;23(11):1183–91.

53. Perings S, Stöckl G, Kelm M, *et al.* Effectiveness and tolerability of ivabradine with or without concomitant beta-blocker therapy in patients with chronic stable angina in routine clinical practice. *Advances in Therapy.* 2016;33(9):1550–64.

54. Köster R, Kaehler J, Meinertz T, *et al.* Treatment of stable angina pectoris by ivabradine in every day practice: The REDUCTION study. *American Heart Journal.* 2009 Oct;158(4):e51- e57.

55. Tagliamonte E, Cirillo T, Rigo F, *et al.* Ivabradine and bisoprolol on doppler-derived coronary flow velocity reserve in patients with stable coronary artery disease: Beyond the heart rate. *Advances in Therapy.* 2015 Aug;32(8):757–67.

56. Ruzyllo W, Tendera M, Ford I, *et al.* Antianginal efficacy and safety of ivabradine compared with amlodipine in patients with stable effort angina pectoris: A 3-month randomised, double-blind, multicentre, noninferiority trial. *Drugs.* 2007;67(3):393–405.

57. Parker JO. Chronic angina pectoris: Inadequacies of current therapy. *American Journal of Geriatric Cardiology.* 2004;13(5):261–6.

58. Balla C, Pavasini R, Ferrari R. Treatment of angina: Where are we?. *Cardiology.* 2018;140(1):52–67.

59. Steg PG, Ferrari R, Ford I, *et al.* Heart rate and use of beta-blockers in stable outpatients with coronary artery disease. *PloS One.* 2012 May 3;7(5):e36284.

60. Daly CA, Clemens F, Sendon JL, *et al.* Inadequate control of heart rate in patients with stable angina: Results from the European heart survey. *Postgraduate Medical Journal.* 2010 Apr;86 (1014):212–7.

61. Ibrahim NE, Gaggin HK, Turchin A, *et al.* Heart rate, beta-blocker use, and outcomes of heart failure with reduced ejection fraction. *European Heart Journal: Cardiovascular Pharmacotherapy.* 2019 Jan 1;5(1):3–11.

62. Tardif JC, Ponikowski P, Kahan T. Efficacy of the I(f) current inhibitor ivabradine in patients with chronic stable angina receiving beta-blocker therapy: A 4-month, randomized, placebo-controlled trial. *European Heart Journal.* 2009 Mar;30(5):540–8.

63. Werdan K, Ebelt H, Nuding S, *et al.*Ivabradine in combination with beta-blocker improves symptoms and quality of life in patients with stable angina pectoris: Results from the ADDITIONS study. *Clinical Research in Cardiology.* 2012 May;101(5):365–73.

64. Zarifis J, Grammatikou V, Kallistratos M, *et al.* Treatment of stable angina pectoris with ivabradine in everyday practice: A Panhellenic, prospective, noninterventional study. *Clinical Cardiology.* 2015 Dec;38(12):725–32.

65. Glezer M, Vasyuk Y, Karpov Y. Efficacy of ivabradine in combination with beta-blockers versus uptitration of beta-blockers in patients with stable angina (CONTROL-2 Study). *Advances in Therapy.* 2018 Mar;35(3):341–52.

66. Koester R, Kaehler J, Meinertz T. Ivabradine for the treatment of stable angina pectoris in octogenarians. *Clinical Research Cardiology.* 2011 Feb;100(2):121–8.

67. Müller-Werdan U, Stöckl G, Ebelt H, *et al.* Ivabradine in combination with beta-blocker reduces symptoms and improves quality of life in elderly patients with stable angina pectoris: age-related results from the ADDITIONS study. *Experimental Gerontology.* 2014 Nov;59:34–41.

68. Tendera M, Borer JS, Tardif JC. Efficacy of I(f) inhibition with ivabradine in different subpopulations with stable angina pectoris. *Cardiology.* 2009;114(2):116–25.

69. Borer JS, Tardif JC. Efficacy of ivabradine, a selective I(f) inhibitor, in patients with chronic stable angina pectoris and diabetes mellitus. *American Journal of Cardiology.* 2010 Jan 1;105(1):29–35.

70. Werdan K, Ebelt H, Nuding S, *et al.* Ivabradine in combination with beta-blockers in patients with chronic stable angina after percutaneous coronary intervention. *Advances in Therapy.* 2015;32(2):120–37.

71. Zarifis J, Grammatikou V, Kallistratos M, *et al.* Antianginal efficacy of Ivabradine in patients with history of coronary revascularization. *Angiology.* 2017 Jan;68(1):10–8.

72. Mangiacapra F, Colaiori I, Ricottini E, *et al.* Heart Rate reduction by IVabradine for improvement of ENDothELial function in patients with coronary artery disease: The RIVENDEL study. *Clinical Research in Cardiology.* 2017;106(1):69–75.

73. Fox K, Ford I, Steg PG, *et al.* Ivabradine for patients with stable coronary artery disease and left-ventricular systolic dysfunction (BEAUTIFUL): A randomised, double-blind, placebo-controlled trial. *Lancet.* 2008 Sep 6;372(9641):807–16.

74. Fox K, Ford I, Steg PG, *et al.* Relationship between ivabradine treatment and cardiovascular outcomes in patients with stable coronary artery disease and left ventricular systolic dysfunction with limiting angina: A subgroup analysis of the randomized, controlled BEAUTIFUL trial. *European Heart Journal.* 2009 Oct;30(19):2337–45.

75. Borer JS, Swedberg K, Komajda M, *et al.* Efficacy profile of ivabradine in patients with heart failure plus angina pectoris. *Cardiology.* 2017;136(2):138–44.

76. Fox K, Ford I, Steg PG, *et al.* Ivabradine in stable coronary artery disease without clinical heart failure. *New England Journal of Medicine.* 2014 Sep 18;371(12):1091–99.

77. Giavarini A, de Silva R. The role of ivabradine in the management of angina pectoris. *Cardiovascular Drugs and Therapy.* 2016;30(4):407–17.

78. Tendera M, Chassany O, Ferrari R, *et al.* Quality of life with ivabradine in patients with angina pectoris: The study assessing the morbidity–mortality benefits of the *If* inhibitor ivabradine in patients with coronary artery disease quality of life substudy. *Circulation: Cardiovascular Quality and Outcomes.* 2016 Jan;9(1):31–8.

Heart Rate and Heart Failure

Dr. I Sathyamurthy, Dr. Rajeev Agrawala

Learning Objectives

At the end of this chapter one should be able to:

- Epidemiology of heart failure
- Heart failure types and clinical course
- High RHR and its impact on HFrEF
- Management of high RHR–HFrEF perspective
- Take home summary

EPIDEMIOLOGY OF HEART FAILURE

Heart failure (HF) is a clinical condition resulting in impairment of ventricular filling, or the ejection of blood caused due to structural and functional defects in the myocardium.[1] HF is a developing issue worldwide with serious consequences and a common pathway to several heart diseases.[2]

Global Scenario of Prevalence and Incidence

HF is a life-threatening disease and is considered a global health priority. Currently, around 26 million people worldwide are living with HF. The outlook for such patients is poor, with survival rates worse than those for bowels, breast, or prostate cancer HF also results in several premature deaths. Around one person in five develops HF in economically developed countries. Globally, around 17–45% of hospitalized patients die within 1-year of admission, and most of them die within 5 years of admission.[3] According to population statistics, the epidemiologic HF burden may have significantly decreased between 2000 and 2010. However, in nationwide surveys, this trend could not be established. Therefore, Lippi G *et al.* in 2017 conducted an electronic search in the Global Health Data Exchange (GHDx) registry, using the keyword "heart failure" to provide a brief investigation of the worldwide epidemiological HF burden. It was observed that the worldwide occurrence of HF is estimated at 64.34 million cases. Furthermore, results suggested that Years Lost due to Disability (YLDs) of HF have persistently increased during the past 28 years (Fig. 5.1). The prevalence is greater in the female sex, and YLDs are more in men. The effect of HF varied considerably to an ~4% increase in the old-age population. This rise has stayed constant in the last 10 years. More accurately, investigation data showed that the HF burden was increased by 3.1% in the last 10 years in the low-to-middle Socio-

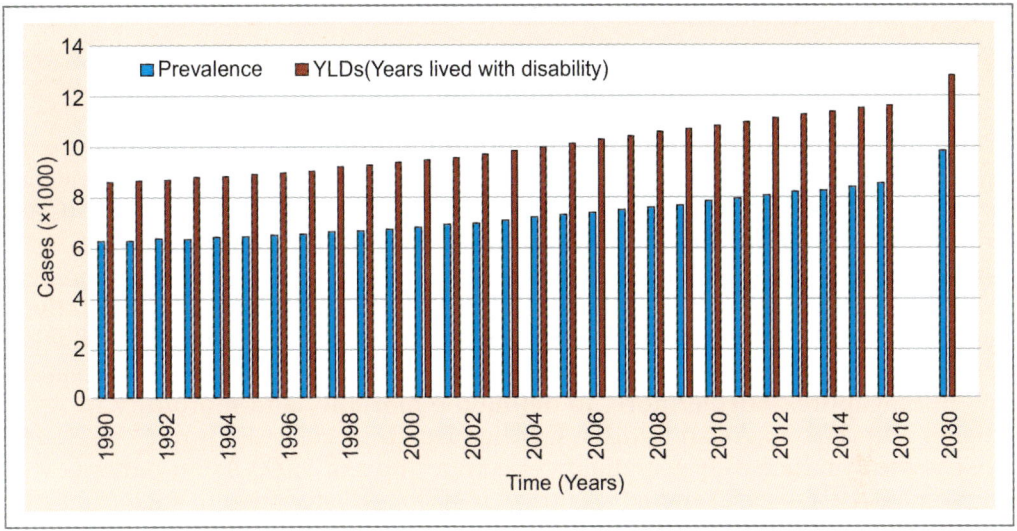

Fig. 5.1: Last 28-year trend and current scenario of worldwide epidemiology of HF[4]

Demographic Index (SDI) regions. These findings revealed that by the year 2030 the HF occurrence will rise above 50% in low-to-middle SDI regions, although it will decline to ~27% in high SDI countries.[4]

Data on outcomes in patients with HF were mostly from North America and Europe. There is very little data obtained from Africa, Asia, and South America. As per facts from the Low-to-Middle-Income Countries (LMIC), the death rate in patients with HF in LMIC is greater than that in High-Income Countries (HIC). However, reasons for variation in outcomes between regions remain unclear. Therefore, in HF patients, the global mortality variation was examined by a prospective cohort study conducted by Dokainish H *et al.* in 2017. The study analyzed the outcomes of the International Congestive Heart Failure (INTER-CHF) prospective cohort study. A total of 5,823 patients with HF were included in this registry. Baseline demographic and clinical characteristics of patients were followed up at 6 months and 1 year from enrolment to record symptoms, medications, and outcomes. Results revealed that the overall mortality was 16.5%. Within one year, 858 deaths were seen and cardiac deaths. The variations in mortality between regions could be the result of health-care infrastructure, quality, and access, or environmental, and genetic factors.[5]

Significant advances in medical therapy have dramatically improved outcomes in chronic HF, yet HF remains a mounting public health concern. The improvement in mortality has been accompanied by a striking increase in morbidity and above 1 million hospitalizations have occurred for acute decompensated heart failure (ADHF). In patients aged >65 years, it is considered the most common discharge diagnosis. The characteristics and management of a patient hospitalized with ADHF are poorly defined despite the great occurrence of this syndrome. Several registries in outpatient settings for HF have been applied; however, similar studies were not conducted in patients hospitalized with ADHF. The Acute Decompensated Heart Failure National Registry (ADHERE™)[6] was developed as a large, observational, national, multicenter study of patient characteristics and consequences of patients hospitalized with ADHF to better define and improve the care of these patients. Demographic characteristics and medical history of 62,018 patients were collected.

Among patients registered in the ADHERE database, 78% admitted for an acute episode of congestive HF initially presented to the emergency department (ED), while only 21% were admitted directly to an inpatient unit. Results revealed that patient outcomes varied tremendously. Mortality was considerably greater in men as compared to women (4.5% *vs* 3.9%; *p* = 0.0042). This was caused by the greater incidence in men of systolic dysfunction [25% of men had left ventricular ejection fraction (LVEF) >40% *vs* 45% of women; *p* <0.0001] and coronary artery disease (CAD) (66% *vs* 53%; *p* <0.0001), which harbored a worse prognosis.[6,7]

In Asia, HF is the main health problem, and its prevalence appears to be even greater compared to Western countries, ranging between 1.3% and 6.7%. Currently, in China, there are 4.2 million people with HF with an assessed incidence of 1.3%, while in Southeast Asia, 9 million people have HF with a prevalence of 6.7% in Malaysia and 4.5% in Singapore.[5] Furthermore, to define the mortality and morbidity in Asian patients with HF, an Asian Sudden Cardiac Death in Heart Failure (ASIAN-HF) registry was conducted. It was the prospective study of 5,000 Asian patients with symptomatic HF (stage C) and left ventricular systolic dysfunction (LVSD) (EF ≤40%) from 44 centers in 11 Asian nations. Results revealed that all-cause mortality (ACM) was found to be 9.6%. A significant regional difference in patient characteristics, treatment, and the death rate was also observed. Asian patients with HF with reduced ejection fraction (HFrEF) had worse consequences than those with HF with preserved ejection fraction (HFpEF), despite being younger. Also, it was seen that in Southeast Asia, patients were almost twice as likely to die in the first year of follow-up and had the highest rate of comorbidities when compared to patients from South and Northeast Asia.[8]

In HF patients, comorbidities are very common which complicate treatment and outcomes. A certain pattern of cardiac structural and functional changes in HF are linked with these comorbidities. Certainly, around the world, patients with age-related multimorbidity are becoming the norm instead of the exception. It occurs mainly in Asia, where nearly two-thirds of patients have multimorbidity along with HF. Thus, Tromp J *et al.* in 2017 analyzed the statistics of 6,480 patients with chronic HF from the ASIAN-HF registry to identify the patterns of multimorbidity in Asian patients with HF and their relationship with patients' Quality of Life (QoL) and health outcomes. In the entire cohort, 5 multimorbidity groups of relatively equal size (*n* = 1,048 ± 1,759) were identified, each characterized by a different combination of comorbidities as shown in Fig. 5.2. Results revealed that the worst QoL in 1-year and serious symptoms

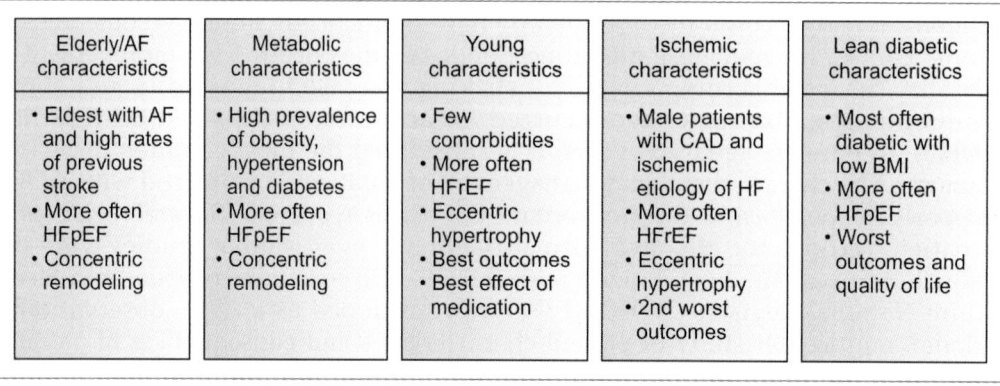

Elderly/AF characteristics	Metabolic characteristics	Young characteristics	Ischemic characteristics	Lean diabetic characteristics
• Eldest with AF and high rates of previous stroke • More often HFpEF • Concentric remodeling	• High prevalence of obesity, hypertension and diabetes • More often HFpEF • Concentric remodeling	• Few comorbidities • More often HFrEF • Eccentric hypertrophy • Best outcomes • Best effect of medication	• Male patients with CAD and ischemic etiology of HF • More often HFrEF • Eccentric hypertrophy • 2nd worst outcomes	• Most often diabetic with low BMI • More often HFpEF • Worst outcomes and quality of life

Fig. 5.2: Concept figure summarizing the most important findings of this study[9]

of HF were detected in lean diabetic group patients. Adjusting for confounders the lean diabetic [Hazard Ratio (HR): 1.79, 95% CI: 1.46 ± 2.2], elderly/atrial fibrillation (AF) (HR: 1.57, 95% CI: 1.26 ± 1.96), ischemic (HR: 1.51, 95% CI: 1.22 ± 1.88), and metabolic (HR: 1.28, 95% CI: 1.02 ± 1.60) groups had greater rates of the primary combined outcome compared to the young group. These data showed that more broad approaches are needed in phenotyping patients with HF and multimorbidity.[9]

HF Scenario in India

HF is a major health problem with considerable morbidity and mortality across the globe. The prevalence of HF keeps on rising in the vast majority of the countries despite improvements in medical care. India is currently in the midst of an epidemiological transition, leading to a rapid increase in the occurrence of cardiovascular (CV) risk factors, cardiovascular disease (CVD), and HF. According to some investigators, the total HF burden in India is close to 20 million, making it one of the largest HF populations in the world. Currently, there is very little data available about HF in India despite this enormous burden.[10]

The hospital-based registries of HF provide key information on patient characteristics, prevailing treatment practices, and survival data. In India, sparse clinical and demographic data on HF is a main concern. Medanta HF registry[10], National HF registry[11], Trivandrum Heart Failure Registry (THFR)[12] which enrolled 1205 patients, and the INDia Ukieri Study (INDUS)[13] are the major HF registries reported in India.

Medanta HF registry was conducted at Medanta (The Medicity, a large, tertiary-care institute in the National Capital Region of India). The study included all the patients with HFrEF during the period early 2014 to mid-2017. Records of all the patients registered at Medanta Heart Failure Clinic (MHFC) were reviewed. The mean age of the participants (n = 5,590) was 59.1 ± 11.8 years with 83.0% males. Mean LVEF was 30.0 ± 6.6%, and Coronary Artery Disease (CAD) was the dominant cause of HF, accounting for 77.8% of the whole population. Most patients (81.8%) received guideline-directed medical therapy along with beta-blocker (BB). The one-year ACM was 17.6%.[10]

Whereas the first organized HF registry in India was THFR. It followed the 2012 European Society of Cardiology (ESC) guideline for identification of HF, which included echocardiographic evaluation. The presentation, management, and 90-day outcomes of HF patients were determined. A total of 1,205 cases (834 men, 69%) were included. Results showed that (CAD) (72%) was the utmost common HF etiology. HFpEF is defined as patients with echocardiography-derived EF ≥45% constituted 26% of the population. The median hospital stay was 6-day with an in-hospital death rate of 8.5% (95% CI: 6.9–10.0). Also, the 90-day all-cause death rate was 2.43 deaths per 1000 person-days. Treatment as per guidelines was provided to 19 and 25% of patients throughout hospital admission and at discharge, respectively. When compared to published data from other registries, the patients hospitalized with HF in the THER were younger, more likely to be men, had a higher prevalence of CAD, reported longer length of hospital stay, and higher mortality.[12]

However, Chaturvedi V et. al. in 2016 conducted the INDUS study to determine the HF prevalence in a rural community in addition to tertiary hospital care settings in North India. All adults (>20 years) with chronic breathlessness were evaluated with a standardized questionnaire by trained health care workers. Results revealed that among 10,163 patients, chronic breathlessness was present in 128 (1.3%). HF was detected in 9% ($n = 12$) of patients. Among them, 67% ($n = 8$) had preserved LVSF and 33% ($n = 4$) had LVSD. Therefore, the occurrence of HF in this common community was 1.2/100. Also, it was observed that 20.4% of patients had HF among 500 consecutive patients. The predominance of HF was 22.5% under 30 years and 14.9% over 50 years indicating the younger population of HF. The assessed prevalence was 1% of the population in India. The assessed mortality causing HF was 0.1–0.16 million individuals per year.[13]

By the end of 2030, the count of HF patients would rise by 25% as the burden of HF is rapidly increasing. The current estimates about the occurrence of HF in India vary widely from 1.3 to 23 million. The incidence of HF in India differs from the West, and the following are the points that describe how the Indian HF patients differ.[14]

- At a younger age, Indian patients present with HF than patients in the West, e.g. the mean age in the THFR, Medanta Registry, and the INTER-CHF (Indian subset) study was 61.2, 58.9, and 56 years, respectively, as compared to 72.4 years in the ADHERE Registry of the USA.
- More males seek healthcare than females in India as the male to female ratio is also different in India (70:30 as per the THFR and 83:17 in the Medanta Registry) compared to the USA and Africa (almost 50:50).
- The predominance of risk factors likewise varies among India and the West, e.g. Diabetes Mellitus (DM) is significantly more pervasive among Indians than those in the West, according to the THFR information.
- In Indian patients, the prognosis of HF is worse than those in the West. The in-hospital mortality detected in the THFR (8.4%) was almost double compared to that present in the ADHERE registry (4%) of the USA. As per the INTER-CHF study, the 1-year mortality of HF is high in India, i.e. 37%. When compared to the West, the maximum number of Indian patients are from low socio-economic strata, who have to spend out-of-pocket for their treatment.[14]

Sparse clinical and demographic data on HF is a concern in India. The result from the registries explained above shows that HF patients in India are younger by 10 years, and the main burden lies in less than 65 years of age, as compared to the patients from HIC. Though, none of them represent data from diverse geographic areas in India. Between the various states and regions of India, significant disparities in health burden are well-documented. Thus, National Heart Failure Registry (NHFR) was initiated to bridge this gap and collected representative data. It provides crucial information on prevailing etiology, distribution, and current practices in the treatment of HF.

NHFR is an ongoing multicentric study of HF patients from 53 centers across India. Patients with acute decompensated HF were enlisted from January 2019 to December 2019 in this registry. From all the enlisted patients, socioeconomics, clinical lab, and other analytic information at baseline were recorded. Also, complete information was gathered from participants about treatment practices and the use of therapy as per guidelines. This registry intends to obtain the in-hospital, 3 months, 6 months, and 1-year result information on mortality, the reason for death, and frequent hospitalization events. The outcomes of this registry are on the way as this study is still ongoing.[11]

Take Home Pearls

- In fact, HF is a complex disease and the main cause of morbidity and mortality in developed and developing countries.

- The incidence of HF is increasing because of the aging population even if the occurrence of HF is stable.
- Data from LMIC indicate that mortality in patients with HF in these countries is greater than that in HIC.
- HF occurrence is a primary medical issue in Asia when compared to western countries.
- India is currently in the midst of an epidemiological transition, resulting in a rapid increase in the incidence of CV risk factors, CVD, and HF.
- In India, HF patients are younger by 10 years, and the maximum of the burden lies below 65 years of age. Also, CAD is the most widely recognized HF etiology.

HEART FAILURE TYPES AND CLINICAL COURSE

Heart failure (HF) is a perplexing disorder in which the heart cannot perform its circulatory function with proper effectiveness because of structural and/or functional changes. No single classification system is available for HF. Figure 5.3 presents the commonly followed classification systems in HF management. Key differences in the HFrEF and HFpEF patient profiles are mentioned in Table 5.1. According to LVEF, it is categorized into three parts: HFrEF, HF with mid-range EF (HFmrEF), and HFpEF. Whereas based on time course, it is categorized as acute and chronic HF. Furthermore, the most commonly used HF classification systems in clinical studies are the NYHA Functional Classification. Each class defines a patient's symptoms during physical

Table 5.1: HFrEF *vs* HFpEF—salient differences[14]

Features	Basic pathophysiology	Gender	Age	Past-history and comorbidities	LV hemodynamics	Impact of vasodilators	Impact on myocardium
Heart failure with reduced ejection fraction (HFrEF)	Reduction of left ventricular systolic function	Men > women	Younger (compared to HFpEF)	History of myocardial infarction (MI) and dilated cardio-myopathy (DCM) is more common	Dilated with eccentric remodeling	Improves left ventricular systolic performance	Myocardial stress/injury is more pronounced
Heart failure with preserved ejection fraction (HFpEF)	Alteration of left ventricular filling	Women> men	More often older	History of hypertension, atrial fibrillation and valvular heart disease (VHD) is more common. impact of co-morbidities may be more profound	Concentric remodeling (with or without left ventricular hypertrophy) is present in many, left ventricular end-diastolic volume is not increased relative to the stroke volume	Have little impact on left ventricular systolic performance	Myocardial inflammation and fibrosis are more prominent

activities. Classifying HF based on a person's functions is a strong factor in the patient's outcome. The classes I to IV used in this system with I indicating less severity and higher numbers indicating greater severity as defined in Fig. 5.3.[14]

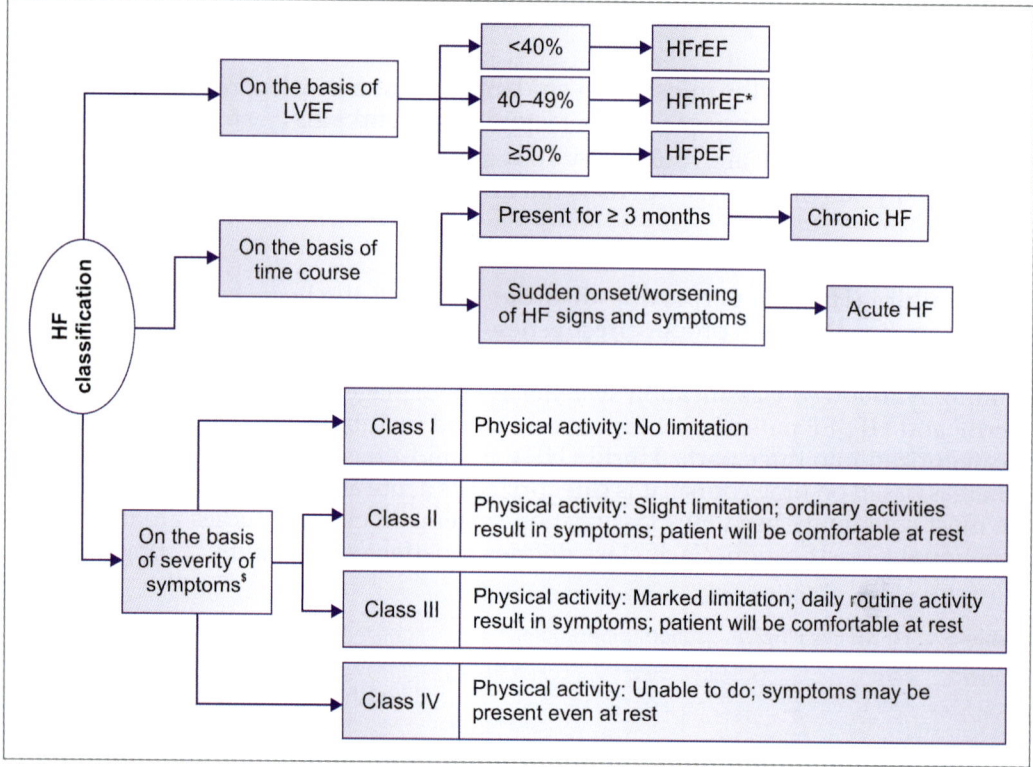

Fig. 5.3: Different classification systems for HF[14]

HF: Heart failure; LVEF: Left ventricular ejection fraction; HFrEF: Heart failure with reduced ejection fraction; HFmrEF: Heart failure with mid-range ejection fraction; HFpEF: Heart failure with preserved ejection fraction.

*It is referred to as a grey zone as the protocol and treatment for this group is not clear.

$New York Heart Association classification

Whereas other terms that are generally used in HF are given below:

- **Stable HF:** During treatment, if HF patient does not show any major change in the symptoms and HF signs persist for at least a month, then the patient's condition is mentioned as "stable".

- **Decompensated HF:** If the condition of a previously "stable" HF patient worsens unexpectedly, it is called "decompensated".

- **New-onset/de novo HF:** A patient with new-onset/de novo HF may present with symptoms in an acute or subacute (gradual) fashion.

- **Advanced HF:** It refers to patients with severe cardiac dysfunction, recurrent decompensation, and severe symptoms despite optimal standard medical therapy.[14]

Etiology of HF

The etiology of HF is diverse within and among world regions. Various CV conditions and inherited imperfections, and systemic diseases can cause HF. HF patients can have mixed etiologies and vary considerably between high-income and developing countries (HIDC) (Fig. 5.4). HF has an estimated 17 primary etiologies, as per the Global Burden of Disease (GBD) Study. Many patients will have several different pathologies—CV and non-CV—that conspire to cause HF. Among HF cases, more than two-thirds be attributed to cause four basic conditions: CAD, chronic obstructive pulmonary disease (COPD), rheumatic heart disease (RHD), and hypertensive heart disease. Identification of these diverse pathologies should be part of the diagnostic workup, as they may offer specific therapeutic opportunities.[15,16]

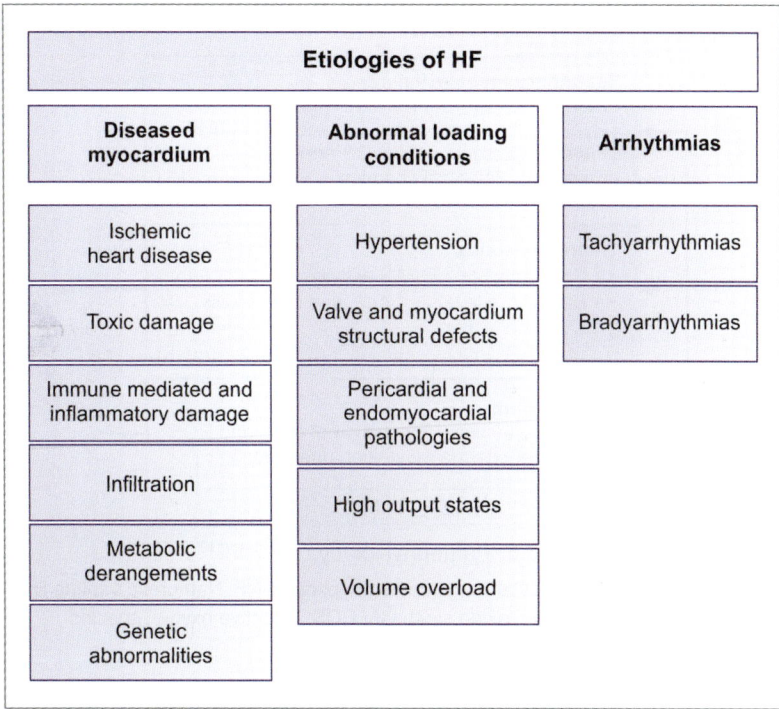

Fig. 5.4: Etiologies of HF[16]

According to the GBD study age-standardized estimates (2010), nearly a quarter (24.8%) of all deaths in India are attributable to CVD. CAD and stroke constitute the major CVD mortality in India (83%), with CAD being predominant. The prevalence of CAD in 1960 in urban India was 2% and increased 7-fold to ≈14% by 2013. Similarly, it was more than quadrupled in rural areas, from 1.7 to 7.4% between 1970 and 2013.[17] Furthermore, to determine that in India, IHD is the contributor to HF, Seth S *et al.* conducted the Acute Failure Registry (AFAR) Study. The study included a total of 90 patients (mean age 53.5 ± 17.7 years). Male patients (63%) with LVSD were present in the majority. Results showed that in this cohort, CAD (53.9%) was the principal reason for HF, following idiopathic cardiomyopathy (18.5%), and then RHD (10.8%). These findings showed that CAD etiology is predominant in India.[18]

Pathophysiology of HFrEF

There is a very complex relationship present between the initial insult and the development of HFrEF. Symptoms of HF and sudden cardiac death are caused due to downstream lethal effects at the myocardial, endothelial, and neurohormonal levels. Initial myocardial injury results in compensatory up-regulation of the sympathetic nervous system (SNS) and the renin-angiotensin-aldosterone system (RAAS). Although this can be valuable in the present moment to keep up myocardial contractility and CO, the ongoing initiation of these systems prompts pernicious auxiliary impacts, including LV rebuilding, myocardial fibrosis, and apoptosis Vasoconstriction can also be a consequence of pathological endothelin and cytokine up-regulation. Finally, the activation of these systems results in worsening HF (Fig. 5.5).[19]

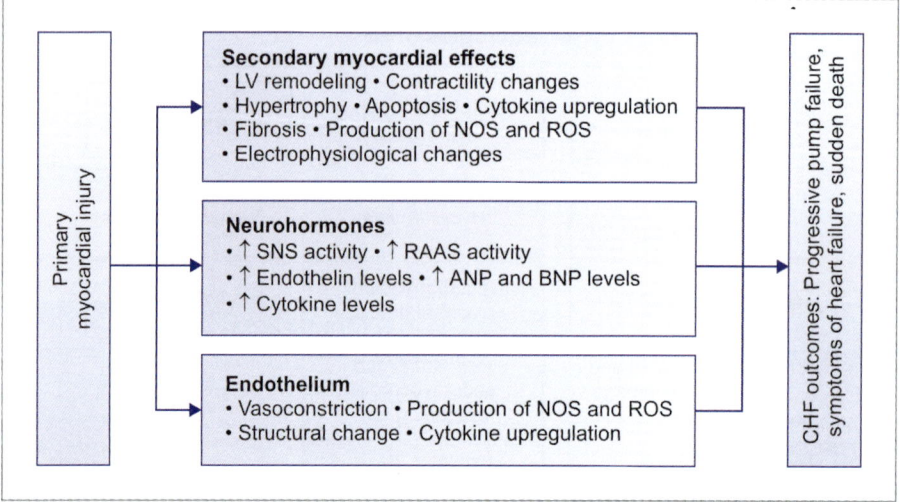

Fig. 5.5: Pathophysiology of HFrEF[19]

ANP: Natriuretic peptide A (also known as atrial natriuretic peptide); BNP: Natriuretic peptide B; CHF: Congestive heart failure; NOS: Nitric oxide synthase; ROS: Reactive oxygen species

Clinical Course of HF and its Management

The clinical course of HF is considered as progressive deterioration with bouts of (often unpredictable) acute or subacute decompensation from fluid overload, over-diuresis, non-adherence, infection, or other intercurrent illness. Sudden death may occur at any time due to arrhythmia, but commonly there is gradual death from pump failure or, in a substantial proportion of death from other CV or non-CV causes. However, most people with HF are not admitted for acute decompensated HF. But comorbidities and/or more general deterioration are addressed tangentially or not at all by disease-specific guidelines and management protocols.[20] HF carries five-year mortality of around 50%. Mortality figures cover significant heterogeneity of outcome, which varies with setting at diagnosis (primary *vs* secondary care), first or subsequent hospital admission, diagnostic criteria (particularly whether and to what extent ejection fraction is reduced), comorbidities (particularly diabetes and cognitive impairment), and degree of implementation of evidence-based therapies.[20]

Prognostic Predictors of Death and Hospitalization in HFrEF

Prognosis Markers: HFrEF has been linked with a poorer prognosis compared to diastolic HF. Thus, information of prognosis markers for mortality of HFrEF is significant to help caregivers in making an informed decision on the type of therapy, as well as in planning resource allocation in healthcare facilities. Prognosis markers have been traditionally associated with worsening symptoms, the severity of diastolic dysfunction, and the presence of CV and non-CV comorbidities. The 2016 ESC HF guidelines identified many different markers for a worse prognosis in HFrEF patients (Table 5.2).[21]

HFrEF is related to epidemiological profiles, for example, older age, male sex, and low financial status, and considered as significant risk factors for the advancement of HFrEF. Worsening symptoms, as per the New York Heart Association (NYHA) functional class, has a direct link with the development of HFrEF and are considered as predictive markers for worsening HFrEF.[23] There are so many interpreters of mortality, but high RHR is one of the important clinical interpreters and linked with HF outcomes.

Table 5.2: Predictors of worse prognosis in HFrEF patients[21]

Predictors of an ominous prognosis	Patient demographics	Clinical markers	Severity of ventricular dysfunction	Biomarkers (for cardiac damage/dysfunction, neurohormonal activation and/or inflammation)	Cardiovascular comorbidities	Extra-cardiac comorbidities	Clinical events
Description	Older age, male sex, low socio-economic status	NYHA III-IV, limited exercise tolerance, reduced functional state or poor quality of life, pulmonary congestion, splanchnic congestion, peripheral edema, jugular venous dilation and hepato-megaly, high resting heart rate and frailty	Depressed LVEF, LV-dilatation, severe diastolic LV-dysfunction, mitral regurgitation, aortic stenosis, LV hyper-trophy, left atrial dilatation, RV dysfunction, pulmonary hypertension and ventricular dyssynchrony	Low sodium, high natriuretic peptides, high plasma renin activity, high aldosterone and catecho-lamine, high endo-thelin-1, high adreno-medullin, and high vasopressin	AF, ventricular arrhythmia, non-revas-cularizable CAD, previous stroke/transient ischemic attack, peripheral artery disease	Diabetes, anemia, iron deficiency, chronic obstructive pulmonary disease, renal failure, liver dysfunction, sleep apnea, cognitive impairment, and depression	Non-adherence with treatment, HF-related hospi-talization, aborted cardiac arrest and implantable cardioverter defibrillator shocks

A high resting heart rate (RHR) is of prognostic relevance not only in elderly people with no apparent heart disease but also in a broad spectrum of CVDs, including chronic HFrEF and acute/decompensated HFrEF along with chronic HFpEF and acute/decompensated HFpEF. It was considered that both sympathetic and RAAS overactivity is mainly responsible for the link between RHR and HF. The reasons for this association are increased oxygen consumption, decreased myocardial perfusion, and consequently decreased cardiac performance (reduced cardiac distensibility and impaired LVDF), hemodynamic changes (increased pre-and afterload), and ultimately pro-arrhythmic effect. An additional mechanism, which explains the relationship between RHR and death rate in HF is inflammation, endothelial dysfunction, and higher oxidative stress.[22,23]

Take Home Pearls

- HF is a disorder in which the heart is unable to perform circulatory function due to systolic or diastolic changes.
- NYHA functional categorization of HF is one of the most widely used classification systems in practice and clinical studies.
- Among all HF cases, about two-thirds of cases constitute four underlying conditions: CAD, COPD, RHD, and hypertensive heart disease.
- Myocardial injury can cause an up-regulation of the RAAS and SNS.
- Worsening symptoms have a direct link with the development of HFrEF, and are considered to be predictive signs for worsening HFrEF.
- The link between RHR and HF is mainly due to sympathetic and RAAS overactivity.

HIGH RHR AND ITS IMPACT ON HFrEF

RHR is a very assessable biological parameter with potential predictive capacity for HF and CVD. In the common population, elevated RHR is associated with CV outcomes, risk factors like obesity and diabetes, hypertension, CAD, CAD with impaired LV function, and chronic HF. Thus, it affects diagnosis throughout the CV continuum. Among patients experiencing HF, RHR is a variable risk factor to prevent rehospitalization for HF. However, the studies that determine the relation between RHR and HF have included adults with CVD, or conduction disorders such as AF, or adults using antiarrhythmics.[24] Therefore, to describe the association between RHR and incident HF and CV mortality, and to observe whether these associations might be attributable to systemic inflammation and endothelial dysfunction, Nanchen *et al.* conducted a prospective study (the PROSPER study). The study included a total of 4,084 adults (aged 10–82 years). Included patients had known CV risk factors, without pre-existing HF or BBs. RHR values were grouped into thirds of their distribution, as predefined beforehand. It was done separately for women and men because women have higher RHR than men, and the links between gender-specific HR thirds and the endpoints were studied using age- and multivariate-adjusted Cox proportional hazards models, with the lowest HR group as the reference group. During a follow-up of 3.2 years, episodes of HF hospitalization and CV mortality as per RHR, along with C-Reactive-Protein (CRP), Interleukin-6 (IL-6), tissue Plasminogen Activator (tPA), and von Willebrand factor (vWf) were examined. Results revealed that mean HR was 67 bpm and 70 bpm for men and women, respectively. CRP, IL-6, tPA, and vWf levels were all positively related to HR. HR was linked with HF hospitalization [Hazard

Ratio (HR): 1.78 for highest *vs* lowest distribution third, 95% CI: 1.21–2.63, p = 0.003] and CV mortality (HR: 1.74, 95% CI: 1.23–2.47, p = 0.002) after multivariate adjustment. Further adjustment for both IL-6 and vWf levels reduced HR to 1.60 (95% CI: 1.08–2.38, p = 0.020) for HF and to 1.50 (95% CI: 1.04–2.15, p = 0.028) for CV mortality. These outcomes confirm the close connection between RHR and systemic inflammation, beyond fundamental determinants of HR, such as gender or height, environmental aspects.[25] Moreover, to observe whether higher RHR is related to the rise in HF among adults without pre-existing heart disease or HR-modifying medication use in the general population, Nanchen D *et al.* studied 4,768 men and women aged ≥55 years from the population-based Rotterdam Study. It was found that during 14.6 years of follow-up, 656 participants developed HF, and the HF risk was more in men with greater RHR. For each rise of 10 beats per minute (bpm), the multivariable-adjusted hazard ratios in men were 1.16 (95% CI: 1.05–1.28; p = 0.005) in the time-fixed HR model and 1.13 (95% CI: 1.02–1.25; p = 0.017) in the time-dependent HR model. In men (n = 1,829), HR was ≤68 bpm), 69 to 78 bpm, and ≥79 bpm for the first, second, and third tertile, respectively. In women (n = 2,939), these rates were ≤72, 73 to 80, and ≥81 bpm, respectively. The risk of HF was more in men with greater RHR based on pulse palpation or ECG beyond other cardiac risk factors.[26]

Being related to sympathetic overactivity, atherosclerosis, and plaque vulnerability, RHR-mediated arterial stress has gained much emphasis on potential mechanisms of CVD progression and clinical manifestations. Numerous prior studies described the association between RHR and LV dysfunction and/or HF in epidemiological studies and patients with CAD. On the other hand, some clinical trials have explored the link between RHR and LV dysfunction and/or HF among asymptomatic individuals with no CVD history. Sufficient cardiac output is provided by RHR and LV stroke volume. During the early phases of LV dysfunction, and progression toward HF, subtle reduction of LV function might therefore be accompanied by a compensatory increase in RHR, even before the elevated HR is identified as marker of excessive neuroendocrine activation. To observe the association between baseline RHR and incidence of HF and global and regional LV dysfunction, Opdahl *et al.* conducted a Multi-Ethnic Study of Atherosclerosis (MESA) trial. This trial included a total of 6,814 men and women. According to Cox analysis with each 1-bpm increase in RHR, there was a 4% greater adjusted relative risk for incident HF [Hazard Ratio (HR): 1.04; 95% CI: 1.02 to 1.06; p <0.001). As per adjusted multiple regression models, RHR was positively related to declining circumferential strain (εcc) and decrease in EF, even when all CAD events were excluded from the model. Outcomes from the MESA trial revealed that elevated RHR was linked with augmented risk for incident HF in asymptomatic participants, and was related to the development of regional and global LV dysfunction independent of subclinical atherosclerosis and CAD.[27]

High HR has been linked with an adverse diagnosis, but most studies emphasize persons with known CVD or observed an inadequate number of outcomes. Jennifer E *et al.* conducted a study to observe the association of HR with both fatal and non-fatal outcomes. The study included a total of 4,058 participants (mean age 55 years, 56% women). With multivariable adjustment for clinical risk factors and physical activity a Cox model was performed. A total of 708 participants established incident CVD (303 HF, 343 CAD, and 216 stroke events), 48 were given a permanent pacemaker, and 1,186 died. HR was related to incident CVD [hazard ratio (HR): 1.15 per 1 SD (11 bpm) rise in HR, 95% CI: 1.07 to 1.24, p = 0.0002], particularly HR (HR: 1.32, 95% CI: 1.18 to 1.48,

p <0.0001). Higher HR was related with higher all-cause (HR: 1.17, 95% CI: 1.11 to 1.24, p <0.0001), and CV mortality (HR: 1.18, 95% CI: 1.04 to 1.33, p = 0.01). These findings revealed that higher HR is at eminent long-term risk for CV events, in particular, HF and all-cause death.[28]

Patients with stable CAD have high event rates, despite modern treatments. Patients with LVSD have even greater rates of mortality. Large studies with long-term follow-up have shown a high HR is an independent predictor of all-cause and CV mortality in CAD patients. The placebo arm of the BEAUTIFUL (morbidity mortality EvAlUaTion of the I_f inhibitor Ivabradine in patients with coronary disease and LV dysfunction) study provided a large population with CAD and LVSD were well-treated in terms of CV prevention. BEAUTIFUL included men and women aged greater than 55 years with CAD, LVEF of less than 40%, and end-diastolic short-axis internal dimension larger than 56 mm. Fox et al. in 2008 performed a subgroup analysis of BEAUTIFUL to check the hypothesis that elevated RHR at baseline is a marker for subsequent CV death and morbidity. In this study, the association of baseline RHR with CV outcomes was analyzed using Cox proportional hazard models. Results revealed that patients with HR of 70 bpm or greater had increased risk for CV death (34%, p = 0.0041), admission to hospital for HF (53%, p <0.0001), admission to hospital for MI (46%, p = 0.0066), and coronary revascularization (38%, p = 0.037). For every increase of 5-bpm, there were increases in CV death, admission to hospital for HF, admission to hospital for MI, and coronary revascularization. Also, the analysis proposes that the rise in HF outcomes rises continuously above 70 bpm. These results revealed that in patients with CAD and LVSD, elevated HR detects those at greater risk of CV outcomes and outcomes related to coronary events.[29,30]

One possible link between decrease HR and survival is the LV function improvement secondary to the induced reduction of ischemia. It is identified that β-blockade-induced benefit in HF is associated with Baseline Heart Rate (BHR) and treatment-induced HR reductions. Therefore, the mechanism of β-blockade was studied to identify the best responders to such treatment. Lechat et al. assessed the relationships between BHR, HR Changes at 2 months (HRC), nature of cardiac rhythm, and results in Cardiac Insufficiency Bisoprolol Study II (CIBIS II). As per the multivariate analysis of CIBIS II, BHR and HRC were both linked to the lowest BHR, survival, and hospitalization for worsening HF, and the greatest HRC. Also, Bisoprolol-induced survival perfection was found significant. These findings showed that BHR and HRC are significantly interrelated to diagnosis in HF.[31]

The outcomes mentioned above clearly suggest that a decrease in HR could improve CV outcomes in HF. Moreover, to confirm this hypothesis, Bohm et al. conducted a systolic heart failure treatment with the I_f inhibitor Ivabradine Trial (SHIFT), investigating the influence of isolated HR reduction on clinical results in HF. Patients were divided into groups to receive placebo (n = 3,264) and Ivabradine (n = 3,241), and hospital admission for worsening HF was considered as the primary composite endpoint. Results revealed that patients with the greater HR ($\geq$87 bpm, n = 682, 286 events) were at more than two-fold greater risk for the primary composite endpoint than were patients with the lowest HR [70 to <72 bpm, n = 461, 92 events; hazard ratio (HR): 2.34, 95% CI: 1.84–2.98, p <0.0001]. Ivabradine helps in HR reduction, as shown by the neutralization of the management effect after 28 days [hazard ratio (HR): 0.95, 0.85–1·06, p = 0.352]. This analysis confirmed that high HR is a risk factor, in HF and Ivabradine improves CV outcomes by lowering HR.[32]

The recent findings of the SHIFT have confirmed the significance of HR in HF with lessen LVEF, but whether higher RHR also has predictive significance in HF patients and preserved LVEF, representing one-third to one-half of the patients with HF, is still less well-documented. The CHARM (Candesartan in Heart failure: Assessment of Reduction in Mortality and Morbidity) program registered 7,599 patients with HF regardless of LVEF and measured the consequence of the angiotensin-receptor blocker Candesartan on CV mortality and morbidity. The study aimed to observe the relationship between RHR at baseline and fatal and nonfatal CV outcomes and death rate in a broad spectrum of patients with HF and to conclude whether the link between HR and outcomes were affected by LVEF or underlying cardiac rhythm. In this program, patients were divided into groups by tertiles of baseline HR, and Cox proportional hazard models were used to explore the link between HR and pre-specified consequences in the whole population. Results revealed that worse outcomes were observed in patients with the highest HR tertile. Also, HR and outcomes showed a similar relationship through LVEF categories and were not affected by BBs. Thus, revealing that RHR is a significant indicator of outcome in patients with stable chronic HF without AF, irrespective of LVEF, or BB use.[33]

The beneficial effects of HR control in HF and particularly LVSD is well understood and are multifaceted. Epidemiological studies determine that high RHR was the predictor of HF. During LV systolic impairment, when the HR is uncontrolled, increased strain is present on the myocardium to meet physiological oxygen demand. Due to this, the heart is at risk of collagen accumulation and ultimately LV cardiac remodeling. In turn, this has a prohibitive influence on the heart by decreasing the EF and the stroke volume in addition to increasing the end-diastolic volume, resulting in reduced functionality (Fig. 5.6).[34]

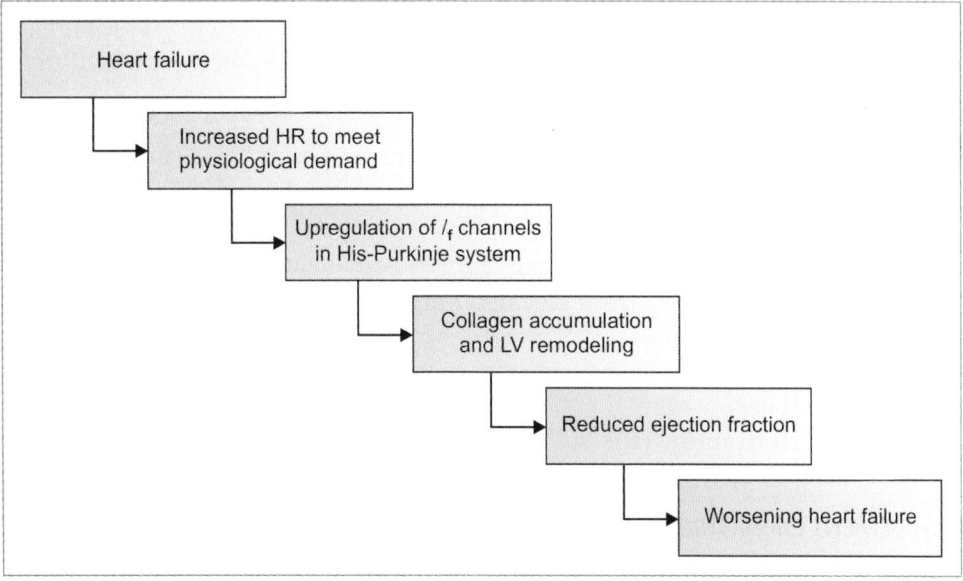

Fig. 5.6: Effect of raised HR in HF.[34] HR: Heart rate, LV: Left ventricular

HR Control in Indian HF Patients

HF is a common CV disorder with increasing prevalence. Several studies on the use of pharmacological therapy and devices have resulted in increasing the use of evidence-based therapy for HF. It is mainly an ailment of the elderly in western countries whereas, in India, it affects a younger age group.[35,36] As per the THFR registry, the occurrence of CAD is comparatively higher than other registries (prevalence ranges from 40 to 60%). India is rapidly progressing with demographic and epidemiological transitions, causing a substantial rise in the CAD burden.[37] While as per consensus recommendation by Mishra *et al.* the preferred HR should be less than 70 in HF patients, but as per results from several epidemiological studies in HF patients in India, the scenario is different, where patients with HR are not in control. According to outcomes from the Indian Heart Study (IHS), Indians have an average RHR of 80 bpm, which is higher than the desired rate of 72-bpm.[38] Indian population shows increased RHR because of increased sympathetic overactivity (SO). Increased sympathetic activation may be central to the progression of HF.[39]

Patients with systolic HF frequently have symptoms despite receiving standard treatment. Despite guideline-recommended treatment that includes Angiotensin-Converting Enzyme Inhibitors (ACEIs) or Angiotensin Receptor Blockers (ARBs) and BBs for all patients, along with diuretics, nitrates, and aldosterone antagonists when required mortality is high with as many as 40% succumbing in a year. Further, almost all patients have shortness of breath, nearly half orthopnea, and about one-third suffer from paroxysmal nocturnal dyspnea, which together suggests a very poor QoL. It may be due to adverse effects of BBs such as bronchospasm, hypotension, and rebound tachycardia, which often limits their use at recommended doses in the majority of patients. The principal action of BB is to decrease HR. The evidence that these agents morbidity and mortality in HF, exert a favorable effect on LV remodeling, and reduce the risk of sudden death have raised the possibility that HR reduction could be related to these benefits, suggesting the need for other HR reducing drugs that are relatively free of side effects.[40] In India, the doses to which BBs can be titrated are very low (carvedilol average doses of 12.5 mg), and the mean HR of patients with HF is very high. Therefore, in these patients, other drugs should be added besides BBs, if they are symptomatic and have HR beyond 70 bpm with an EF <35%.[41]

Take Home Pearls

- RHR is a measurable biological parameter with potential predictive capacity for HF and CVD.
- RHR is a modifiable risk factor to prevent rehospitalization for HF.
- Patients with a greater HR are at elevated long-term risk for CV events, particularly HF and all-cause death.
- RHR is a major predictor of consequence in a patient's HF without AF, irrespective of LVEF, or BB use.
- The average RHR in India is 80 bpm, which is greater than the desired rate of 72 bpm. Indian population shows increased RHR because of increased SO.

MANAGEMENT OF HIGH RHR–HFrEF PERSPECTIVE

The main aim of management in patients with HF is to develop their functional capability, clinical status, QoL, and decrease mortality. Understanding the cause of HF allows one to attain the objectives of management. The fact that several drugs for HF have shown detrimental effects on long-term outcomes, despite showing beneficial effects on shorter-term surrogate markers, has led regulatory bodies and clinical practice guidelines to seek mortality/morbidity data for approving/recommending therapeutic interventions for HF. Though, it is now known that preventing HF hospitalization is considered important if a mortality excess is ruled out. Initial and ongoing assessments of individuals with HF ought to incorporate an evaluation of symptoms and their functional outcomes. These evaluations fill in as the reason for settling on treatment choices, monitoring the impacts of treatment, and altering treatment as proper. Diminishing indications and improving function are two of the essential objectives of HF treatment and represent important patient-centric outcomes for HF care. Successful management of HF involves non-pharmacological management and pharmacological management.[14,42]

Non-Pharmacological Management of HFrEF Patient

Non-pharmacological management of HF is as significant as the drugs and devices used to manage HF. All patients need support and dietary advice regarding the conservation of optimal weight. As obesity increases the load on the heart, especially during physical activity; therefore, weight reduction through restriction of dietary fat and calories is imperative for obese people. For CAD patients and raised lipids, a low-fat diet may delay the recurrence of significant CV events. Similarly, salt intake should be restricted, as it may aggravate a patient's condition. In HF patients, less dietary sodium intake of 2,000 mg per day alone may provide substantial hemodynamic and clinical benefits. Also, it was known HF patients often have intense thirst, which causes excessive fluid intake and hyponatremia. Therefore, fluid intake should be restricted where possible, to about 1 liter a day, and during periods of hot weather, diarrhea, vomiting, or fever, fluid intake may be increased or the dose of diuretic reduced. Bed rest is a significant part of the treatment of acute HF or decompensated chronic HF, though early mobilization is important. Otherwise, regular and moderate physical activity for the condition of the patient should be exhilarated. Dynamic exercise activities such as walking, cycling, swimming, bowling, gardening, etc. should be continued at a pace that is comfortable for the patient. Exercise instruction should be included in the HF program. Exercise training assistance has been proved to improve the practical status and may help diminish morbidity and death rates in individuals with stable HFrEF. As even moderate usage of alcohol intake may be related to decreasing ventricular systolic function, alcohol use should be discouraged. It was known that smoking increases the risk of many CV, pulmonary, and other problems, including cancers, and thus, should be eluded at all costs.[43]

Individual's self-care education is a helpful non-pharmacological component to HF care. It might decrease the probability of non-adherence with prescribed therapeutic strategies and lead to early detection of worsening clinical status and subsequent therapy. HF disease management programs, in which patient education is an integral component, have been demonstrated to be compelling in improving self-care and diminishing readmissions.

Vaccination (pneumococcal vaccination and influenza vaccination) also plays an important role in the management of HF. Improved vaccination rates may decrease the occurrence of respiratory infections, modify the natural history of chronic HF and thereby prevent HF exacerbations, hospitalization, excess cost, and associated morbidity/mortality.[44]

Implantable cardioverter-defibrillator (ICD) therapy prevents sudden cardiac death (SCD) due to ventricular tachyarrhythmias in select patients with HFrEF. However, frequent or inappropriate shocks from an ICD can prompt diminished QoL. Patients may contrast in the eagerness to have an ICD embedded dependent on their inclinations for quality and length of life. Given the critical dangers and advantages of ICD implantation, qualified patients ought to be completely educated regarding this treatment choice.[42]

Cardiac resynchronization therapy (CRT) has been shown to improve survival and symptoms among symptomatic patients with HF and LVEF ≤35%, LBBB, and QRS duration ≥150 ms. CRT implantation is recommended as it improves both quantity and QoL, unlike ICDs, where there is no symptomatic benefit.[42]

Pharmacological Management of HFrEF Patient

Pharmacological treatment is the keystone of HF management. Neurohormonal antagonists [ACEIs, Mineralocorticoid/aldosterone Receptor Antagonists (MRAs), and BBs] improve survival in patients with HFrEF and are recommended for the treatment of every HFrEF patient if not contraindicated. ACEIs decrease mortality in patients with HFrEF and are recommended in all symptomatic patients. ACEIs should be up-titrated to the maximum tolerable dosage to attain suitable inhibition of the RAAS. ACEIs are prescribed in patients with asymptomatic LVSD to lessen the risk of HF development and death.[14,16]

MRAs (Spironolactone and Eplerenone) act by blocking the aldosterone receptors. Spironolactone or Eplerenone are suggested in all symptomatic patients (despite management with ACEI and BB) with HFrEF and LVEF ≤35%, to decrease mortality and HF hospitalization. But care should be taken when MRAs are used in patients with impaired renal function. Regular checks of serum potassium levels and renal function should be done.

ARB (for example, Candesartan, Valsartan) was recommended as a substitute for ACE inhibitors. Long-term treatment with ARBs has additionally been appeared to decrease morbidity and death rate, particularly in ACE inhibitor-intolerant individuals. Candesartan reduces CV mortality. Valsartan showed an effect on hospitalization for HF in patients with HFrEF receiving background ACEIs. EMA studied the ACEI/ARB combination for HFrEF, which proposed that benefits compensate risks only in patients in whom other treatments are inappropriate. Therefore, ARBs are given to HFrEF patients who cannot tolerate an ACEI. The major risk associated with the utilization of ARBs is hyperkalemia owing to the hindrance of potassium excretion, going from 2 to 5% in preliminaries to 24 to 36% in populace based registries. The ACEI/ARB combination should be given only to symptomatic HFrEF patients receiving a BB who are not able to tolerate an MRA and must be used under strict supervision.[14,16,42]

Angiotensin Receptor-Neprilysin Inhibitor (ARNI) is a new class of drug which prevents both RAAS and the neutral endopeptidase system. Sacubitril-Valsartan is the only drug approved to be used in this class. Sacubitril is a Neprilysin Inhibitor (NI), while Valsartan is an ARB. Concerning the decrease in mortality, Sacubitril-Valsartan is superior to ACEI (Enalapril). For patients on ARNI, N-terminal pro-Brain Natriuretic Peptide (NT-pro-BNP), but not BNP, is a suitable biomarker to monitor overall disease status. In patients with persistent indicative HFrEF NYHA class II or III who endure an ACE inhibitor or ARB, substitution by an ARNI is prescribed to additionally diminish morbidity and death rate.[14,16,42]

BBs also improve survival rate and diminish hospitalization for a patient with HFrEF. Treatment with BBs ought to be started when a patient is determined to have decreased LVEF and does not have prohibitively low SBP, fluid overload, or recent treatment with an IV positive inotropic agent. BBs have additionally been proved to decrease the indications of HF, improve the clinical status of patients, and diminish future clinical deterioration. There is consensus that BBs and ACEIs should be given together once the HFrEF is diagnosed. Several studies revealed the positive effects of therapy with BBs in HFrEF, including the CIBIS II, Carvedilol Prospective Randomized Cumulative Survival (COPERNICUS), Metoprolol CR/XL Randomized Intervention Trial in CHF (MERIT-HF), and the Study of the Effects of Nebivolol Intervention on Outcomes and Rehospitalization in Seniors (SENIORS) with heart failure. Similar to ACEIs, BBs should be started at a low-dose, and dosages should be increased in the course.[14,16,42]

In patients having signs of congestion, these medicines should be used along with diuretics. Diuretics should be modified as per the patient's clinical status.[16]

Benefits of HR Decrease in HF

HR reduction can improve contractility, perhaps by reducing energy expenditure, decreasing myocardial oxygen consumption, and improving the relation between energy requirements and energy availability. Therefore, HR-slowing therapies may hold a particular advantage in CVD patients. Indeed, guidelines from the European Society of Cardiology and the European Society of Hypertension for the management of CVD already recommend recognition of HR as a CV risk factor.[45] The benefits of slowing the HR are likely to be the result of a combination of factors as shown in Fig. 5.7. HR reduction improves the relationship between force and frequency at the level of failing myocytes, with consequent positive inotropism. HR reduction also causes unloading of the ventricle and improves the ventricular pressure-volume curve with a reduction in energy expenditure, resulting in reduced or reversed LV remodeling.[46]

An important relation between RHR and all-cause and CV mortality has been described in several studies and pertain to both the common people and with various CVDs, including hypertension, acute myocardial infarction (AMI), and HF or LV

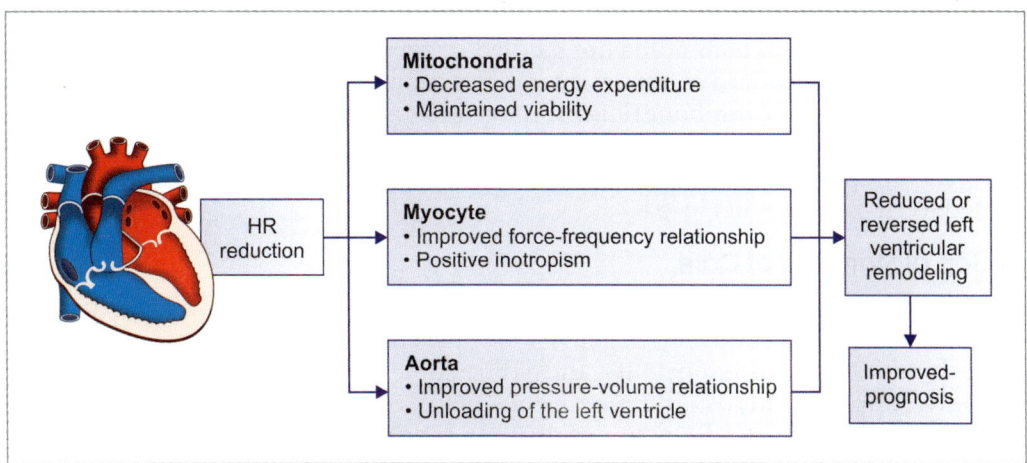

Fig. 5.7: Beneficial effects of HR reduction in HF[46]

dysfunction. Fox K *et al.* in their study, showed the relation of HR management and consequence in HF patients. Here, as for AMI, the relationship was observed between reduction in HR and mortality and agents that increased HR tended to escalate mortality.[47]

Epidemiological trials have also suggested that life expectancy is inversely related to RHR and that the threat of an increase in HF strongly increases with higher RHR. The management of high RHR in HFrEF patients is an ongoing process, which requires lifelong medications. BBs are specified as first-line treatment to decrease mortality in HFrEF patients. This positive effect of BBs may be partially-related to a decrease in HR, and but also, protection of the heart from catecholamines may contribute significantly to the effects of these drugs.[14,48]

However, little is known about patients with elevated HR despite BB therapy.[49] To define the relationship of elevated HR in patients with HFrEF, DeVore *et al.* evaluated the data from the Duke Echocardiography Laboratory Database. Patients were stratified by HR (<70, ≥70 bpm) and compared using generalized linear models specified with gamma error distributions and log-links for costs and proportional hazard models for mortality/hospitalization. Results revealed that of the 722 suitable patients, 582 (81%) were given BBs. The median HR was observed to be 81 bpm (25th, 75th percentile 69–96), and 527 (73%) had HR ≥70 bpm. After multivariable adjustment, HR ≥70 bpm increased 1-year ACM or hospitalization, hazard ratio 1.37 (95% CI: 1.07, 1.75). These outcomes from the large tertiary care center revealed that despite the extensive use of BBs, the HR ≥70 bpm was detected in 73% of patients with HFrEF and related with worse 1-year outcomes.[50]

As per ESC 2016 guidelines and the 2017 focused update to the 2013 ACCF/AHA guidelines, Ivabradine is suggested to be used along with BBs for the management of high RHR in HF patients. It decreases the hospitalization risk for HF in patients with stable, symptomatic chronic HF with LVEF of 35% or less, or has a contraindication for BB therapy. Ivabradine inhibits the I_f current in the sinoatrial node, thus, decreases HR. Ivabradine can be beneficial to reduce HF hospitalization for patients with symptomatic (NYHA class II-III) stable chronic HFrEF (LVEF ≤35%) who are receiving GDEM (Guideline-Directed Evaluation and Management), including a BB at the maximum tolerated dose, with HR of 70 bpm or greater at rest.[16,48,51,52]

Spectrum of Clinical Evidence with Ivabradine in HFrEF

The positive effects of Ivabradine are studied in several randomized and real-world studies, on top of standard of care, as an initial combination with many drugs. Various studies have shown the beneficial impact of Ivabradine on rehospitalization. Ivabradine is also found to improve QoL in several studies. Also, it has positive effects on special populations of HF. The spectrum of clinical evidence with Ivabradine related to HF is shown in Fig. 5.8.

On Top of Standard of Care

Beta-adrenergic blockade has been a mainstay of therapy in chronic HFrEF for more than two decades. Despite their negative inotropic effects, BB therapy has consistently been shown to decrease mortality and HF-related hospitalizations. BB therapy is strongly supported across the major consensus recommendation statements in patients with decrease EF.[39] Several other randomized controlled trials have demonstrated the mortality benefits in HF with drugs such as ACE inhibitors, ARBs, MRAs.[16] It has also been shown that adding Ivabradine to the patients with ongoing

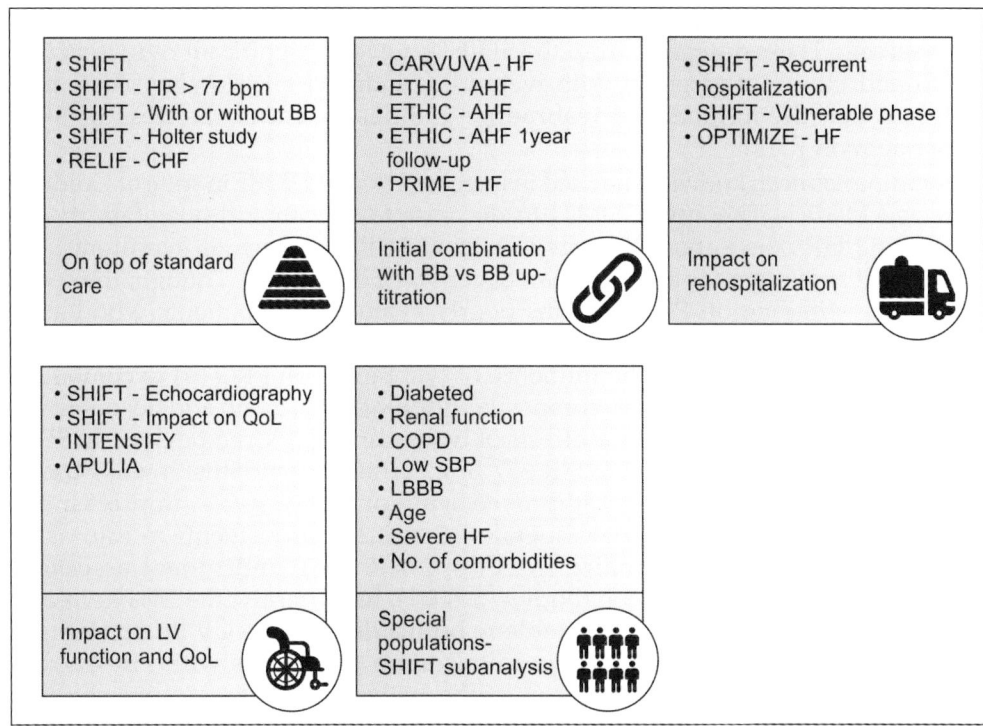

Fig. 5.8: Spectrum of clinical evidence with Ivabradine in HFrEF. CHF: Congestive heart failure; HF: Heart failure; SBP: Systolic blood pressure; BB: Beta-blockers; LBBB: Left bundle branch block

symptoms and having sinus rhythm with the HR of ≥70 bpm reduced CV mortality or, in particular, rehospitalization.

For patients with sinus rhythm and elevated HR and EF ≤35% despite the BB therapy, the ESC guidelines state that Ivabradine therapy can be added, as it can improve the outcomes. Also, in patients who have an intolerance to BBs, Ivabradine can be used as an alternate therapy.[53] The systolic heart failure treatment with the I_f inhibitor ivabradine trial (SHIFT) is the main trial for ivabradine, on top of the standard of care for HF patients. The following are the observational studies based on which it was determined that ivabradine increases the CV outcomes and QoL and also reduces the mortality in patients:

- The SHIFT was a large international clinical phase III trial performed to test the consequence of decrease HR with the I_f inhibitor ivabradine in 6,558 patients with systolic HF, LVEF 35% in sinus rhythm, and with HR at rest ≥70 bpm on maximized guidelines-directed background therapy. Patients were randomized to ivabradine 5 mg twice daily (n = 3,268) vs placebo twice daily (n = 3,290). The primary endpoint was CV mortality or hospitalization for HF. At a baseline, in the Ivabradine group, the usage of BBs was 89% (although only 26% at target dose). Outcomes revealed that at 32 months, mean HR was 67 bpm in the Ivabradine group vs 75 bpm in the placebo group (p <0.050). The CV mortality or HF hospitalization was 14.5% in the ivabradine group vs 17.7% in the placebo group (p <0.0001). This benefit was especially pronounced in patients with a baseline RHR ≥77 bpm. CV mortality was

7.5% *vs* 8.3% ($p = 0.13$), and HF hospitalization was 9.4% *vs* 12.7% ($p < 0.0001$), respectively. These outcomes from the SHIFT showed a significant reduction of CV death and HF hospitalization with ivabradine-induced HR slowing. Also, it was detected that the influence of ivabradine is independent of the dose of BB but dependent on RHR.[54]

- Ivabradine has been known to be used in increase HR and HFrEF in spite of Guideline-Directed Medical Therapy (GDMT) to decrease CV death and hospitalization for worsening HF. The Patient-Reported Outcomes (PROs) such as symptoms, QoL, and global assessment is a global plan of care for HF patients. Though, the specific effect of Ivabradine on PRO remains poorly evaluated. In patients who had HR above the median of 77 bpm (pre-specified analysis), Bouabdallaoui *et al.* performed an analysis (i) to determine the influence of Ivabradine on PRO (ii) to combine the Ivabradine effect on the primary composite endpoint of CV death and hospitalization for HF; and (iii) to reconsider the effects of Ivabradine on LV remodeling. In SHIFT, 51.6% of patients had a baseline HR >77 bpm. After 22.9 months, it was observed that Ivabradine on top of GDMT improved symptoms (28% *vs* 23% improvement in NYHA functional class, $p = 0.0003$), QoL (5.3 *vs* 2.2 improvements in Kansas City Cardiomyopathy Questionnaire (KCCQ), $p = 0.005$), and global assessment considerably more than placebo (both $p < 0.0001$). Importantly, the 25% decrease in the primary endpoint was attributable to both a decrease in CV death (HR: 0.81, $p = 0.0137$) and a decrease in HF hospitalization in patients with HR ≥77 bpm. Improvement in LVEF was detected in the Ivabradine group *vs* placebo when reassessed at 8 months (2.7 ± 8.2 in the Ivabradine group *vs* –0.1 ± 8.9 in the placebo group). These results showed that Ivabradine is on the top of recommended medical therapy on PRO, and strengthen its role in improving results in patients with chronic HFrEF and baseline HR ≥77 bpm.[55]

- Whereas to determine the Ivabradine effect on death rate in patients with HF and a reduced LVEF not receiving a BB, Cleland *et al.* conducted a post hoc analysis of the SHIFT data. Of 6,505 patients valid for this analysis, 685 (10.5%) were not taking a BB, of whom 398 (58.1%) were in NYHA class III or IV, and 476 (69.5%) had CAD. Patients not taking BB had a mean BHR of 84 (SD12 bpm), which had dropped to 68 (SD11 bpm) at 28 days in those who were given Ivabradine and 81 (SD14 bpm) in those who were given the placebo. Results revealed that overall, 552 patients in placebo died compared to 503 patients given Ivabradine (unadjusted HR: 0.91; 95% CI: 0.80–1.02; $p = 0.11$). Amongst patients taking BBs, there were 459 deaths in placebo compared to 432 deaths in ivabradine (unadjusted HR: 0.94; 95% CI: 0.83–1.08; $p = 0.38$). Amongst those not taking BB, there were 93 deaths in those assigned to placebo but only 71 in those assigned to Ivabradine (unadjusted HR: 0.70; 95% CI: 0.52–0.96; $p = 0.026$). These results of SHIFT data revealed that patients who were not prescribed BBs had higher HRs and higher mortality than those prescribed BBs and tended to have a greater benefit from Ivabradine. This retrospective post-hoc analysis is reliable with the assumption that patients with HFrEF in sinus rhythm must receive a BB whenever possible but, when this is not the case, ivabradine may decrease the death rate in the absence of a BB.[56]

- The studies mentioned above clearly explain that ivabradine lowers HR, mortality, and hospitalization. But it is still uncertain that the duration of HF prior to therapy independently influence outcomes or it changes the HR reduction. So, to assess this effect, Bohm *et al.* in 2017 conducted a post-hoc analysis of the SHIFT trial. In this trial, the results and the treatment effect of Ivabradine in patients with HF were examined. Analysis shown that extended period of HF was present in elder patients (62.5 years *vs* 59.0 years; *p* <0.0001), who had more serious disease (NHYA classes III/IV in 56% *vs* 44.9%; *p* <0.0001) and more occurrences of comorbidities [MI: 62.9% *vs* 49.4% (*p* <0.0001); renal dysfunction: 31.5% *vs* 21.5% (*p* <0.0001); peripheral artery disease: 7.0% *vs* 4.8% (*p* <0.0001)] compared with patients with a latest diagnosis. After adjustments, extended HF duration was independently linked with poorer consequences. Also, Ivabradine effects were not dependent on HF duration. Results showed that the HF period predicts results independently of risk indicators such as advanced age, greater severity, and other comorbidities.[57]

- Furthermore, to determine the 24-hour HR lowering effect of Ivabradine in CHF patients, Bohm *et al.* analyzed the predictions from the SHIFT Holter substudy. The 24-hour Holter monitoring was performed at baseline and 8 months after randomization to Ivabradine (*n* = 298) or matching placebo (*n* = 304) titrated maximally to 7.5 mg bid in patients with baseline HR ≥70 bpm. Results revealed that HR over 24-hour reduced by 9.5 ± 10.0 bpm with Ivabradine, from 75.4 ± 10.3 bpm (*p* <0.0001), and by 1.2 ± 8.9 bpm with placebo, from 74.8 ± 9.7 bpm (*p* <0.0001) after 8 months. Ivabradine showed a similar HR decrease in resting office and 24-hour, awake, and sleep recordings, with positive effects on HR variability. Also, it was observed that at 8-month, 21.3% on ivabradine *vs* 8.5% on placebo had ≥1 episode of HR <40 bpm (*p* <0.0001). These findings revealed that ivabradine lowers HR significantly and maintain HR variability in patients with systolic HF, without inducing significant bradycardia, ventricular arrhythmias, or supraventricular arrhythmias.[58]

- Ivabradine is used to control HR in patients with CHF and decreased EF. However, data on its effectiveness and long-term effects are rare. To describe the outcome of long-term treatment (1-year), effectiveness, and safety of ivabradine used in CHF outpatients, Zugck *et al.* conducted a prospective cohort study (RELIF-CHF). The study included a total of 767 CHF patients. They were given ivabradine two times daily, of whom 684 (90%) were still on ivabradine at study end. In 497 patients (65%), BB therapy was also prescribed along with ivabradine. After 1-year, it was observed, HR in ivabradine treated patients was 16 bpm lower when compared to baseline. It is related to substantial improvement in NYHA class and fewer signs of decompensation (36 to 8%). In one year, hospitalized patients decreased from 23% before treatment to 5% with ivabradine therapy. QoL was considerably improved in all aspects. These findings revealed that ivabradine is effective in CHF patients throughout the 1-year of treatment.[59]

Initial Combination with BB *vs* BB Up-titration

Given cumulating results of large scale studies, up-titration of BB and HR reduction achievement are keys to reducing mortality in patients with HFrEF.[60] BB therapy is strongly supported across major consensus recommendation statements in patients with reduced EF. BBs and ACEIs are complementary and can be given together after HFrEF is diagnosed. BB must be given to patients at a low dose and steadily up-titrated to the maximum tolerated dose. BB should be carefully initiated after the patient is stabilized in AHF patients. Across major BB trials in chronic HFrEF, dosages attained in trial participants generally approached target doses. In the CIBIS II study, 42% of patients achieved target dosage, with >50% of patients receiving at least 75% of the target dosage in the maintenance phase. In the US Carvedilol HF Study (USCS), patients achieved 80% of the target dosages. While in the MERIT-HF study, 87% of patients receiving >100 mg daily and 64% receiving the target dose of 200 mg daily, and in the Organized Program to Initiate Lifesaving Treatment in Hospitalized HF Patients (OPTIMIZE-HF) registry, it was observed that less than 10% of patients attained the target dosages of BB at discharge.[16,39]

Current guidelines recommended that BB doses be up-titrated to clinical trial target dosages proven to improve mortality and morbidity as first-line therapy. However, achieved dosages of BB outside of clinical trial settings are typically lower than target; this may be due to side effects limiting titration of BB, additionally to clinician inertia to optimize therapies. Most studies examining HR, BB dosing, and outcomes only examined cross-sectional data, rather than considering secular trends in HR and BB administration. Thus, Ibrahim et al. did a systematic longitudinal evaluation of HR, BB usage, and outcomes among a large population of 6,071 patients with HFrEF in an integrated health network. Results revealed that 27.9% of patients were on ≥50% Guideline-Directed Medical Therapy (GDMT) target BB dose at baseline. After completion of follow-up, 19.4% had HR ≥70 bpm despite receiving ≥50% of the target BB dose. Also, in an adjusted analysis, BHR was found related to all-cause mortality/HF hospitalization [hazard ratio (HR): 1.28 per 15 bpm HR increase; $p < 0.001$]. When compared, hazard ratio for BB dose was 0.97 (per 77.2 mg increase; $p = 0.36$). When assessing patients based on HR and BB dose, a noteworthy variance in the cumulative hazard for ACM or HF hospitalization ($p < 0.001$) was observed. These findings revealed that in a real-world analysis, high RHR was common in HFrEF patients and related to adverse outcomes.[61]

Another trial from a tertiary referral center showed that 53% of patients who had been up-titrated to their maximum tolerated BB dose (or were intolerant of BBs) had HR of >70 bpm, and 20% had an HR of >80 bpm. There is, therefore, a clear scope for additional HR lowering with ivabradine for patients in sinus rhythm who are receiving their maximum dose of BB but still have an HR of 70 bpm or more.[62]

As changed hemodynamic homeostasis of HF patients is related to a rise in HR, and the adverse events in HF are also related to HR. In this context, the BBs' effect on prognosis has been linked to their HR-reducing effect. Ivabradine improves event-free survival in HF patients with and without adequate beta-blockade. Moreover, in CAD patients, ivabradine and BB when given together are more effective than beta-blockade alone in improving exercise tolerance. This raises the question of whether Ivabradine would be an effective add-on treatment to ACE inhibitors and diuretics in HF, allowing up-titration of ACE inhibitors to optimal doses in HF. Therefore, to assess the outcome of carvedilol, ivabradine, or their combination on exercise capacity in patients with HF (CARVIVA HF), Volterrani et al. conducted the trial. In this trial, patients were divided into three groups: Carvedilol up to 25 mg bid ($n = 38$), Ivabradine up to 7.5 mg bid ($n = 41$), and carvedilol/ivabradine up to 12.5/5 mg bid ($n = 42$) was recommended. A decrease in HR was observed in all three groups, but to a significant amount in combination therapy. Better QoL was observed in patients treated with ivabradine and its combination. Thus, it showed that Ivabradine and its combination with Carvedilol are more efficient than Carvedilol alone in improving exercise capacity and QoL. The study also showed that patients allocated to Ivabradine-based therapy are more likely to reach target therapeutic doses than patients receiving carvedilol alone.[63]

Ivabradine has a prognostic benefit and improves the functionality and safety parameters, even in patients with chronic severe systolic HF. Recently, ivabradine not only has a prognostic benefit for HR control but also a prognostic significance for the time required to achieve this control. Therefore, introducing medications initially in the susceptible phase post-hospitalization is important to decrease mortality and rehospitalizations. To define the consequences of the initial co-administration of ivabradine and BBs (intervention group) vs BBs alone (control group) in patients hospitalized with HF and HFrEF, Hidalgo et al. conducted a comparative randomized study. The study included a total of 71 patients, 33 in the intervention group, and 38 in the control group, respectively. Results showed that HR at 28 days (64.3 ± 7.5 vs 70.3 ± 9.3 bpm, $p = 0.01$) and four months (60.6 ± 7.5 vs 67.8 ± 8 bpm, $p = 0.004$) after discharge was considerably lesser in the intervention group.[63] Similarly, outcomes from a one-year follow-up ETHIC-AHF study performed in 71 patients revealed that at one year HR remained considerably lesser in the intervention group (61.8 ± 5.5 vs 68.5 ± 9.3 bpm, $p = 0.01$), and the EF at one year was found considerably greater in the intervention group (48.2 ± 17 vs 41.8 ± 10%, $p = 0.002$).[64] Also, the likelihood of CV death was 26% lesser in the Ivabradine group, although without reaching statistical significance. Both studies showed that the ivabradine and BBs when given in combination are feasible and safe.[65]

Previous studies suggest that the hospital setting provides an important opportunity to initiate GDMT in HFrEF patients. Management with ivabradine in AHF patients had a limited evaluation and less randomized data. Therefore, pre-discharge initiation of ivabradine in the management of heart failure (PRIME-HF) study was performed to report the pre-discharge ivabradine initiation in stabilized AHF patients with EF ≤35%. It was an investigator-initiated, randomized, open-label study of pre-discharge initiation of ivabradine vs usual care. Overall, 104 patients were included in the study. Results showed that at 180 days, 21/52 (40.4%) of patients to pre-discharge initiation were treated with ivabradine compared with 6/52 (11.5%) to usual care, and the pre-discharge initiation group experienced a better decrease in HR through 180 days (mean, −10.0 bpm; 95% CI: −15.7 to −4.3; vs 0.7 bpm; 95% CI: −5.4 to 6.7; $p = 0.011$). Patient-reported outcomes, BB usage/dose, and safety events were similar (all $p > 0.05$). These findings revealed that ivabradine initiation prior to discharge among stabilized HF patients increased ivabradine use at 180 days and lowered HR without reducing BBs or increasing adverse events.[66]

The objective for prescribing BBs and ivabradine both together is due to synergic action at the heart level. BBs decrease HR but they also disturb isovolumic ventricular relaxation and escalate alpha-adrenergic coronary vasoconstriction. Ivabradine protects isovolumic ventricular relaxation because ivabradine does not increase alpha-adrenergic coronary vasoconstriction, as shown by BBs. Furthermore, ivabradine considerably increases stroke volume in patients with severe CHF. The intensification in stroke volume is of clinical relevance, as BBs decrease stroke volume during initiation. This effect of BB could be compensated for by giving ivabradine with lower initial dosages of BBs. Ivabradine reduces LV end-diastolic pressure, which results in a rise in stroke volume and maintenance of cardiac output.[67]

Impact on Rehospitalization

For patients aged >65 years, HF is the most well-known reason for hospital admission. Overall, 80–90% of these hospitalized patients have worsening chronic HF, and only

10–20% have de novo or end-stage HF.[67] Despite current intensive multidrug therapy, persons with HF are frequently admitted to hospital because of exacerbation of their symptoms and, once admitted, are often readmitted.[69] The reported 3-month to 1-year readmission rate has varied between 30 and 50%. Indeed, worsening HF is the most common cause of hospitalization in patients with HF and, when recurrent, presages death. Thus, identifying 'frequent flyers' who are at higher risk for rehospitalization to facilitate transitions of care and the timely implementation of GDMT would be a high priority research area. Frequent flyers define patients with chronic severe HF who have frequent hospital admissions.[70] The clinical course of HF includes a period in which the patient is at greater risk of death or rehospitalization for HF. This period called "vulnerable phase" takes place in the peri-acute HF phase because of microenvironmental deviations in the CV system.[71] The exact duration over which the "vulnerable phase" extends into the post-discharge period is unclear, but limited data suggest that it lasts 2–3 months.[68]

Duration of discharge from the hospital represents the beginning of chronic HF management. Habal et al. in 2014 conducted a study to determine the association of discharge HR with 30-day and 1-year mortality and hospitalization consequences in a cohort of 9,097 patients with HF discharged from hospital. Discharged HR was divided into groups such as 40 to 60, 61 to 70, 71 to 80, 81 to 90, and >90 bpm. A significant increase in all-cause 30-day mortality with adjusted odds ratios (OR) of 1.59 (95% CI: 1.18–2.14; $p = 0.003$) for discharge HR: 81 to 90 bpm and 1.56 (95% CI: 1.13–2.16; $p = 0.007$) for HR >90 bpm when compared with the reference group was observed. One-year ACM (adjusted OR: 1.41; 95% CI: 1.16–1.72; $p <0.001$) and CV death (adjusted OR: 1.47; 95% CI: 1.12–1.92; $p = 0.005$) was greater with discharge HR >90 bpm when compared with the reference group (HR: 40–60 bpm). These results showed that higher discharge HR was linked with more risk of all-cause and CV mortality.[72]

Pulse rate (PR) effect measured during diagnosis and management on outcomes in HFrEF has not been properly determined in a real-world setting. Also, BB use in a real-world situation defining this relation between PR and consequences in HFrEF is not distinguished. Therefore, to describe the association of PR with consequences in HFrEF, Kurgansky et al. conducted an observational study with long-term follow-up using national electronic health record data to assess the assumption that PR measured during diagnosis is related to mortality and hospitalization outcomes in HFrEF patients. An incident HFrEF case was identified. Results revealed that a significant positive, near-linear relationship was found for both baselines and serially measured PR with all-cause mortality. Patients with PR <70 bpm and ≥50% BB target dose had considerably improved mortality outcomes when compared to <50% BB target dose. Also, patients with PR ≥70 bpm who achieved ≥50% BB target dose had significantly more survival than patients with 50% BB target dose. It revealed that high PR during diagnosis and follow-up is strongly related to a higher risk of adverse outcomes in HFrEF patients, independent of the use of BB.[73]

Furthermore, to define the discharge HR and BB dose in patients hospitalized with HF, DeVore et al. analyzed the data from the OPTIMIZE-HF registry. Of the 46,706 hospitalizations involved in the registry, 10,696 met the study criteria. The median HR at discharge was 76 bpm. The main aim was to assess the discharge dose relative to the target dosage. Outcomes revealed that of 10,696 patients, 7,826 (73%) were discharged on a BB. Among patients discharged on BB, 2,886 (37%) patients were discharged on less than 25% of target dosage, 2,639 (34%) on 25 to 49% of target dosage, 1,586 (20%) on 50 to 99% of target dosage, and 715 (9.1%) on 100% of target dosage or greater. These findings revealed that despite management with BB, a considerable number of patients hospitalized with HFrEF had increased HR at discharge.[74]

Despite available therapies and quality development initiatives, early mortality and rehospitalization rates may reach 15 and 30%, respectively, in 90 days post-discharge. Early readmissions are generally linked to congestion, while late readmissions may be linked to progressive HF. Indeed, the discovery of evidence-based treatments and care strategies that especially improve outcomes during the susceptible phase following HF hospitalization has been challenging.[75] Outcomes from the SHIFT study revealed that over about 2-year of follow-up, Ivabradine-treated patients were at significantly lower risk for suffering a second hospitalization for worsening HF than were patients receiving placebo. In addition, treatment with Ivabradine was associated with more days alive out of hospital than with placebo. Also, the risk for suffering a third hospitalization for worsening HF was significantly reduced by ivabradine.[69]

Similarly, Komajda et al. conducted a post-hoc analysis from the SHIFT study examining the effectiveness of Ivabradine in decreasing early consequent rehospitalization following hospitalization for HF. A total of 1,186 patients experienced at least one HF hospitalization. Among these, a total of 334 patients (28%) were rehospitalized within 3-month mostly for CV causes (86%), including HF hospitalization (61%). Ivabradine was related to fewer all-cause hospitalizations at 1-month [Incidence Rate Ratio (IRR): 0.70, 95% CI: 0.50–1.00, p <0.05], 2-month (IRR: 0.75, 95% CI: 0.58–0.98, p = 0.03), and 3-month (IRR: 0.79, 95% CI: 0.63–0.99, p = 0.04. A trend for a decrease in CV and HF hospitalizations were also observed in the patients.[76]

For further determination on the evidence of Ivabradine in HFrEF, Lopatin et al. studied the effect of combined BB and Ivabradine *vs* BBs alone on short- and long-term mortality. A retrospective examination was conducted on 370 hospitalized HF patients with HR ≥70 bpm (150 BB + Ivabradine, 220 BB alone) in the Optimize Heart Failure Care Program. Results showed fewer deaths and HF hospitalizations at 1 month, 3 months, 6 months, and 12 months in patients on BB + Ivabradine *vs* BBs alone. More patients achieved ≥50% target doses of BBs with BB + Ivabradine at 12 months than on admission (82.0% *vs* 66.6%, p = 0.0001). These results showed that BB + Ivabradine combination treatment was related to a substantial decrease in overall mortality and rehospitalization over the consequent 12 months.[77]

Impact on LV Function and QoL

HF significantly diminishes HRQoL, particularly in the regions of physical functioning and vitality. The absence of progress in HRQoL after release from the hospital is a powerful indicator of rehospitalization and fatality. Other determinants of poor HRQoL incorporate depression, more youthful age, higher BMI, greater manifestation burden, lower SBP, low perceived control, and uncertainty about prognosis.[42] HF and LVSD are common conditions, with prevalence in the common people over the age of 45 of at least 2.3% and 1.8%, respectively. The diagnosis of HF patients and LVSD is very poor, effectively malignant, with a median survival of only 1.7 years in men and 3.2 years in women. Few studies with comparative normative results indicate that HF worsens QoL more than other chronic diseases and those women may suffer worse impairment.[78] Continuing symptoms and poor HRQoL indicate that comorbidities may be a significant cause of health and non-CV comorbidities may be associated with

HF-related symptoms.[79] Cardiac remodeling is dominant to the cause of HF and is a well-known prognostic factor in HF patients. The therapeutic effects of beta-blockade, ACE inhibition, and cardiac resynchronization treatment have been related to their valuable effects on cardiac remodeling.[80]

Moreover, to assess the effects of selective HR decrease with Ivabradine on LV remodeling and function, Tardif JC et al. analyzed results from the SHIFT echocardiography substudy. A total of 611 patients' data was included (304 Ivabradine, 307 placebos) for substudy, and echocardiographic data at baseline and 8 months was available only for 411 patients (Ivabradine 208, placebo 203). Results revealed that Ivabradine management decrease LV End Systolic Volume Index (LVESVI) (primary substudy endpoint) vs placebo. Ivabradine also improved LV End Diastolic Volume Index (LVEDVI) and LVEF. The occurrence of the SHIFT primary composite outcome was greater in patients with LVESVI above the median (59 mL/m^2) at baseline (HR: 1.62, 95% CI: 1.03–2.56, $p = 0.04$), and the results indicate a noteworthy decrease in LV volumes and a rise in LVEF during 8-month treatment.[80]

Also, to observe the Ivabradine effect on HR along with health and QoL improvement, different studies were performed such as INTENSIFY, APULIA, and SHIFT. In one study, Ekram I et al. evaluated whether a decrease in HR with Ivabradine can lead to increased HRQoL. In patients with systolic HF treated with recommended therapy, HRQoL was determined by Kansas City Cardiomyopathy Questionnaire (KCCQ) containing the following dimensions: Overall Summary Score (OSS) and Clinical Summary Score (CSS), analyzed at baseline, and 4, 12, and 24 months, and last post-baseline visit. A total of 1,944 patients (968 Ivabradine, 976 placebos) were assessed. Outcomes revealed that Ivabradine reduced HR by 10.1 bpm and improved KCCQ for CSS and 2.4 for OSS. Also, it was seen that health-related QoL at follow-up was better in the Ivabradine group as compared to placebo.[81]

Similarly, in the INTENSIFY study, Zugck C[82] et al. determined the effectiveness and tolerability of Ivabradine and its impact on QoL in chronic systolic heart failure (CHF) patients for 4 months. A total of 1,956 CHF patients were included in the study. In CHF patients, treatment with Ivabradine, RHR, HF symptoms (NYHA class, signs of decompensation), LVEF, Brain Natriuretic Peptide (BNP) values, QoL, and concomitant medication with focus on BB therapy was documented at baseline, after 4 weeks, and after 4 months. As concomitant medication 77.8% were receiving BBs. Other medications included ACE inhibitors or ARBs (83%), diuretics (61%), aldosterone antagonists (18%), and cardiac glycosides (8%). Insufficient HR lowering with a BB was the most common reason for prescribing Ivabradine, documented in 74.6% of patients, followed by decreased exercise capacity in 43.6% and intolerance to high doses of BBs in 40.5%. About 90.4% of patients started with 5 mg, 9.3% with 2.5 mg, and 0.2% with 7.5 mg twice daily. Mean HR of patients was decreased by Ivabradine from 85 ± 11.8 bpm to 72 ± 9.9 bpm after 1 month and 67 ± 8.9 bpm after 4 months at baseline. BNP concentrations were tracked in a subgroup, and values exceeding 400 pg/mL were noted in 53.9% of patients. The mean value of the European QoL-5 dimensions (EQ-5D) QoL index was 0.64 ± 0.28. Also, patients with signs of decompensation decreased to 5.4%, and the proportion of patients with BNP levels [400 pg/mL dropped to 26.7%, accompanied by a shift in NYHA classification towards lower grading (24.0% and 60.5% in NYHA I and II, respectively). EQ-5D index improved to 0.79 ± 0.21. Results showed that Ivabradine efficiently decreases HR and symptoms in CHF patients in daily clinical practice.[82]

Whereas in the APULIA study, Riccioni G[83] et al. assessed the QoL in 221 consecutive CHF patients, randomized into two groups (IVA group: 110 patients; BB group: 111 patients). Nobody was hospitalized during the 1-month study period for CV or other diseases. Results showed that after 1-month of therapy, all treatments in both groups significantly reduced HR, but IVA demonstrated a more significant (p <0.001) decrease in HR compared with BB treatment.[83]

These outcomes from the above studies demonstrated that Ivabradine efficiently decreased HR in CHF patients and helped in the improvement of health and QoL.

Special Population—SHIFT Sub-analysis

HF is a complex clinical syndrome characterized by structural and functional damage of ventricular filling. An increase in cardiac and non-cardiac comorbidities with the advancement of age leads to poor prognosis and alters the response to management in HF. While comorbidities are consistent predictors of morbidity and mortality in HF, their interrelationships with symptoms, functional limitations, and overall health have not been explored.[79,84] SHIFT sub-analysis was used, which is one of the large population's studies, used to examine the effect of Ivabradine in patients with comorbidities such as diabetes, worsening renal function, chronic obstructive pulmonary disease (COPD), systolic blood pressure (SBP), left bundle branch block (LBBB) and severe HF, symptoms, functional limitations, and patient-rated health. Comorbid diabetes, which is present in 20–40% of HF patients, is related to poor outcomes in HF, and vice-versa. Both HF and DM cause the deterioration of renal function, which adversely affects outcomes. DM increases the risk of all-cause mortality, morbidity, and HF hospitalization in HF patients.[84] Therefore, to evaluate the safety and efficacy of Ivabradine in patients with chronic systolic HF and diabetes, Komajda et al. conducted a post-hoc analysis in the SHIFT trial. The primary composite endpoint (PCE) was CV death or HHF. Outcomes revealed that Ivabradine decreases the PCE in patients with and without diabetes (adjusted HR: 0.80, 95% CI: 0.68–0.94 and HR: 0.84, 95% CI: 0.75–0.95, respectively; interaction p was non-significant) vs placebo, and adverse events were significantly more frequent in patients with diabetes (78%) than without (74%) (p <0.001). Thus, comorbid diabetes in chronic HF worsens the diagnosis of systolic HF patients, and regardless of diabetic status, Ivabradine is effective and safe in these patients.[85]

Another comorbid condition causing worsening of HF is renal dysfunction. It is present in approximately 40% of patients with HF. According to meta-analyzes, patients with renal dysfunction have a substantially greater risk of mortality compared to patients having a normal renal function. Voors et al. examined the SHIFT trial to define the association between HR and renal function. A total of 6,505 patients were enrolled in the SHIFT. Follow-up measurements were available in 6,160 patients. Worsening renal function (WRF) was defined as a creatinine increase of ≥0.3 mg/dL and ≥25% from the baseline value. Results showed that WRF was related to a greater risk of the primary composite endpoint of hospitalization for worsening HF or CV death [hazard ratio (HR): 1.38, p <0.001] and of ACM (HR: 1.42, p <0.001). Ivabradine use was related to a reduction in primary composite endpoint in patients both with (HR: 0.82, p = 0.023) and without renal dysfunction (HR: 0.81, p <0.001) at baseline (p for interaction = 0.89). Thus, revealing that in chronic stable SHF patients, HR is directly linked with WRF risk, however, HR decrease by Ivabradine had a neutral effect on renal function during 2 years of follow-up. The beneficial CV effects of Ivabradine were comparable in patients with and without renal dysfunction.[86]

Furthermore, it was known that both CHF and COPD are well-described causes of morbidity and mortality. However, some reports have verified that they frequently coexist, with important prognostic and therapeutic implications. Tavazzi *et al.* performed an analysis of the SHIFT trial to assess (i) the clinical profile of CHF and COPD patients, the usage of drugs in these patients, and the predictive effect of this comorbidity (ii) the comparative effectiveness of a new HR-reducing agent (Ivabradine) in patients with and without COPD, as bradycardic BBs are beneficial in chronic HF patients and COPD is a major barrier to the use of these drugs. It was observed in the study that the primary endpoint and its component, hospitalization for worsening HF, were more common in COPD patients [HR: 1.22 (p = 0.006), and 1.34 (p = 0.001)] respectively, but the relative risk was reduced similarly by Ivabradine in both COPD (14, and 17%) and non-COPD (18% and 27%) patients (p interaction = 0.82, and 0.53, respectively). A similar effect was noted also for CV death. In the Ivabradine group, bradycardia happened more frequently, with a similar occurrence in patients with or without COPD. It determines the link between COPD and HF results in a worse prognosis, and COPD was considered as a barrier to the optimization of BB therapy. Ivabradine was found to be safe and can be prescribed along with BBs in COPD.[87]

Low SBP was also found to be connected with the poor results in HF and complicates management. CHF patients between 15 and 25% also have low SBP <120 mmHg and are at greater risk of in-hospital and post-discharge mortality and morbidity. To conclude the effectiveness and safety of Ivabradine in the SHIFT population, Komajda *et al.* conducted a post-hoc analysis. The analysis included a total of 2,110 patients with SBP <115 mmHg, 1,968 with 115≤ SBP<130 mmHg, and 2,427 with SBP ≥130 mmHg. Younger patients had low SBP, had lower EF when compared to other patients. The study determined that Ivabradine had a similar relative risk reduction of the composite outcome in the three SBP groups. Also, same results were observed for CV mortality (p interaction = 0.91), hospitalization, ACM (p interaction = 0.90), and HF mortality (p interaction = 0.18). Ivabradine is beneficial for HF patients with low blood pressure and elevated HR.[88]

Likewise, it was known that the broadening of the QRS complex because of diminished propagation of interventricular conduction as in LBBB, increases morbidity and mortality in patients with chronic HF. HR reduction with Ivabradine improves outcomes in patients with systolic HF. Therefore, Reil *et al.* conducted a study to define the consequence of LBBB on outcomes in patients with systolic HF and the link between LBBB and the effect of Ivabradine treatment. Patients (n = 6,505) were distributed into groups with (n = 912) or without (n = 5,593) LBBB at baseline, and according to tertiles of HR (70–73, 74–80, and ≥81 bpm). The effect of LBBB, HR, and Ivabradine on the primary endpoint (CV death or HF hospitalization) was examined. As per results, LBBB increased the primary endpoint by 65%, HF hospitalization by 86%, ACM by 49%, and CV mortality by 49% (all p = 0.001). No interaction was observed between the effect of HR on outcomes and LBBB (p = 0.83 for the primary endpoint); thus, LBBB raises the risk for all HRs. Ivabradine was observed to be safe in LBBB. Its effect was directionally similar to that in patients without LBBB but did not reach statistical significance, probably due to lack of power to test this effect because of a few numbers of LBBB patients.[89]

The incidence of CHF progressively increases with growing age and CV morbidity. The care of patients with HF is complex due to cardiac and non-cardiac comorbidities, disabilities, and frailty. Comorbidities increase hospitalization in HF, and non-CV comorbidities lead to preventable hospitalizations. Bohm *et al.* in 2015 evaluated the effect of comorbidities on mortality and morbidity and investigated whether the influence of Ivabradine was affected by comorbidities. Results showed that more comorbidities were present in older patients, women, patients with more advanced HF. CV death were significantly increased (p <0.0001) with comorbidity load. For Ivabradine, the hospitalization rate was lesser at all comorbidity loads. These findings concluded that cardiac and non-cardiac comorbidities considerably affect CV outcomes. A decrease in HR with Ivabradine was continued at all comorbidity loads.[90]

In CHF, HR at baseline influences the Ivabradine's effect on CV outcomes. Therefore, to determine what should be the target HR achieved in HF for improved outcomes, Bohm *et al.* analyzed an Ivabradine effect as per the SHIFT study. Participants of the SHIFT study was divided by BHR ≥75 or <75 bpm. The effect of Ivabradine was investigated for the primary composite endpoint (CV death or HF hospitalization) and other endpoints. Results showed that Ivabradine decrease the primary endpoint, ACM, CV mortality, HF death, and HF hospitalization in ≥75 bpm group. Also, it was observed that Ivabradine-associated risk reductions are related to both HRs achieved and magnitude of HR reduction; patients achieving <60 bpm or displaying a >10 bpm reduction have the best prognosis.[91]

Take Home Pearls

- In patients with CAD and raised lipids, a low-fat diet may delay the recurrence of significant CV events.
- Neurohormonal antagonists (ACEIs, MRAs, and BBs) improve survival in HFrEF patients and are recommended for the management of every patient with HFrFF unless contraindicated or not tolerated.
- HR reduction improves the relationship between force and frequency at the level of failing myocytes, with consequent positive inotropism.
- Elevated HR of 70 bpm or greater despite BB use may represent a new management target in patients in sinus rhythm with HFrEF.
- Ivabradine can be favorable to reduce HF hospitalization for patients with symptomatic (NYHA class II-III) stable chronic HFrEF (LVEF ≤35%).

TAKE HOME SUMMARY

HF is a final common pathway to various heart diseases, and it is a growing problem worldwide with serious consequences where there are limited resources. Right now, around 26 million people globally suffer from HF. Despite improvements in overall healthcare, ironically, the incidence of HF continues to rise in most countries. India is currently in the midst of an epidemiological transition, causing a rapid increase in the prevalence of CV risk factors, CVD, and HF. Data from several registries showed that HF patients in India are younger by 10 years, and the majority of the burden lies below 65 years of age, as compared to the patients from high-income countries. High RHR is related to adverse clinical outcomes in HF patients, and HR reduction is an independent predictive factor in these patients. The management of high RHR in HFrEF patients is a continuing process that requires lifelong medications. BBs and other guideline-recommended HF therapies, including Ivabradine have a vital role in improving outcomes in HFrEF. Target dosages of BBs in HF in clinical studies are rarely achieved due to poor tolerability. As per ESC 2016 guidelines and the 2017 focused update to the 2013 ACCF/AHA guidelines, Ivabradine has been suggested to be used along with BBs for the management of high RHR in HF patients. The beneficial effects of Ivabradine were studied in several randomized and real-world studies, on top of standard of care, as an initial combination with many drugs, and the outcomes of these studies have shown its beneficial impact in improving HR, HF, rehospitalization, or QoL. Ivabradine has a prognostic benefit for HR control as well as prognostic significance for the time required to achieve this control. Likewise, it has been established in several studies that Ivabradine complements the mechanism of action of other drugs.

REFERENCES

1. Inamdar AA, Inamdar AC. Heart failure: Diagnosis, management and utilization. *Journal of Clinical Medicine*. 2016 Jul;5(7):62.
2. Adebayo SO, Olunuga TO, Durodola A, *et al*. Heart failure: Definition, classification, and pathophysiology–A mini-review. *Nigerian Journal of Cardiology*. 2017;14(1):9–14.
3. Ponikowski P, Anker SD, AlHabib KF, *et al*. Heart failure: Preventing disease and death worldwide. *ESC Heart Failure*. 2014 Sep;1(1):4–25.
4. Lippi G, Sanchis-Gomar F. Global epidemiology and future trends of heart failure. *AME Medical Journal*. 2020 June;5:1–6.
5. Dokainish H, Teo K, Zhu J, *et al*. Global mortality variations in patients with heart failure: Results from the International Congestive Heart Failure (INTER-CHF) prospective cohort study. The *Lancet Global Health*. 2017 Jul 1;5(7):E665–E672.
6. Fonarow GC, Corday E, ADHERE® Scientific Advisory Committee. Overview of acutely decompensated congestive heart failure (ADHF): A report from the ADHERE registry. *Heart Failure Reviews*. 2004 Jul;9(3):179–85.
7. Yancy CW, Fonarow GC, ADHERE® Scientific Advisory Committee. Quality of care and outcomes in acute decompensated heart failure: The ADHERE Registry. *Current Heart Failure Reports*. 2004 Sep;1(3):121–8.
8. Lam CS, Anand I, Zhang S, *et al*. Asian sudden cardiac death in heart failure (ASIAN-HF) registry. *European Journal of Heart Failure*. 2013 Aug;15(8):928–36.
9. Tromp J, Tay WT, Ouwerkerk W, *et al*. Multimorbidity in patients with heart failure from 11 Asian regions: A prospective cohort study using the ASIAN-HF registry. *PLoS Medicine*. 2018 Mar 27;15(3):e1002541.
10. Chopra VK, Mittal S, Bansal M, *et al*. Clinical profile and one-year survival of patients with heart failure with reduced ejection fraction: The largest report from India. *Indian Heart Journal*. 2019;71(3):242–8.
11. Harikrishnan S, Bahl A, Roy A, *et al*. National Heart Failure Registry, India: Design and methods. *Indian Heart Journal*. 2019 Dec;71(6):488–91.
12. Harikrishnan S, Sanjay G, Anees T, *et al*. Clinical presentation, management, in-hospital and 90-day outcomes of heart failure patients in Trivandrum, Kerala, India: The Trivandrum Heart Failure Registry. *European Journal of Heart Failure*. 2015 Aug;17(8):794–800.
13. Chaturvedi V, Parakh N, Seth S, *et al*. Heart failure in India: The INDUS (INDia Ukieri Study) study. *J Pract Cardiovasc Sci*. 2016;2(1):28–35.
14. Mishra S, Mohan JC, Nair T, *et al*. Management protocols for chronic heart failure in India. *Indian Heart Journal*. 2018;70(1):105–27.
15. Ziaeian B, Fonarow GC. Epidemiology and aetiology of heart failure. *Nature Reviews Cardiology*. 2016 Jun;13(6):368–78.
16. Ponikowski P, Voors AA, Anker SD, *et al*. 2016 ESC guidelines for the diagnosis and treatment of acute and chronic heart failure: The Task Force for the diagnosis and treatment of acute and

chronic heart failure of the European Society of Cardiology (ESC) Developed with the special contribution of the Heart Failure Association (HFA) of the ESC. *European Heart Journal*. 2016 Jul 14;37(27):2129–200.

17. Prabhakaran D, Jeemon P, Roy A. Cardiovascular diseases in India: Current epidemiology and future directions. *Circulation*. 2016 Apr 19;133(16):1605–20.

18. Seth S, Khanal S, Ramakrishnan S, *et al.* Epidemiology of acute decompensated heart failure in India: The AFAR study (Acute failure registry study). *Journal of the Practice of Cardiovascular Sciences*. 2015 Jan 1;1(1):35–8.

19. Bloom MW, Greenberg B, Jaarsma T, *et al.* Heart failure with reduced ejection fraction. *Nature Reviews Disease Primers*. 2017 Aug 24;3:17058.

20. Greenhalgh T, A'Court C, Shaw S. Understanding heart failure; explaining telehealth—a hermeneutic systematic review. *BMC Cardiovascular Disorders*. 2017 Dec 1;17(1):156.

21. Albakri A. Systolic heart failure: A review of clinical status and meta-analysis of diagnosis and clinical management methods. *Open Access Text*. 2018 Nov 28.

22. Mueller-Werdan U, Stoeckl G, Werdan K. Advances in the management of heart failure: The role of ivabradine. *Vascular Health and Risk Management*. 2016;12:453–70.

23. Tadic M, Cuspidi C, Grassi G. The influence of sex on left ventricular remodeling in arterial hypertension. *Heart Failure Reviews*. 2019 Nov 1;24(6):905–14.

24. Böhm M, Bewarder Y, Kindermann I, *et al.* Optimization of heart failure treatment by heart rate reduction. *International Journal of Heart Failure*. 2020 Jan;2(1):1–11.

25. Nanchen D, Stott DJ, Gussekloo J, *et al.* Resting heart rate and incident heart failure and cardiovascular mortality in older adults: Role of inflammation and endothelial dysfunction: The PROSPER study. *European Journal of Heart Failure*. 2013 May;15(5):581–8.

26. Nanchen D, Leening MJ, Locatelli I, *et al.* Resting heart rate and the risk of heart failure in healthy adults: The Rotterdam Study. *Circulation: Heart Failure*. 2013 May;6(3):403–10.

27. Opdahl A, Venkatesh BA, Fernandes VR, *et al.* Resting heart rate as predictor for left ventricular dysfunction and heart failure: The Multi-Ethnic Study of Atherosclerosis. *Journal of the American College of Cardiology*. 2014 Apr 1;63(12):1182–9.

28. Ho JE, Larson MG, Ghorbani A, *et al.* Long-term cardiovascular risks associated with an elevated heart rate: The Framingham Heart Study. *Journal of the American Heart Association*. 2014 Jun;3(3):e000668.

29. Fox K, Ford I, Steg PG, *et al.* Heart rate as a prognostic risk factor in patients with coronary artery disease and left-ventricular systolic dysfunction (BEAUTIFUL): A subgroup analysis of a randomised controlled trial. *Lancet*. 2008 Sep 6;372(9641):817–21.

30. Fox K, Ford I, Steg PG, *et al.* Ivabradine for patients with stable coronary artery disease and left-ventricular systolic dysfunction (BEAUTIFUL): A randomised, double-blind, placebo-controlled trial. *Lancet*. 2008 Sep 6;372(9641):807–16.

31. Lechat P, Hulot JS, Escolano S, *et al.* Heart rate and cardiac rhythm relationships with bisoprolol benefit in chronic heart failure in CIBIS II Trial. *Circulation*. 2001 Mar 13;103(10):1428–33.

32. Böhm M, Swedberg K, Komajda M, *et al.* Heart rate as a risk factor in chronic heart failure (SHIFT): The association between heart rate and outcomes in a randomised placebo-controlled trial. *Lancet*. 2010 Sep 11;376(9744):886–94.

33. Castagno D, Skali H, Takeuchi M, *et al.* Association of heart rate and outcomes in a broad spectrum of patients with chronic heart failure: Results from the CHARM (Candesartan in Heart Failure: Assessment of Reduction in Mortality and morbidity) program. *Journal of the American College of Cardiology*. 2012 May 15;59(20):1785–95.

34. Rushworth GF, Lambrakis P, Leslie SJ. Ivabradine: A new rate-limiting therapy for coronary artery disease and heart failure. *Therapeutic Advances in Drug Safety*. 2011 Feb;2(1):19–28.

35. Reddy S, Bahl A, Talwar KK. Congestive heart failure in Indians: How do we improve diagnosis and management?. *Indian Journal of Medical Research*. 2010 Nov;132(5):549–60.

36. Huffman MD, Prabhakaran D. Heart failure: Epidemiology and prevention in India. *National Medical Journal of India*. 2010;23(5):283–8.

37. Harikrishnan S, Sanjay G, Anees T, *et al.* Clinical presentation, management, in-hospital and 90-day outcomes of heart failure patients in Trivandrum, Kerala, India: The Trivandrum Heart Failure Registry. *European Journal of Heart Failure.* 2015 Aug;17(8):794–800.

38. Kaul U, Verberk W, Suvarna V, *et al.* India Heart Study—IHS. *Indian Heart Journal.* 2019 Nov; 71:S80–S81.

39. Bhatt AS, DeVore AD, DeWald TA, *et al.* Achieving a maximally tolerated β-blocker dose in heart failure patients: Is there room for improvement? *Journal of the American College of Cardiology.* 2017 May 23;69(20):2542–50.

40. Rao MS, Mandal SC. Epidemiologic surveillance on quality of life in patients with systolic heart failure after treatment with the selective heart rate inhibitor ivabradine. *Journal of the Practice of Cardiovascular Sciences.* 2017 Jan;3(2):100.

41. Seth S, Ramakrishnan S, Parekh N, *et al.* Heart failure guidelines for India: Update 2017. *Journal of the Practice of Cardiovascular Sciences.* 2017;3(3):133–8.

42. Heidenreich PA, Fonarow GC, Breathett K, *et al.* 2020 ACC/AHA Clinical performance and quality measures for adults with heart failure: A report of the American College of Cardiology/ American Heart Association Task Force on performance measures. *Circulation: Cardiovascular Quality and Outcomes.* 2020 Nov;13(11):HCQ. 0000000000000099.

43. Pinto B, Rathi C, Dedhia A. 211 Heart Failure in Young and Elderly–Management strategies.

44. Saleem KA. Pharmacotherapy of chronic heart failure with reduced ejection fraction (HFrEF). *International Journal of Research and Review.* 2020 Feb;7(2):434–48.

45. Borer JS, Khan W. Heart rate in heart failure: A novel cardiovascular risk factor. *Medicographia.* 2011;33:394–400.

46. Ferrari R, Fox K. Heart rate reduction in coronary artery disease and heart failure. *Nature Reviews Cardiology.* 2016 Aug;13(8):493–501.

47. Fox K, Borer JS, Camm AJ, *et al.* Resting heart rate in cardiovascular disease. *Journal of the American College of Cardiology.* 2007 Aug 28;50(9):823–30.

48. Hasenfuss G. Benefit of heart rate reduction in heart failure. *Current Heart Failure Reports.* 2010 Dec;7(4):156–8.

49. DeVore AD, Mi X, Mentz RJ, *et al.* Discharge heart rate and β-blocker dose in patients hospitalized with heart failure: Findings from the OPTIMIZE-HF registry. *American Heart Journal.* 2016 Mar;173:172–8.

50. DeVore AD, Schulte PJ, Mentz RJ, *et al.* Relation of elevated heart rate in patients with heart failure with reduced ejection fraction to one-year outcomes and costs. *American Journal of Cardiology.* 2016 Mar 15;117(6):946–51.

51. Yancy CW, Jessup M, Bozkurt B. 2017 ACC/AHA/HFSA focused update of the 2013 ACCF/ AHA guideline for the management of heart failure: A report of the American College of Cardiology/American Heart Association: Task force on clinical practice guidelines and the Heart Failure Society of America. *Circulation.* 2017;136(6):e137–e161.

52. Sathyamurthy I, Newale S. Ivabradine: Evidence and current role in cardiovascular diseases and other emerging indications. *Indian Heart Journal.* 2018 Dec;70 Suppl 3(Suppl 3):S435-S441.

53. Cavusoglu Y, Altay H, Ekmekçi A, *et al.* Practical approaches for the treatment of chronic heart failure: Frequently asked questions, overlooked points and controversial issues in current clinical practice. *Anatolian Journal of Cardiology.* 2015 Oct;15 Suppl 2:1–60.

54. Swedberg K, Komajda M, Böhm M, *et al.* Ivabradine and outcomes in chronic heart failure (SHIFT): a randomised placebo-controlled study. *Lancet.* 2010 Sep 11;376(9744):875–85.

55. Bouabdallaoui N, O' Meara E, Bernier V, *et al.* Beneficial effects of ivabradine in patients with heart failure, low ejection fraction, and heart rate above 77 bpm. *ESC Heart Failure.* 2019 Dec;6(6):1199–207.

56. Cleland JG, Robertson M, Ford I, *et al.* 246 Effect of Ivabradine on Mortality in Patients with heart failure and a reduced left ventricular ejection fraction not receiving a beta-blocker: An analysis from SHIFT. *European Heart Journal.* 2017 Aug;38(suppl_1).

57. Bohm M, Komajda M, Borer JS, *et al.* SHIFT Duration of chronic heart failure affects outcomes with preserved effects of heart rate reduction with ivabradine: Findings from SHIFT. *European Journal of Heart Failure.* 2018 Feb;20(2):373–81.

58. Böhm M, Borer JS, Camm J, *et al.* Twenty-four-hour heart rate lowering with ivabradine in chronic heart failure: Insights from the SHIFT Holter substudy. *European Journal of Heart Failure.* 2015 May;17(5):518–26.

59. Zugck C, Störk S, Stöckl G, *et al.* Long-term treatment with ivabradine over 12 months in patients with chronic heart failure in clinical practice: Effect on symptoms, quality of life and hospitalizations. *International Journal of Cardiology.* 2017 Aug 1;240:P258–P264.

60. Izumida T, Imamura T, Nakamura M, *et al.* How to consider target heart rate in patients with systolic heart failure. *ESC Heart Failure.* 2020 Oct;7(5):3231–4.

61. Ibrahim NE, Gaggin HK, Turchin A, *et al.* Heart rate, beta-blocker use, and outcomes of heart failure with reduced ejection fraction. *European Heart Journal: Cardiovascular Pharmacotherapy.* 2019 Jan 1;5(1):3–11.

62. Cowie MR. Ivabradine: The start of a SHIFT in heart failure treatment. *Interventional Cardiology.* 2013;5(1):415–26.

63. Volterrani M, Cice G, Caminiti G, *et al.* Effect of Carvedilol, Ivabradine or their combination on exercise capacity in patients with Heart Failure (The CARVIVA HF trial). *International Journal of Cardiology.* 2011 Sep 1;151(2):218–24.

64. Hidalgo FJ, Anguita M, Castillo JC, *et al.* Effect of early treatment with ivabradine combined with beta-blockers versus beta-blockers alone in patients hospitalised with heart failure and reduced left ventricular ejection fraction (ETHIC-AHF): A randomised study. *International Journal of Cardiology.* 2016 Aug 15;217:7–11.

65. Hidalgo FJ, Carrasco F, Castillo JC, *et al.* Early therapy with beta blockers plus ivabradine versus beta blockers alone in patients hospitalised with heart failure and reduced ejection fraction (ETHIC-AHF study): Results at one-year follow-up. *International Journal of Clinical Cardiology.* 2017;4(1):093.

66. Mentz RJ, DeVore AD, Tasissa G, *et al.* PredischaRge initiation of Ivabradine in the ManagEment of Heart Failure: Results of the PRIME-HF Trial. *American Heart Journal.* 2020 May;223:98–105.

67. Volterrani M, Iellamo F. Complementary and synergic role of combined beta-blockers and ivabradine in patients with chronic heart failure and depressed systolic function: A new therapeutic option?. *Cardiac Failure Review.* 2016 Nov;2(2):130–6.

68. Greene SJ, Fonarow GC, Vaduganathan M, *et al.* The vulnerable phase after hospitalization for heart failure. *Nature Reviews Cardiology.* 2015 Apr;12(4):220–9.

69. Borer JS, Böhm M, Ford I, *et al.* Effect of ivabradine on recurrent hospitalization for worsening heart failure in patients with chronic systolic heart failure: The SHIFT Study. *European Heart Journal.* 2012 Nov;33(22):2813–20.

70. Ambrosy AP, Lee KK. Applying data science approaches to identify frequent flyers in heart failure: Rise of the machines. *European Journal of Heart Failure.* 2019 Mar;21:319–21.

71. Lopatin YM, Rosano GM. Treatment of patients in the vulnerable phase (at discharge or early after discharge). *International Cardiovascular Forum Journal* 2017; 10.

72. Habal MV, Liu PP, Austin PC, *et al.* Association of heart rate at hospital discharge with mortality and hospitalizations in patients with heart failure. *Circulation: Heart Failure.* 2014 Jan;7(1):12–20.

73. Kurgansky KE, Schubert P, Parker R, *et al.* Association of pulse rate with outcomes in heart failure with reduced ejection fraction: A retrospective cohort study. *BMC Cardiovascular Disorders.* 2020 Dec;20(1).

74. DeVore AD, Mi X, Mentz RJ, *et al.* Discharge heart rate and β-blocker dose in patients hospitalized with heart failure: Findings from the OPTIMIZE-HF registry. *American Heart Journal.* 2016 Mar;173:172–8.

75. Vaduganathan M, Patel RB, Greene SJ, *et al.* Targeting the vulnerable phase of heart failure: Initiate novel therapies in stable patients prior to hospitalization. *European Journal of Heart Failure.* 2016 Sep;18(9):1190–2.

76. Komajda M, Tavazzi L, Swedberg K, *et al*. Chronic exposure to ivabradine reduces readmissions in the vulnerable phase after hospitalization for worsening systolic heart failure: A post-hoc analysis of SHIFT. *European Journal of Heart Failure*. 2016 Sep;18(9):1182–9.

77. Lopatin YM, Cowie MR, Grebennikova AA, *et al*. Optimization of heart rate lowering therapy in hospitalized patients with heart failure: Insights from the Optimize Heart Failure Care Program. *International Journal of Cardiology*. 2018 Jun 1;260:113–7.

78. Hobbs FD, Kenkre JE, Roalfe AK, *et al*. Impact of heart failure and left ventricular systolic dysfunction on quality of life. A cross-sectional study comparing common chronic cardiac and medical disorders and a representative adult population. *European Heart Journal*. 2002 Dec;23(23):1867–76.

79. Lawson CA, Solis-Trapala I, Dahlstrom U, *et al*. Comorbidity health pathways in heart failure patients: A sequences-of-regressions analysis using cross-sectional data from 10,575 patients in the Swedish Heart Failure Registry. *PLoS Medicine*. 2018 Mar 27;15(3):e1002540.

80. Tardif JC, O'Meara E, Komajda M, *et al*. Effects of selective heart rate reduction with ivabradine on left ventricular remodelling and function: Results from the SHIFT echocardiography substudy. *European Heart Journal*. 2011 Oct;32(20):2507–15.

81. Ekman I, Chassany O, Komajda M, *et al*. Heart rate reduction with ivabradine and health related quality of life in patients with chronic heart failure: Results from the SHIFT study. *European Heart Journal*. 2011 Oct;32(19):2395–404.

82. Zugck C, Martinka P, Stöckl G. Ivabradine treatment in a chronic heart failure patient cohort: Symptom reduction and improvement in quality of life in clinical practice. *Advances in therapy*. 2014 Sep;31(9):961–74.

83. Riccioni G, Masciocco L, Benvenuto A, *et al*. Ivabradine improves quality of life in subjects with chronic heart failure compared to treatment with β-blockers: Results of a multicentric observational APULIA study. *Pharmacology*. 2013;92(5–6):276–80.

84. Mehrotra S, Sharma TM, Bahl A. Impact of comorbidities in heart failure–prevalence, effect on functional status, and outcome in indian population: A single-center experience. *Journal of Clinical and Preventive Cardiology*. 2019;8(4):166–72.

85. Komajda M, Tavazzi L, Francq BG, *et al*. Efficacy and safety of ivabradine in patients with chronic systolic heart failure and diabetes: An analysis from the SHIFT trial. *European Journal of Heart Failure*. 2015 Dec;17(12):1294–301.

86. Voors AA, van Veldhuisen DJ, Robertson M, *et al*. The effect of heart rate reduction with ivabradine on renal function in patients with chronic heart failure: An analysis from SHIFT. *European Journal of Heart Failure*. 2014 Apr;16(4):426–34.

87. Tavazzi L, Swedberg K, Komajda M, *et al*. Clinical profiles and outcomes in patients with chronic heart failure and chronic obstructive pulmonary disease: An efficacy and safety analysis of SHIFT study. *International Journal of Cardiology*. 2013 Dec 10;170(2):182–8.

88. Komajda M, Böhm M, Borer JS, *et al*. Efficacy and safety of ivabradine in patients with chronic systolic heart failure according to blood pressure level in SHIFT. *European Journal of Heart Failure*. 2014 Jul;16(7):810–6.

89. Reil JC, Robertson M, Ford I, *et al*. Impact of left bundle branch block on heart rate and its relationship to treatment with ivabradine in chronic heart failure. *European Journal of Heart Failure*. 2013 Sep;15(9):1044–52.

90. Böhm M, Robertson M, Ford I, *et al*. Influence of cardiovascular and noncardiovascular co-morbidities on outcomes and treatment effect of heart rate reduction with ivabradine in stable heart failure (from the SHIFT Trial). *American Journal of Cardiology*. 2015 Dec 15;116(12):1890–97.

91. Böhm M, Borer J, Ford I, *et al*. Heart rate at baseline influences the effect of ivabradine on cardiovascular outcomes in chronic heart failure: Analysis from the SHIFT study. *Clinical Research in Cardiology*. 2013 Jan;102(1):11–22.

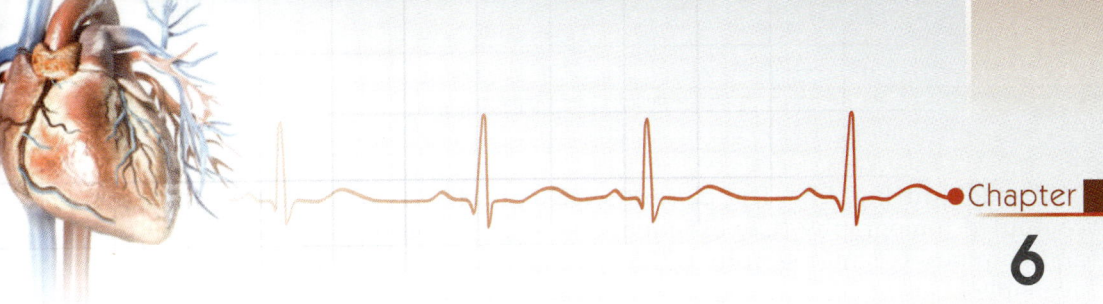

Heart Rate and other Clinical Scenarios

Dr. Brian Pinto

Learning Objectives

At the end of this chapter one should be able to:

- Heart rate (HR) in other cardiovascular (CV) and non-CV scenarios
- HR modulation in CVD beyond CAD and HFrEF
- HR modulation in non-CV conditions
- Take home summary

HEART RATE (HR) IN OTHER CARDIOVASCULAR (CV) AND NON-CV SCENARIOS

HR is regulated by the autonomic nervous system (ANS) and reflects the metabolic demands of the body. In turn, coronary blood flow and myocardial oxygen consumption are also affected by high HR. It is related to CV outcomes in all the stages of the CV continuum, besides in patients with other CV disorders such as supraventricular tachycardia, valvular diseases, cardiogenic shock, and non-CV disorders such as pulmonary, cerebrovascular, renal disease, sepsis, cancer, and erectile dysfunction. Thus, HR can be considered as a potential risk factor and therapeutic target in other conditions beyond heart failure (HF) and coronary artery disease (CAD). Nevertheless, the HR-risk association suggests testing the concept of HR reduction in other conditions like acute illness, including cardiogenic shock, or chronic conditions, such as pulmonary disease, erectile dysfunction, provided that patients are stable enough to tolerate HR reduction. Since the latter conditions are frequent comorbidities in chronic heart failure (CHF), it is interesting to observe that HR reduction reduces outcomes in patients with different comorbidity loads.[1]

Recently, analysis of heart rate variability (HRV) has been developed as a valued non-invasive tool to determine autonomic status. It has become progressively clear that several CV disorder states are related to typical deviations in HRV. For instance, HF is categorized by HRV changes indicative of sympathetic activation and vagal withdrawal. The same is true for other CV and non-CV conditions. Moreover, HRV has a prognostic value, and pharmacological interventions may improve HRV, in particular the vagal components.[2] For instance, decreased HRV in mitral stenosis patients with sinus rhythm suggests increased sympathetic activity in patients susceptible to atrial fibrillation (AF), whereas a noticeable rise of HRV in AF patients suggest that the ventricular rhythm has a respiratory linked periodicity, and major parasympathetic activity may modify the intrinsic behavior of the atrioventricular

(AV) node during AF.[3] The patient's HR and HRV play a vital role in cardiac computed tomography (CT) examinations, e.g. CT coronary artery calcium (CAC) and coronary CT angiography (CTA), because of the limit of temporal resolution available in current CT systems.[4] An elevated HR may impair left ventricular (LV) diastolic filling (with a decrease in stroke volume), compromise coronary blood flow, and increase myocardial oxygen demand in patients with sepsis.[5] Throughout the early sepsis, HR changes were predictive for 48-hour mortality. In the first 4-hour of sepsis, a rise in HR ≥50 bpm indicates death with sensitivity and specificity of 88%.[6] Higher resting heart rate (RHR) in significant aortic regurgitation (AR) was independently associated with mortality and provided incremental value to guideline-recommended surgical triggers. Thus, higher RHR in AR is not benign and should be integrated into therapeutic considerations.[7] Therefore, HR modulation is important in many CV conditions/procedures and non-CV conditions beyond HF and CAD (Fig. 6.1).

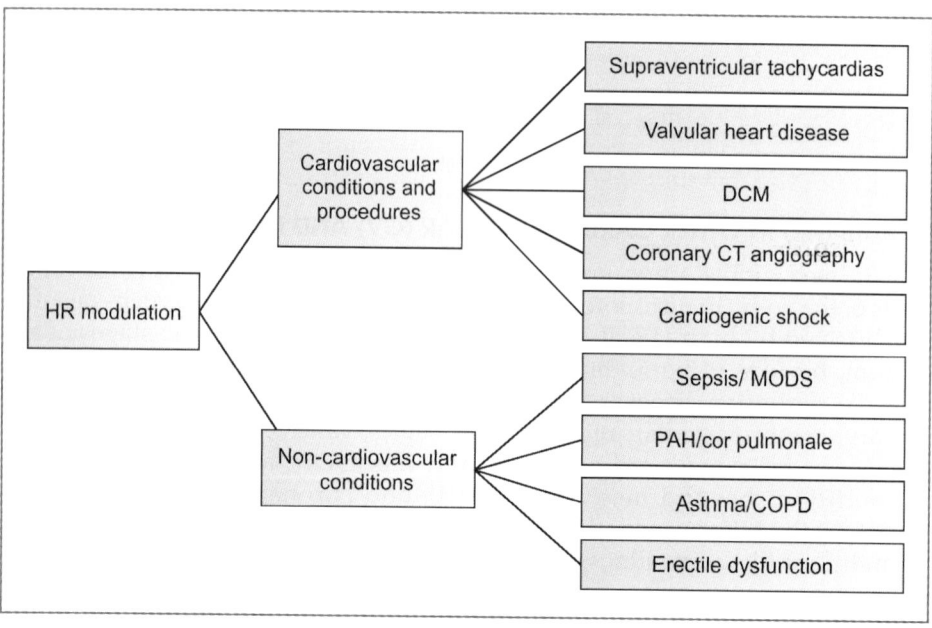

Fig. 6.1: HR modulation in other CV and non-CV conditions. DCM: Dilated cardiomyopathy; CT: Computed tomography, PAH: Pulmonary arterial hypertension; COPD: Chronic obstructive pulmonary disease; MODS: Multiple organ dysfunction syndrome

Take Home Pearls

- HR reveals the metabolic demands of the body and is controlled by the ANS.
- HR is related to CV consequences in all the steps of the CV continuum, besides in patients with pulmonary, cerebrovascular, renal disease, sepsis, cancer, and erectile dysfunction.
- Various CV and non-CV disorders related to high HR requiring HR variation other than CAD and HF.

HR MODULATION IN CVD BEYOND CAD AND HF WITH REDUCED EJECTION FRACTION (HFrEF)

An elevated HR is an indicator of CV risk in stable CAD patients. A high RHR is a marker of risk in patients with HF, asymptomatic LV Systolic Dysfunction (LVSD), stable CAD, and in subjects with CV risk factors. Indeed, a rise in HR indicates various pathophysiological variations that cause adverse cardiac events. These adverse cardiac events include an increase of oxidative stress, plaque instability, endothelial dysfunction, higher myocardial oxygen consumption, decrease in diastole duration with consequent reduction of coronary perfusion, remodeling and hypertrophy of LV, reduction of LV filling duration, and decrease of myocardial contractility. By counteracting these unfavorable mechanisms, HR modulation may improve symptoms and outcomes.[8]

Also, HR modulation is necessary for patients with other CV conditions such as supraventricular tachycardia (SVT), valvular diseases, cardiogenic shock. SVT is a fast HR (tachycardia) commonly occurred when electrical impulses produced at or over the AV hub is out of synch. At the point when an individual goes into this arrhythmia, the heartbeat at the rate of at least 100 beats per minute (bpm) and can be as high as 300 bpm. Individuals with SVT may go into this arrhythmia now and again unrelated to exercise, stress, or other basic reasons for fast HR.[9] Also, decreased HRV is a reflection of enhanced sympathetic overdrive and decreased vagal activity, which has a strong association with the cause of ventricular arrhythmias in common people and especially in cardiac patients.[10] Thus, HR modulation is necessary for patients with other CV disorders such as SVT, valvular diseases, cardiogenic shock. Here, we are going to discuss HR modulation in various CV conditions beyond HF and CAD.

Supraventricular Tachycardias (SVTs)

Supraventricular arrhythmias are very common and patients are usually symptomatic, needed treatment with drugs and electrophysiological procedures. The term 'SVT' literally indicates tachycardia (atrial rates >100 bpm at rest), the mechanism of which includes tissue from the His bundle or above. The SVT occurrence is 2.25/1,000 persons, and the incidence is 35/100,000 person-years in common people. Females have a two times higher risk of evolving SVT as compared to males. Aged individuals have a five times higher risk of developing SVT as compared to younger persons. Patients with lone paroxysmal SVT are younger, have a more rapid SVT rate, and have prior arrival of symptoms based on a range of factors and may result in palpitations, fatigue, light-headedness, chest discomfort, dyspnea, and altered consciousness. Usually, SVT has been used to define all types of tachycardias other than ventricular tachycardia (VT) and AF. Thus, it comprised of tachycardias, for example, AV re-entry because of accessory connections, which is not, in essence, a supraventricular rhythm (Fig. 6.2).[11]

Management recommendations should be considered in the perspective of frequency and extent of the SVT, along with clinical signs, for instance, symptoms or adverse effects. Diltiazem, verapamil, and oral beta-blockers (BBs) are used in the ongoing treatment of patients with symptomatic SVT. Sotalol is used for ongoing treatment in patients who do not prefer catheter ablation. Oral amiodarone is used in patients in whom BBs, diltiazem, dofetilide, flecainide, propafenone, sotalol, or verapamil are contraindicated. Oral digoxin is recommended in ongoing treatment in patients with symptomatic SVT who do not prefer catheter ablation.[12]

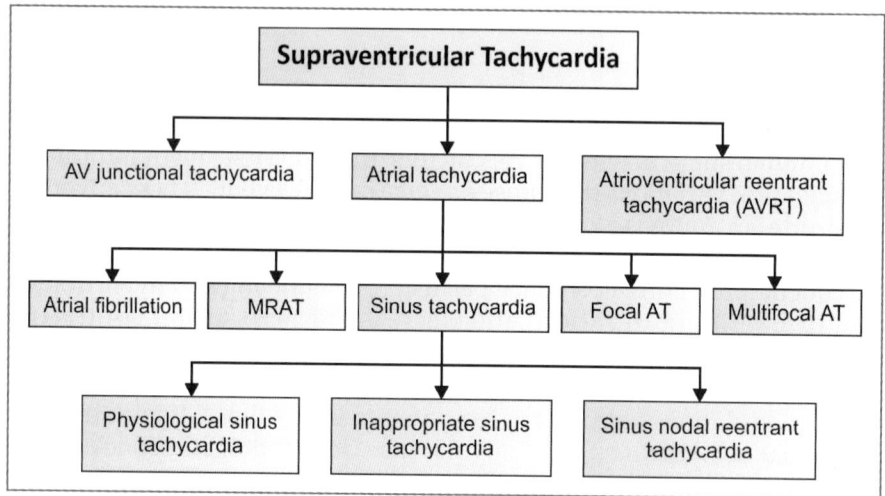

Fig. 6.2: Conventional classification of SVT. AT: Atrial tachycardia; AV: Atrioventricular

Unlike common tachyarrhythmias such as AF, treatment options for inappropriate sinus tachycardia (IST), persistent sinus tachycardia (PST), postural orthostatic tachycardia syndrome (POTS), and other uncommon tachyarrhythmias are less clear. These tachycardias are more common in younger adults, particularly women, who have poorly understood pathophysiologic mechanisms, and significantly lower quality of life (QoL). Furthermore, treatment options with standard rate-slowing medications (e.g. BBs) are useless, poorly tolerated, or both. Therefore, the efficacy and tolerability of Ivabradine for HFrEF and ischemic heart disease (IHD) have prompted studies evaluating its use as a treatment option for several tachycardias.[13]

Inappropriate Sinus Tachycardia (IST)

IST is a clinical syndrome deficient in prescribed analytic criteria. It is generally described as an elevated RHR [hazard ratio (HR): >90–100 bpm] with an inflated response to physical or emotional stress and a clear sinus mechanism.[14] It is a chronic medical condition and linked with significant loss of QoL. Clinical manifestations range from patients who are asymptomatic to suffering incapacitating incessant tachycardia. Common complaints include palpitations, light-headedness, presyncope, syncope, orthostatic intolerance, chest pain/pressure, dyspnea, and exercise intolerance. Noncardiac symptoms are frequent as well, such as anxiety, depression, abdominal discomfort, myalgia, and headache. An Icelandic study of randomly sampled patients from insurance registries for hypertension estimated the prevalence of IST to be 1.16%, with no difference between IST and the control group in age, gender, and physical activity.[16]

IST has been assumed to be relatively uncommon among the general people, but no earlier studies concerning the occurrence of IST are present. The disease is not related to structural heart disease. Patients with this clinical syndrome are young, 20–45 years old and over 90% of patients are female. Also, there is a disproportionate occurrence of IST in health care professionals, such as cardiac nurses and physiotherapists. The explanation for these findings is lacking, but it can be selection bias. Recently, Lopera *et al.* reported four elderly females (aged 61–71 years) with long-standing IST, representing them as a unique subgroup within the IST patient population. Thus, IST included a wide spectrum of patient populations, such as elderly and younger subjects.[17]

The primary cause of IST is yet to be completely understood. However. Though, the causes can be divided into two groups: either as an intrinsic increase in sinus node automaticity or an extrinsic cause (sympathovagal imbalance, decreased parasympathetic tone, increased sympathetic receptor sensitivity, and impaired neurohormonal modulation). Among extrinsic causes is evolving proof that immunoglobulin G (IgG) anti-β receptor antibodies activate positive chronotropic action by prompting long-lasting increment in cyclic adenosine monophosphate (cAMP), which facilitates calcium influx and depolarization causing constant activation of the β-adrenergic receptor without desensitization.[16] The latest study discovered a familial form of IST linked with a gain-of-function mutation in the Hyperpolarization-activated Cyclic Nucleotide-gated channel 4 (HCN4) pacemaker channel causing greater sensitivity to the second messenger cAMP, which further causes a rise in the sympathetic drive.[16]

The management of IST is complex and remains a considerable challenge mostly because IST is a multifaceted condition. HR control does not always cause the elimination of symptoms. Treatment includes non-pharmacological and pharmacological interventions and lifestyle alteration.[16] Management options are very less in IST. Initially, it is recommended to decrease caffeine and other stimulant intakes, engage in regular exercise activities, and maintain adequate fluid and salt intake. The use of β-adrenergic blockers is not preferred because they are linked with various adverse effects. Benzodiazepines may be helpful, but this drug class has not been assessed carefully.[18] The European Society of Cardiology (ESC) 2019 guidelines recommend Ibutilide (IV), or IV or oral (in-hospital) Dofetilide for the alteration of atrial flutter. Ibutilide (IV) is recommended for acute therapy of focal AT. Recently ESC 2019 guidelines have recommended Ivabradine alone or in combination with a BB in symptomatic patients with IST.[11]

Pharmacologic HR reduction can be attained by BBs or non-dihydropyridine calcium channel blockers (CCBs). However, both classes of drugs are nonspecific inhibitors of pacemaker activity in the sinoatrial (SA) node resulting in cardiac and systemic side effects including negative inotropy, AV block, hypotension, bronchospasm, fatigue, depression, and sexual dysfunction. Ivabradine is a specific and selective inhibitor of the HCN channels, which generate a funny current (I_f), also called a pacemaker current. HCN channels, especially isoform HCN4, are highly expressed in the SA node and are the utmost important channels involved in pacemaker activity. Inhibition of HCN channels causes a decline of I_f and therefore prolongs the spontaneous diastolic depolarization of SA node cells resulting in a reduced HR without negative effects on inotropy, AV conduction, or blood pressure (BP).[16]

Ivabradine acts by preventing the I_f current results in a decrease in HR and improvement in signs and QoL.[16] It is a first-in-class selective and specific inhibitor of the I_f current, a hyperpolarization-activated current that regulates the pacemaker activity of the SA node. By inhibiting I_f, Ivabradine slows spontaneous firing of pacemaker cells causing a dose-dependent reduction in HR.[8] Multiple studies, including randomized trials, have reported its efficacy in IST.[13] Though Ivabradine is currently indicated only in the treatment of chronic heart failure (CHF) and chronic stable angina pectoris, its effect has been studied in other conditions, which have been discussed in this chapter. Boeken U *et al.* 2019 conducted a study to assess the effects and side-effects of ivabradine in patients with IST after heart transplantation (htx). Between 10/2010 and 9/2018, 115 patients underwent htx. Ivabradine was administered in 50 patients immediately after htx along with BBs in 20 patients. Mean HR was decreased from 115.7 ± 13.3 bpm at baseline to 89.0 ± 10.1 bpm before hospital discharge (p <0.05) and to 81.2 ± 7.6 bpm at first follow-up. The percentage of HR reduction correlated with initial HR and was more pronounced compared to patients with only metoprolol. The findings of the study revealed that patients with IST after htx can be successfully cured with ivabradine. Reducing the RHR, IST does negatively influence cardiac contractility and conductance.[13]

Patients with IST cured with ivabradine showed both HR normalization and QoL improvement. Benezet-Mazuecos J conducted a study evaluate the long-term effect of Ivabradine on HR control and clinical status in patients detected with IST. Twenty-four patients (18 women, 41 ± 13-year-olds) were diagnosed with IST according to current guidelines criteria. The patients were prescribed 5–7.5 mg of ivabradine twice a day. Twenty-four-hour Holter recordings and the SF-36 health survey were done at 6 months to estimate both HR control and clinical status. Holter recordings before and after 6 months on treatment showed a significant reduction in the average maximal HR of 155 ± 18 bpm vs 132 ± 16 bpm, mean HR of 97 ± 6 bpm vs 79 ± 8 bpm (mean daytime HR of 103 ± 8 bpm vs 84 ± 10 bpm) and minimal HR of 58 ± 12 bpm vs 48 ± 7 bpm (Wilcoxon analysis, p <0.05). The SF-36 mean score showed a significant improvement on Ivabradine treatment (57 ± 23 vs 76 ± 20), with better physical and mental status scores (56 ± 25 vs 74 ± 22 and 58 ± 24 vs 78 ± 18, respectively) (Wilcoxon analysis, p <0.001). Patients were advised to stop management after one year to re-examine the situation. Only two patients (20%) stayed on IST criteria. Ivabradine treatment showed both HR normalization and QoL improvement. After 1-year, stopping ivabradine unpredictably revealed that HR remained within the normal limits in 80% of the patients.[19]

IST is described by an increased HR at rest and an extravagant HR response to physical activity or emotional stress. BBs and CCBs are first-line therapy but at times are poorly tolerated because of side effects. Ivabradine is currently indicated only in the management of CHF and chronic stable angina pectoris, but its effect has also been studied in IST. Calo L et $al.$ in 2010 performed a study to estimate the effectiveness and safety of ivabradine in IST patients. The study enrolled a total of eighteen sequential symptomatic patients affected by IST. A total of sixteen patients finished the study. Holter ECG evaluation revealed a substantial decrease of medium HR (p <.001) and maximal HR (p <.001, basal vs 3–6 months; p = .02, 3 vs 6 months). Minimal HR slightly decreased at 3 months and then stabilized (p = .49, 3 vs 6 months) despite an increased drug dose. The stress test presented a substantial decrease at rest (p <.001) and maximal HR (p <.05), signifying an increased tolerance to physical stress, which was confirmed by a progressive increase of maximal load reached (>100 W) during the stress test at 3 months (75%) and 6 months (85%). The study indicated that Ivabradine is an effective and safe substitute to CCBs and BBs for the management of IST.[20]

Furthermore, to evaluate the effect of Ivabradine treatment on the prevention of tachycardia episodes in patients with IST, Grigoryan S et $al.$ in 2018 conducted a prospective controlled study. A total of 51 patients (39 women and 12 men) with IST without structural heart disease (mean age 33.3 ± 9.7) were enrolled and distributed into two groups. The first group was prescribed ivabradine (Group A) daily dose of

10 mg, and the second group has administrated bisoprolol (Group B) daily dose of 5 mg for 36 weeks. The obtained results showed shown that the baseline data of daily maximum and mean HR in both groups was 166 ± 5 bpm, 95 ± 4 bpm, and 172 ± 3 bpm, 96 ± 3 bpm accordingly. After 36 weeks of management with Ivabradine, these indices were considerably decreased in the first group 104 ± 11 bpm, 72 ± 12 bpm; $p < 0.01$. The follow-up during 36 weeks had revealed that the tachycardia episodes (primary endpoint) in the Ivabradine group decreased by 12% compared to group Bisoprolol, where episodes decreased by 3.6%. The outcomes of the trial confirmed that the long-term treatment with both ivabradine and bisoprolol significantly decreases the initial values of HR, but ivabradine decreases the frequency of IST recurrence.[13]

Some patients can have persistent sinus tachycardia without any underlying illness or structural heart disease and are classified as having IST.[21] PST is often present in patients (pts) with Lung Cancer (LC) due to hypoxia, inflammation, bronchodilators. On the other side, Ivabradine is successfully used to decrease tachycardia in stable angina and HF, but its effect has also been studied in PST.[13] Tase A et al. conducted a retrospective study in 2016 to investigate the long-term impact of Uninterrupted Ivabradine Treatment (UIT) on PST in LC patients. A total of 144 consecutive pts with LC of any type and at any stage was retrospectively analyzed, treated with UIT for PST for 48 months. HR significantly lowered in UIT pts vs the control group. The most spectacular decrease of HR with UIT was in the group of pts with HR 111–120 bpm. This effect remained stable in the long-term follow-up, while BP, cardiac conduction (ECG), myocardial contractility (LVEF) was not affected. No aggravation of dyspnea, wheezing, or sibilant rales were observed in the UIT group. The study revealed that UIT appears to be a safe and feasible long-term therapeutic option for treating PST in LC pts. UIT is considered an alternative to BBs in this clinical setting, by reducing the RHR without impairing cardiac parameters and airway physiology.[13]

Postural Orthostatic Tachycardia Syndrome (POTS)

POTS are a disorder in which the ANS fails to compensate for upright body position. It is characterized by an extreme increase in HR (tachycardia) to a rate of more than 120 bpm after standing (5~30 min). Patients with POTS show various signs ranging from mild to severe. The most common primary condition is cerebral hypoperfusion caused due to extreme tachycardia, neurological dysfunction. These symptoms include diaphoresis, light-headedness, tremor, palpitations, fatigue, exercise intolerance, near syncope, and recurrent syncope in an upright position. POTS patients may also suffer from mental clouding ("brain fog"), blurred vision, shortness of breath, early satiety, nausea, headache, and chest discomfort. Other signs include anxiety, flushing, postprandial hypotension, lower back pain, aching neck and shoulders, cold hands (and often feet and nose), and hypovolemia.

The incidence of POTS is unidentified. In clinical practice, it is probably about 5–10 times as common as orthostatic hypotension (OH). Robertson et al. have described that nearly 500,000 Americans may suffer from POTS. If this occurrence is employed, there could be over 200,000 Japanese suffering from POTS. Almost 75 to 80% of POTS patients are women; thus, the typical POTS patient is somewhere between menarche and menopause. The reasons for its female majority are uncertain, though women are more susceptible to orthostatic stress. Relations with the menstrual cycle are not recognized yet, however, some female patients reported an increase of symptoms in the premenstrual phase. Recently interpreted that POTS was first described in adults, but as per pediatric cases, POTS is a common form of orthostatic intolerance (OI) during upright tilt in adolescents with Chronic Fatigue Syndrome (CFS). In adults with CFS, approximately 25% of patients exhibit typical signs of POTS.[22]

Changing diet, improved eating habits, and increasing liquid intake benefits people with POTS. Eating small meals reduces the severity of postprandial hypotension as the amount of blood required for digestion is decreased. It is also helpful in POTS patients with hypovolemia. Sodium chloride 0.9% infusion has been useful in decreasing symptoms in POTS patients and improving QoL. Freitas et al. stated that sodium chloride 0.9% infusion was most efficient between a variety of treatments, producing a decrease in HR and decreasing systolic BP variability in POTS patients. BBs are beneficial in management for POTS patients as they possess beta-receptor super-sensitivity, high noradrenaline levels and/or hyper-adrenergic states. Though BBs may worsen hypotension and decrease renin levels. Thus, BBs should be used with caution in patients with low BP and/or plasma renin. Several GPs combine salt tablets with Fludrocortisone to confirm its efficiency, though this must be determined by salt intake. Sometimes, pyridostigmine bromide is used to treat POTS as it increases the outcome of acetylcholine by preventing its breakdown. Pyridostigmine bromide enhances the agonist activity and overcomes the blockage of these receptors. Therefore, it is useful for POTS patients of post-viral, paraneoplastic, or autoimmune forms. Ivabradine, a sinus node blocker, improves the symptoms in POTS patients as there is a presence of sinus tachycardia in some POTS patients. Ivabradine may be better than BBs as it decreases the HR without negative inotropic effects, sexual disturbance, and vasodilation, which is usually related to BB.[23]

According to ESC 2019 guidelines, a regular and progressive exercise program should be performed. The consumption of ≥2–3 L of water and 10–12 g of sodium chloride daily may be recommended. ESC 2019 guidelines recommended Midodrine, low-dose non-selective BB, or Pyridostigmine. Ivabradine may be considered, but Ivabradine has not been approved in India or elsewhere in the world for the given condition.[11] Recently, ivabradine is recommended only in the treatment of CHF and chronic stable angina pectoris, but its effect has also been studied in other conditions.

Some studies identify and evaluating the usage of ivabradine to treat POTS. Barzilai M et al. conducted a study in which Ivabradine's effect on the hemodynamics and sympathovagal balance in POTS patients were assessed. It was an open-label trial, without a placebo control, enrolled a total of eight patients with POTS. Patients were prescribed a single oral dose of 7.5 mg ivabradine. Description of symptoms, autonomic function tests, hemodynamic, and HR and BP variability was examined in a supine position. Ivabradine reduced the HR of POTS patients at rest by 4 ± 1 bpm ($p < 0.05$). HR reduced from 118 ± 4 bpm to 101 ± 5 bpm ($p < 0.01$) in 5 minutes head-up tilt. The study revealed that ivabradine is an effective medication for decelerating the HR of POTS patients at rest and during tilting, without showing any adverse effects. Furthermore, ivabradine exerts its effects without inducing the sympathovagal balance.[24]

Ivabradine is selective I_f channel blocker that reduces HR without disturbing other CV functions. It was presented to improve signs in patients with postural tachycardia syndrome (POTS) as per various case reports and case series. Ruzieh M et al. conducted a retrospective study that enrolled patients who were identified with POTS and received ivabradine as part of their treatment were examined. Forty-nine patients (47 females, 95.9%) received ivabradine. The average age was 35.1 ± 10.35 years. The symptoms observed were palpitations and light-headedness, and both improved significantly, with 88.4% and 76.1% response rate, respectively. A total of 38 patients reported improvement in their symptoms. Also, ivabradine resulted in an objective decrease in sitting and standing HR (78.1 ± 10.7 *vs* 72.5 ± 7.6, *p*-value: 0.01) and (107.4 ± 14.1 *vs* 95.1 ± 13.7, *p*-value: <0.001), respectively, with no significant change in BP. Outcomes revealed that Ivabradine is efficient in managing patients with POTS. Nearly 78% of this cohort reported a significant improvement in symptoms with no major adverse effects.[25]

Valvular Heart Disease (VHD)

VHDs as a group are among the most expected reasons for HF. They are also potentially lethal, particularly in patients who have been conservatively managed because of sudden death in patients having VHDs, which is very common even in the absence of other risk factors.[26] VHDs are the primary cause of morbidity and mortality in India. Rheumatic heart diseases (RHD) continue to be the dominant form in developing nations. Data obtained by echocardiography, some autopsy, and surgical pathology are the rich source of studying the incidence of VHD. The incidence of RHD varies among different nations. In developed countries, there is a decrease in the incidence of rheumatic fever and the prevalence of RHD, but in developing countries, RHD has continued to be a major health concern. In India, the occurrence of rheumatic fever and RHD among school children is 2–11 per 1,000 with a mean of 6 per 1,000. The ICMR has conducted three school-based surveys in children 5 to 14 years in age over 40 years between 1970 and 2010. The first survey from 1972 to 1975 was in schools at Agra, Alleppey, Bombay (Mumbai), Delhi, and Hyderabad. The second survey from 1984 to 1987 was in schools at Vellore, Delhi, and Varanasi. The third study enrolled children from 10 centers in the country located at Jodhpur, Shimla, Jammu, Kochi, Chandigarh, Indore, Wayanad, Mumbai, Vellore, and Dibrugarh. It had a wider coverage, but not of the entire country. In the first study (1972–1975), 133,000 children were evaluated, and the prevalence of RHD varied from 0.8 to 11/1,000, overall, 5.3/1,000. The second study (1984–1987) included 53,786 children, and the prevalence ranged from 1.0 to 5.6/1,000 overall 2.9/1,000. The third and the largest study enrolled 176,904 school children with a prevalence varying from 0.13 to 1.5/1,000 (Overall 0.9/1,000) in the 5 to 14 years age range. The data suggest a decrease in RHD from 5.3 to 2.9 to below 1.0/1,000 between 1970 and 2010. In a study on 118,212 school children, a heart murmur was observed in 389 normal children of 4–18 years in age. Echo evaluation identified 61 children with RHD giving an incidence of 0.5/1,000 children in Uttar Pradesh. The studies from Punjab, Gujarat, Rajasthan, Uttar Pradesh, and Tamil Nadu have found the prevalence ranged from 0.67 to 4.54/1,000 children.[27]

Although the aortic and mitral valves are most commonly implicated, the tricuspid and pulmonic valves can also be dysfunctional, leading to adverse outcomes.[26] Structural VHD may deteriorate the clinical status of patients with HF. Patients with HF with VHD are at higher risk of events, including sudden cardiac death.[27] A detailed understanding of the several valvular disorders is essential in the treatment of patients with VHD. It is also important to know the role of the therapeutic interventions *vs* the natural history of the disease in the assessment of outcomes.[29] Non-invasive diagnostic modalities, for instance, echocardiography, cardiac magnetic resonance, and exercise tolerance testing deliver quantitative, qualitative, and prognostic data.[30] Patients with symptomatic valve lesions should be referred to specialist assessment. In most cases, medical therapy serves as a link to definitive mechanical or surgical therapy.[31]

Among different mechanisms affected or modified by aortic-valve disease, the autonomic regulation, as evaluated by HRV, has been mainly examined in patients manifesting severe aortic valve stenosis. HRV is the interval variations between consecutive heartbeats. These variations in the HR are controlled by many mechanisms such as interaction with the respiratory cycle, the baroreflex mechanism, and the ANS modulation of the sinus node. Other HRV indices based on power spectrum analysis estimate the contribution of the sympathetic and parasympathetic modulation on the HRV fluctuations at different frequencies.[32] Although assessing autonomic modulation is difficult, HRV measurements are clinically useful in evaluating CV responsiveness to modifications in ANS controls.[33]

Aortic Stenosis (AS)

AS is the most common valve disease in high-income countries, and it is set to become a major health care burden with an aging population. It is categorized by fibro-calcific-remodeling of the valve leaflets, which causes narrowing of the aortic valve opening and a hypertrophic response of the left ventricle, which results in heart failure, syncope, angina, and finally death.[34] Aortic valve surgery and transcatheter aortic valve replacement are the unique treatments that reduce mortality, but 33% of patients reject invasive treatment.[35] Statins have been the most extensively studied medical treatment in AS. As per experimental data, statin therapy decreases osteoblast activity and cholesterol deposition in valve leaflets.

Lipoprotein (a) (Lp[a]) has also been found to be as a potential therapeutic target in AS. Results from a genome-wide study including 6,942 participants identified as rs10455872 single-nucleotide polymorphism in the LPA locus revealed that coding for Lp(a) was observed to be considerably related with aortic valve calcification. It suggests a causal role for this mutation in the pathogenesis of AS. Likewise, the latest post hoc sub-analysis of the ASTRONOMER trial (Aortic Stenosis Progression Observation: Measuring Effects of Rosuvastatin) presented that elevated levels of Lp(a) were related not only with rapid progression of AS but also with considerably poorer clinical outcomes after multivariable adjustment. Other lipid-lowering therapies such as recombinant apolipoprotein A-1 Milano, an anti-inflammatory molecule that reverses cholesterol transport, demonstrated interesting results regarding aortic valve calcification reduction and Aortic Valve Area (AVA) improvement in an animal model. Usually, antihypertensive agents were contraindicated in AS because any decrease in post-valvular cardiac afterload could cause severe diastolic hypotension, which leads to an imbalance in myocardial supply and demand. Systemic hypertension increases the diastolic transvalvular pressure gradient. This augmented pressure gradient is identified by the valve leaflets that undergo remodeling with increased collagen deposition, inflammation, and endothelial dysfunction. Antihypertensive therapy is the only treatment option in patients with AS according to current guidelines. The American Heart Association/American College of Cardiology guidelines recommended treating hypertension in patients with asymptomatic AS of any severity, with emphasis on careful titration and BP monitoring.

Renin-Angiotensin-Aldosterone System (RAAS) inhibition was the most studied antihypertensive therapy in AS because it decreases AS progression, reduces myocardial remodeling, and exerts protective effects on the vasculature. RAAS inhibition reduces cardiomyocyte hypertrophy and myocardial fibrosis to a larger extent than other vasodilators for a given decrease in systolic BP. It suggests that RAAS inhibition has pleiotropic effects on the myocardium that go beyond afterload reduction.

Furthermore, it was also observed in studies that patients with stable AS having low LVEF react to nitroprusside with an enhanced cardiac index. In patients with AS, nitrate derivatives also improve endocardial perfusion and diastolic function. Emerging therapeutic agents that have been studied in experimental models of AS and small human case series with promising results include the phosphodiesterase type 5 (PDE5) inhibitor sildenafil.[36]

Ivabradine can also be used for the treatment of AS, though it is currently indicated only in the treatment of chronic heart failure and chronic stable angina pectoris. It has better outcomes when compared to BBs and considered as a substitute for patients with AS who are intolerant to BBs. Ivabradine has negative chronotropic effects and the absence of inotropic effects that results in replacing BB with Ivabradine in patients with severe AS.[37] A prospective interventional case-control study compared the hemodynamic and clinical effects between BB treatment and the substitution by Ivabradine in patients with symptomatic severe AS who dismissed invasive treatment. Patients who have angina or known Stable Coronary Artery Disease (SCAD) were in sinus rhythm and LV Ejection Fraction (LVEF) greater than 55%. The study was completed in 10 patients. A baseline echocardiogram, electrocardiogram, six minute walk test (6MWT) was made. Afterward, the BB was withdrawn and pts began Ivabradine 2.5 mg bid increasing the dose on day 15th to 5 mg bid. One month after beginning Ivabradine, the same studies were repeated. No significant changes were observed in HR (62.5 bpm vs 61 bpm, $p = 0.26$), and LV end-diastolic diameter (4.93 cm vs 4.78 cm, $p = 0.87$), but improved significantly LVEF (69% vs 73.45%, $p = 0.028$), systolic volume (87.39 ml vs 95.82 ml, $p = 0.007$), cardiac output (5.17 l/m vs 5.69 l/m, $p = 0.047$) and 6MWT distance (251 mts vs 333 mts $p = 0.049$). Ivabradine had shown to be a safe and more appropriate treatment than BBs.[35]

Similarly, another prospective interventional case-control study analysis was conducted to evaluate the possible hemodynamic and clinical benefits after reducing HR with Ivabradine. A prospective interventional case-control study was conducted in patients with symptomatic AS who dismissed invasive treatment, all of them were in sinus rhythm and preserved ejection fraction. No patient had BBs in-home treatment. A baseline echocardiogram, electrocardiogram, laboratory, and 6MWT were made. Afterward, patients began with Ivabradine 2.5 mg bid, increasing the dose on day 15th to 5 mg bid. One month after beginning Ivabradine the same studies were repeated. The analysis was completed in 18 patients; six patients did not perform the 6MWT with motor problems. Ivabradine reduces significantly HR (78 bpm vs 62 bpm, $p = 0.001$), increased significantly LV end-diastolic diameter (4.68 cm vs 4.91 cm, $p = 0.004$), and improved significantly LVEF (69.1% vs 75.15% $p = 0.01$) and systolic volume (78.05 ml vs 100.74 ml, $p <0.001$. The walk distance was improved significantly (383 m vs 424 m, $p <0.004$). There was no significant benefit in the cardiac output. Ivabradine has been seen to be a safe drug in pts with severe symptomatic AS who dismissed invasive treatment.[38]

HR reduction using ivabradine generated an indirect positive inotropic effect that improves echocardiographic, hemodynamic, and clinical parameters. The reduction of HR with ivabradine was safe and can be used in elderly pts with SSAS who would not undergo Aortic Valve Replacement (AVR). Though Ivabradine is currently indicated only in the treatment of chronic heart failure and chronic stable angina pectoris, its effect has also been studied in aortic stenosis (AS) by Quiroga GC *et al.* The study included 61 patients with severe AS, sinus rhythm, and preserved ejection fraction. Patients were followed-up for 30 days. Demographic data, comorbidities, and medical treatment were recorded. A baseline and at day 30 echocardiogram, electrocardiogram, blood test, Minnesota questionnaire, and 6MWT were done in all patients. The population was distributed into two groups. In Group A Ivabradine was added (2.5 mg bid, increasing the dose on day 15th to 5 mg bid) after baseline tests. In Group B, no intervention was made. The basal status *vs* day 30 status in each group and the differences between both groups (ΔA *vs* ΔB) were compared. Ivabradine reduced significantly HR ($p <0.001$), increases left ventricular end-diastolic diameter ($p = 0.01$), improved LVEF ($p = 0.001$), stroke volume ($p <0.001$), aortic VTI ($p <0.001$) and LV outflow tract VTI ($p <0.001$), the 6MWT distance ($p = 0.001$) and reduced Minnesota questionnaire ($p = 0.01$). When differences between baseline *vs* day 30 status of Group A and B were compared (ΔA *vs* ΔB), patients in Group A showed an increased LVEF, aortic VTI, LVOT VTI, peak and mean gradient, stroke volume, and the 6MWT distance. Outcomes revealed that HR reduction using Ivabradine generated an indirect positive inotropic effect that improves echocardiographic, hemodynamic, and clinical parameters.

The decrease in HR with ivabradine may decrease the occurrence of major CV events. A study was conducted in which data was analyzed of 98 pts with SSAS, sinus rhythm, and preserved LVEF who were rejected or declined an AVR. Group A 49 pts prescribed ivabradine, and Group B 49 pts continued with conventional treatment (51% received BB). The baseline characteristics of the groups were similar, with no significant differences in age, sex, CV risk factors, symptoms, coronary disease, low flow, low gradient, renal failure, anemia, and medical treatment. The total follow-up was 939 (754–1124) days. The reduction of HR with ivabradine decreased death from any cause, hospitalization, and the composite of death from any cause or hospitalization. The study revealed that the reduction of HR with Ivabradine is safe and can be an option for elderly pts with SSAS who would not undergo AVR.[39]

Mitral Stenosis (MS) and Mitral Valve Prolapse (MVP)

MS is a type of VHD consists of constricting the MV orifice. Nowadays, rheumatic fever is considered the most common reason for MS, but the stenosis generally appears clinically significant only after some years. The uncommon causes of MS are calcification of the MV leaflets and congenital heart disease. Other reasons for MS include infective endocarditis, mitral annular calcification, endomyocardial fibroelastosis, malignant carcinoid syndrome, systemic lupus erythematosus, Whipple disease, Fabry disease, and rheumatoid arthritis. Management for MS includes medical therapy, surgical therapy, and percutaneous mitral valvuloplasty. Medical therapy reduces new cases of rheumatic fever, improve symptoms, and lessen the thromboembolic risk.[40]

MVP is a billowing of MV leaflets into the left atrium during systole. Idiopathic myxomatous degeneration is considered the most common reason. MVP is commonly asymptomatic in the absence of substantial regurgitation, even though some patients also experience chest pain, dyspnea, dizziness, and palpitations, according to some studies. Myxomatous degeneration of the MV leaflets and chordae tendineae results in MVP.[41]

MVP patients with no symptoms often require no treatment. MVP patients showing symptoms of chest pain, palpitations should be prescribed BBs such as propranolol. MV repair or MV replacement should be done in patients with severe mitral regurgitation. The ACC/AHA guidelines recommended MV repair before symptoms of congestive HF appear. Till 2007, preceding invasive procedures, the AHA recommended prescribing antibiotics. Asymptomatic patients with MVP are treated predictably with observation and monitoring. Patient reassurance is needed along with consideration of a healthy lifestyle and regular exercise.[40]

Role of Ivabradine in HR Modulation in MS and MVP

HRV may be useful in predicting the prognosis in patients with mitral regurgitation caused due to MVP, a disorder that consistently results in left ventricular hypertrophy (LVH), and dysfunction. Reduced HRV in MS patients with sinus rhythm indicates higher sympathetic activity in patients susceptible to AF, while an increase of HRV in patients with AF may indicate that the ventricular rhythm has a respiratory-related periodicity, and predominant parasympathetic activity may control the intrinsic behavior of the AV node during AF. Therefore, the assessment of HRV is a valuable tool to determine the patients with rheumatic MS who are susceptible to AF.[3]

Patients with MS become symptomatic at a higher HR. Ivabradine should be strongly indicated in the medical management of MS patients where BBs are contraindicated, such as reactive airway disease.[42] Rheumatic MS is a common problem in the young population in most of the developing world. Severe MS is commonly symptomatic and managed by Balloon Mitral Valvuloplasty (BMV) or surgery, while mild to moderate MS is commonly asymptomatic and managed medically. Patients in the latter group may become symptomatic during episodes of exercise and increased HR. As an increase in HR happens generally at the expense of diastole, and in the presence of obstruction at the MV, this causes increased left atrial pressure. Afterward, there is effort intolerance and dyspnea due to a rise in Pulmonary Capillary Wedge Pressure (PCWP).

Theoretically, BBs and CCBs help in controlling tachycardia-related symptoms by improving diastolic filling and preventing a rise in PCWP. Though, the useful effects of these medications may negate due to their negative inotropic effect on the myocardium and neuromuscular system. CCBs can control HR when the patient is in sinus rhythm. Outcomes from various studies with these drugs have been contradictory. Ivabradine currently has been approved for HR control in CHF and chronic stable angina patients. It does not possess the side effects of BBs as it has a selective action on the sinus node. But its effect has also been studied in MS. Parakh J *et al.* in 2012 analyzed the relative efficacy of HR control with Ivabradine or Atenolol and its influence on effort tolerance in patients with mild-moderate MS in normal sinus rhythm. The study included a total of fifty patients with mild-moderate MS in sinus rhythm. Patients were divided into two groups; either receives Ivabradine or Atenolol for 4 weeks. In the first treatment period, 23 patients were given ivabradine, and 27 were given Atenolol. Results revealed that Ivabradine and Atenolol increased the mean total exercise to 500.7 seconds (SD 99.7) and 463.7 seconds (SD 113.1) from a baseline of 410.3 seconds (SD 115.4), respectively. These findings revealed that the ivabradine is more efficient than atenolol for effort-related signs in patients with mild-moderate MS.[43]

Pure HR reduction with ivabradine without undesirable hemodynamic side effects associated with BBs may be better for symptomatic improvement in MS patients with

Normal sinus rhythm (NSR). Dhanger MK *et al.* conducted a study involving a total of 100 MS patients with NSR. Patients were randomized in a ratio of 1:1 to receive either Ivabradine (5 mg BD) or Atenolol (50 mg OD) for 12 weeks. Clinical assessment, TMT, and echo-Doppler evaluation were done to relate the efficacy and side effects of two drugs. The mean dose of ivabradine and atenolol was 6.05 ± 1.25 mg and 60 ± 26.7 mg, respectively, at 12 weeks. The decrease in RHR was the same in both groups. Significant Right Ventricular Systolic Pressure (RVSP) reduction was observed in the ivabradine group but not in the atenolol group. Therefore, ivabradine is a valuable substitute to BBs in the management of patients with symptomatic MS, having efficacy similar to BBs with lower side effects.[44]

Symptoms in MS are HR dependent. A rise in HR reduces the diastolic filling period with the rise in the transmitral gradient. By reducing HR, BBs improve hemodynamics and relieve symptoms, but the uses may be limited by side effects. Thus, a randomized crossover trial was performed by Saggu DK *et al.* to compare the efficacy of ivabradine and metoprolol in patients with mild-to-moderate MS in normal sinus rhythm. A total of 34 patients with mild-to-moderate MS were enrolled in the study. Substantial reduction in baseline and peak exercise HR was detected at the end of follow-up with both drugs. The reduction in MV gradient and pulmonary artery systolic pressure (PASP) was the same after ivabradine and metoprolol treatment. Both drugs improved symptoms and hemodynamic to a similar extent from baseline. Thus, ivabradine can be used efficiently and safely in patients with MS in NSR who are intolerant or contraindicated for BB therapy.[45]

Atenolol or ivabradine can also be used for HR control in moderate MS patients in sinus rhythm. These drugs considerably improve exercise capacity and total exercise duration. The study performed by Rajesh GN *et al.* proved that ivabradine is not better than atenolol for controlling HR. BBs are commonly used in patients with MS to control HR and improve exercise-related symptoms. The study enrolled a total of eighty-two patients with moderate MS. Patients were randomized to prescribe Ivabradine ($n = 42$) 5 mg bid or Atenolol ($n = 40$) 50 mg daily for 6 weeks. On direct comparison, no major change was observed in the improvement of exercise time between the ivabradine and Atenolol group ($p = 0.847$). Also, no considerable change was observed in the LV Myocardial Performance Index (MPI) in both the drug groups.[46]

The conventional medical treatment for MVP involving palpitation due to sinus tachycardia is essentially based on BBs. However, patient compliance with treatment is poor due to the side effects of BBs, such as bronchoconstriction and negative inotropic and hypotensive effects. Therefore, the use of another agent is considered that selectively decreases the HR by preventing the I_f pacemaker current, without the potentially harmful hemodynamic effects of BBs. The I_f current is directly regulated by cAMP, a secondary messenger of the ANS. So, by direct inhibiting I_f current, there is a selective reduction of RHR and tachycardia mediated by an increase in the sympathetic tone. Thus, the study conducted by Cicek D *et al.* evaluated the effects of ivabradine used as a substitute to BBs in MVP patients complaining of palpitations due to sinus tachycardia. The study enrolled 48 MVP patients. After 2 weeks of a wash-out, echocardiographic, electrocardiographic, 24-hour Holter, and routine blood examinations were conducted. Ivabradine treatment was initiated at a dosage of 5 mg bid. After 1 month of treatment, the above-mentioned examinations were repeated. The treatment was completed by 45 patients. No substantial variances were observed between the pre- and post-treatment values of the echocardiographic, hemodynamic, and electrophysiological parameters. However, the symptom periods (164 ± 12 *vs* 114 ± 9; $p = 0.003$) and the maximum (149 ± 18 *vs* 136 ± 16; $p = 0.001$), mean (85 ± 8 *vs* 77 ± 8; $p = 0.002$), and minimum HRs (61 ± 3 *vs* 52 ± 5; $p = 0.001$) recorded by Holter monitoring were considerably decreased. The study revealed that Ivabradine is effective and safe to relieve palpitation symptoms due to sinus tachycardia in patients with MVP.[47]

Dilated Cardiomyopathy (DCM)

DCM is defined as LV dilation and systolic dysfunction in the absence of CAD or abnormal loading conditions proportionate to the extent of LV impairment.[48] Persistent changes in HR affects LV function in both normal and abnormal hearts. Persistent rapid HR was observed associated with a DCM with reduced LVEF and congestive HF in the clinical setting. Transient increases in HR may alter cardiac function. A moderate tachycardia induced by pacing in patients with idiopathic DCM produced a rate-dependent deterioration in LVEF. There is proof that a slow HR benefited LF function in patients with reduced LV function. BB or Amiodarone therapy in patients with decreased LV function was associated with improvement in LVEF and a reduction in resting. The increase in LVEF was more in patients with HF who had a significant notable decrease in RHR after treatment. Patients with idiopathic DCM have a greater increment in LVEF following BB therapy compared with similar remedies in patients with cardiomyopathy due to IHD.[49]

Although a persistent tachycardia was detrimental to cardiac function, the role of RHR in determining cardiac function in patients with reduced cardiac function is unknown. An RHR in the upper range of normal was often present in patients with HF related to normal subjects, and the greater the RHR, the greater the severity of HF. Thus, it might be that an RHR in the higher range of normal in patients with reduced cardiac function could result in a further decrease in LVEF and worsening HF.[49]

Pharmacological therapy is constant with established guidelines for CHF with the introduction of loop diuretics for symptomatic relief, as well as Angiotensin-Converting Enzyme (ACE)-inhibitor and BB therapy. Commencement of an aldosterone antagonist is warranted in patients with moderate or severe LV Systolic Dysfunction (LVSD). Anticoagulation is essential to abrogate the risk of thromboembolism in patients with coexistent CHF and AF.[50] Some studies also revealed the role of Ivabradine in standard treatment in patients with DCM and symptomatic HF, though currently it is only indicated in the treatment of chronic heart failure and chronic stable angina pectoris. By adding Ivabradine in standard therapy improves functional class, exercise tolerance, and LV function in patients with HF. To define the role of Ivabradine in HR manipulation in DCM, Raja DC *et al.* conducted a study. A total of 187 patients with HF (DCM, NYHA II-IV, baseline HR >70/min) were included in the study, of which 125 patients were randomized to standard therapy (BBs, ACEI, diuretics, $n = 62$) or add-on Ivabradine (titrated to maximum 7.5 mg BD, $n = 63$). BBs were titrated in both groups. Results revealed that at 3 months both groups show improvement in NYHA class, 6MWT, Minnesota Living With Heart Failure (MLWHF) scores, and fall in BNP. Though, the extent of variation was seen well in the Ivabradine group. The use of Ivabradine was constant at a 6 months follow-up. The percentage change in HR was considerably more in the Ivabradine group (32.2 *vs* 19.3%, $p = 0.001$) with no difference in BP. RHR <70/min was achieved in 96.8 *vs* 27.9%, respectively, in two groups.[51]

DCM is the most common reason for HF in young adults. It is a disabling syndrome that can severely affect the patient's QoL with poor diagnosis. Thus, Mansour S et al. conducted a study to examine the influence of ivabradine on signs, QoL, effort tolerance, and echocardiographic parameters in patients with idiopathic DCM and NYHA class III or IV HF symptoms. Out of 167 patients, 53 patients were randomly allocated to either guideline-based medical therapy alone (23 patients, control group) or ivabradine as add-on therapy (30 patients) for 3 months with 1-year follow-up. Adding ivabradine considerably decreased the HR from 96 to 72 bpm (p <0.0001 vs control group), with more improvement in echocardiographic LV dimensions, LV volumes, LVEF (p = 0.045), NYHA class symptoms (p = 0.004), exercise tolerance (p = 0.03), and QoL (p = 0.02). The average number of hospitalizations was 1.0 ± 1.4 in the ivabradine group vs 2.1 ± 1.1 in the control group (p = 0.003). Adding ivabradine to standard therapy in HF patients improved symptoms, QoL, echocardiographic parameters, effort tolerance, and reduced hospitalization. This beneficial effect of ivabradine is because of its HR-reducing properties.[52]

DCM represents one-half of all cardiomyopathies in children. Approximately 40% of children undergo cardiac transplantation or die in 5 years of DCM diagnosis, attesting to the significance of HF in this patient population. The study conducted by Bonnet D et al. explored the dose-response relationship of ivabradine in children with DCM. The primary endpoint was ≥20% decrease in HR from baseline. It was a randomized, double-blind, placebo-controlled, phase II/III study with 12 months of follow-up. Children (n = 116) receiving stable HF therapy were randomized to either ivabradine or placebo. After an initial titration period, the dose was adjusted to attain the primary endpoint. LV function (echocardiography), clinical status (NYHA functional class or Ross class), N-terminal pro-B-type natriuretic peptide, and QoL were assessed. The primary endpoint was achieved by 51 of 73 children of the ivabradine group (70%) vs 5 of 41 of the placebo group (12%) at varying doses (odds ratio: 17.24; p <0.0001). NYHA functional class improved better with ivabradine at 12 months than placebo (38 vs 25%; p = 0.24). A trend toward improvement in QoL was observed for ivabradine vs placebo (p = 0.053). The study revealed that ivabradine safely decreased the RHR of children with chronic HF and DCM. Ivabradine therapy improved LVEF, and clinical status and QoL showed favorable trends.[53]

Cardiogenic Shock (CS)

CS is a state of end-organ hypoperfusion associated with HF. Any reason impairing acute LV or right ventricular (RV) function may cause CS. As per the current Intraaortic Balloon Pump (IABP)-SHOCK II trial, 74% of the patients with Cardiogenic shock complicating an acute ST-elevation Myocardial Infarction (CSMI) are treated with norepinephrine, 53% of them with dobutamine, 26% of them with epinephrine, 4% of them with levosimendan, and 4% of them with dopamine. Percutaneous circulatory support devices such as IABP, LV Assist Device (LVAD), or Extracorporeal Life Support (ECLS) create treatment options for selected patients such as CS.[54]

CS is an emergency requiring immediate resuscitative therapy preceding the permanent loss of vital organs. Early restoration of coronary blood is the main intrusion and is the standard treatment for patients with cardiogenic shock because of MI.

The goal of medical therapy is to refurbish cardiac output and inhibit permanent end-organ damage promptly.[55]

- Norepinephrine is chosen over dopamine in patients with severe hypotension or hypotension not responding to other medications. Though, norepinephrine should be used carefully as it can cause tachycardia and increased myocardial oxygen demand in patients with recent MIs.
- Dobutamine is extensively used and has beta-1 and beta-2 agonist properties, which can improve myocardial contractility, lower LV end-diastolic pressure, and increased cardiac output.
- Milrinone has been shown to decrease LV filling pressures.
- Fibrinolytic therapy should be prescribed to patients who are not suitable for either the percutaneous coronary intervention or coronary artery bypass graft if there are no contraindications.
- Patients with MI or ACS are prescribed aspirin and heparin.
- Diuretics reduce plasma volume and edema and thus decreasing cardiac output and BP.[55]

Cardiac dysfunction in patients with cardiogenic shock is usually initiated by MI or ischemia. When the myocardial function is low, several compensatory mechanisms are triggered to increase HR and contractility to increase preload. These compensatory mechanisms can deteriorate the situation during the development of cardiogenic shock. A rise in HR increases myocardial oxygen demand and worsens ischemia. Vasoconstriction raises myocardial afterload, further weakening cardiac performance, and increasing myocardial oxygen demand. It further worsens ischemia and begins a vicious cycle that will result in death if continual. The meta-analysis performed by the Fibrinolytic Therapy Trialists Collaborative Group demonstrated a decrease in mortality rate from 36.1 to 29.7% when thrombolytic therapy was used in patients with initial systolic BP less than 100 mmHg. In patients with initial HRs greater than 100 bpm, the mortality rate decreased from 23.8 to 18.9%.[56]

Ivabradine is a selective sinus node inhibitor indicated in patients with symptomatic chronic HF on stable guideline-recommended HF therapy including, correct dosages of BBs. Tachycardia, especially in the context of inotropic therapy, maybe deleterious resulting in increased myocardial oxygen consumption and reduction in the diastolic filling. As ivabradine is currently indicated only in the treatment of chronic heart failure and chronic stable angina pectoris, it has also been studied in cardiogenic shock (CS). Chiu MH *et al.* in 2019 conducted a study to determine the safety and tolerability of ivabradine for a decrease in HR in CS patients. Five patients (four non-ischemic and one ischemic) with severe LV dysfunction, CS, and sinus tachycardia were invasively monitored during treatment with inotropic and/or vasopressor therapy. All patients tolerated ivabradine during the 48 hours. At 24 hours after initiation (*vs* baseline), a reduction in HR (91.6 ± 6.4 *vs* 106 ± 6.8 bpm, $p = 0.04$), pulmonary arterial occlusion pressure (24 ± 5 *vs* 30 ± 4 mmHg, $p = 0.04$), and right atrial pressure (9 ± 4.3 *vs* 17 ± 6 mmHg, $p = 0.0002$) was observed. No significant change was detected with mean arterial pressure or thermo dilution-derived cardiac index. Inotropic support was stopped effectively in all five patients (88 ± 30 h) with BB therapy. The findings of the study revealed that ivabradine is safe, and it can be used to decrease HR in patients previously intolerant of BB.[57]

The usage of ivabradine in cardiogenic shock is currently contraindicated. However, studies have recommended increasing HR may be deleterious for patients with HFrEF because of an inverted Bowditch-Treppe response. Limited case series have recommended the use of ivabradine in decompensated HFrEF may be beneficial. Chiu MH *et al.* showed a case series of patients who presented with severely decompensated HFrEF and received inotropic support and concomitant ivabradine. Four patients with HFrEF presenting with elevated sinus HR and cardiogenic shock. Ivabradine 2.5 mg 12 hours was initiated and subsequently titrated with continued monitoring with baseline, 24 hours, and the latest obtained parameters recorded. Ivabradine was tolerated in all cases, with a mean dosage of 6 mg q12h. Mean HR and pulmonary wedge pressure fell 20 and 32%, respectively, from baseline to the last measurement, while stroke volume increased with an overall improvement in cardiac index. No changes were noted in mean arterial BP. All patients experienced an effective wean of inotropic support in 48 hours and were discharged alive on BB and ACE inhibitor treatment. In this small series of patients with cardiogenic shock, BB intolerance, and elevated sinus HR, ivabradine was added without any deleterious hemodynamic effect and associated with early clinical improvement.[58]

Coronary CT Angiography (CCTA)

CCTA is a non-invasive method to image the heart and coronary arteries for which image quality is best with HR <60 bpm during the scan.[13] The patient's HR and HRV play an essential role in cardiac CT examinations, e.g. CT CAC and CCTA, due to the limit of temporal resolution available in current CT systems. A study to assess the effect of HR on the quality of CTA exams obtained with 16-channel multidetector row CT (MDCT) demonstrated a significant negative correlation between mean HR and image quality. Besides mean HR, significant differences in HR (e.g. from 41 to 100 bpm during scanning, equivalent to an R–R interval ranging from 1463 to 600 ms resulted in misregistration of ECG-gated data and severe discontinuities in the reconstructed cardiac images. Also, variation in the HR resulted in significant discontinuities in the CT images. Thus, most vendors offer an ECG editor that allows the operator to adjust the synchronization and thereby reduce artifacts caused by short-term deviations of the patient's HR. Although the primary disease is the main factor influencing an individual patient's HR and its variability, HR and HRV may be influenced by many other factors under the clinical conditions that exist during a cardiac CT exam. These include breath-holding during the scan, the injection of intravenous contrast media, the usage of BBs or nitroglycerin, and patient demographics (age, gender, etc.).[4]

BBs are generally used to achieve short-term HR reduction during the scan; several trials have also investigated Ivabradine for this purpose.[13] Ivabradine it is currently indicated only in the treatment of CHF and chronic stable angina pectoris, but its effect has also been studied in other conditions like coronary CT angiography (CCTA). Adile KK *et al.* in 2012 conducted a study to examine the role of oral ivabradine as an HR reducing agent in patients undergoing CT coronary angiography (CTCA). Ivabradine mainly contributes to sinus node pacemaker activity and has no major direct CV effects such as a decrease in PB and impairment of cardiac conduction. A total of 100 sequential patients were investigated who had been referred for CTCA for the assessment of CAD. Patients had been prescribed two pre-medication protocols: oral metoprolol or oral ivabradine. Ivabradine was significantly more effective than metoprolol in lowering the HR; the mean percentage reduction in HR with ivabradine *vs* Metoprolol was 23.89 + 6.95% *vs* 15.20 + 4.50%, respectively ($p = 0.0001$). The outcomes of the study showed that ivabradine is a potentially attractive alternative to currently used drugs for the decrease in HR in patients undergoing CTCA.[59]

CCTA is increasingly seen as a first-line investigation in patients with suspected CAD. HR control improves the image quality and diagnostic precision of CCTA. Typically, BBs are administered to induce sinus bradycardia. Sinus bradycardia may also be induced by ivabradine. The study conducted by Guler EC *et al.* assumed that ivabradine would be an effective substitute to metoprolol in decreasing HR in CCTA patients in a real-world setting. A retrospective analysis was conducted, including patients who were given an ivabradine-based (IB) *vs* a metoprolol only (MO) protocol to attain a target HR ≤65 bpm. A total of 5,955 consecutive patients were involved in the analysis: 3,211 were imaged in an era of a MO strategy and 2,744 CCTA following an IB strategy. A total of 2,676 patients had HRs >65 and received HR lowering medication: 1,958 patients had MO, and 718 received IB protocol. Target HR of ≤65 bpm was achieved in 77% of MO and 89% of IB patients (*p* <0.01). A novel single-dose IB protocol to control HR for CCTA was more effective in attaining target HR than a MO strategy. The use of ivabradine, however, sustained a 1.6-fold increase in the time delay from medication administration and imaging compared to a MO protocol.[60]

Take Home Pearls

- Ivabradine showed both HR stabilization and QoL perfection in patients with IST.

- A decrease in HR with Ivabradine is safe and can be an alternative for elderly patients with SSAS who would not perform aortic valve replacement.

- DCM is one of the most common reasons for HF and sudden death. Ivabradine safely decreased the RHR of children with DCM.

- A low and stable HR is an essential condition for the attainment of optimal image quality and diagnostic precision with CTCA.

HR MODULATION IN NON-CV CONDITIONS

Other non-CV comorbidities have a negative effect on patients' symptoms and are related to the poor diagnosis.[61] HR variation is also essential in these disorders. Other non-CV conditions include sepsis, multiple organ dysfunction syndrome (MODS) in sepsis/septic shock, COPD, pulmonary arterial hypertension (PAH), and erectile dysfunction.

Sepsis

In intensive care units, sepsis is considered one of the main reasons for death.[5] It is a medical emergency that can result in end-stage organ dysfunction and death. The global epidemiological burden of sepsis is, though, difficult to determine. It is assessed that globally every year more than 30 million people are affected by sepsis, which results in possibly 6 million deaths yearly.[62]

Significance of HR Modulation in Sepsis

Tachycardia is a trademark of sepsis with various possible determining factors, including fever, hypovolemia, sympathetic tone, and/or exogenous catecholamines. Though the HR response to sepsis may be an adaptive response to retain oxygen delivery, tachycardia was also reported as an independent risk factor for mortality in severe sepsis and septic shock, irrespective of body temperature. An increase in HR may damage LV diastolic filling, increase myocardial oxygen demand, and compromise coronary blood flow.[5]

No evidence-based guidelines were present for the early treatment of severe sepsis and septic shock preceding the year 2001. Beal and Cerra predicted that with rapid and appropriate resuscitation of shock, conversion of sepsis to multiple organ dysfunctions could be prevented. An essential part of the initial treatment of sepsis is the quick beginning of suitable antibiotic therapy and source control.[43] BBs are effective in controlling HR in septic shock, with advantageous effects on hemodynamics and diagnosis.[62] However, BBs possess negative inotropic and hypotensive effects, which make the clinical routine usage difficult especially in patients with LV systolic dysfunction.

Ivabradine is a pure HR-lowering drug without having any negative effects on inotropic function and arterial load. It has positive effects on endothelial function, inflammation, and microvascular perfusion. Similarly, ivabradine improves clinical outcomes in patients with chronic LVSD and tachycardia.[62] It prevents the pacemaker current to decrease the risk of HF hospitalization and CV death in symptomatic patients with a reduced LVEF ≤35% and sinus rhythm ≥70 bpm. The HCN channels create the pacemaker current I_f in the SA node cells of the heart (Fig. 6.3). Ivabradine can further slowdown the pacemaker activity of human atrial cardiomyocytes and thus efficiently decrease HR even in the presence of endotoxin.[63] Currently, it is indicated only in the treatment of CHF and chronic stable angina pectoris.

Further, a retrospective observational trial was performed. The study included a total of twenty-three patients. Among them, 43.5% with septic shock, 21.7% with cardiogenic shock, and 21.7% with mixed shock were involved. There was a substantial reduction in CR of 21% (p <0.0001), and manifestations of tissue perfusion such as norepinephrine dose, urine output, central venous oxygen saturation, cardiac

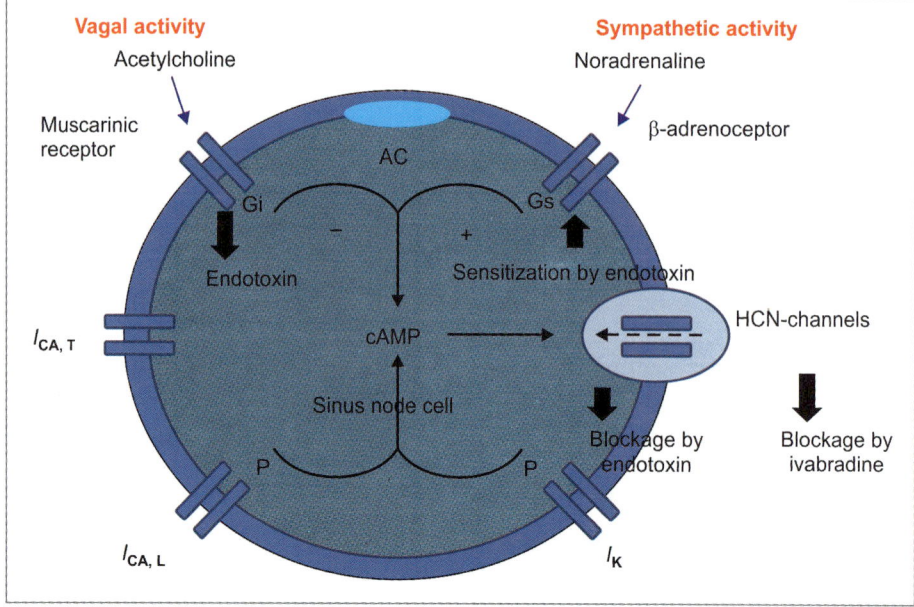

Fig. 6.3: Effects of endotoxin

output, and systemic vascular resistance, and all improved considerably. Perfection in the clinical and biochemical constraints of tissue perfusion was detected with the usage of ivabradine in patients in shock and tachycardia, independently of deviations in cardiac output.[64]

The effects of ivabradine have also been assessed in patients with sepsis and/or MODS, though it was currently indicated only in the treatment of CHF and chronic stable angina pectoris. A total of 50 patients with sepsis and/or MODS with an HR of at least 90 bpm were enrolled in the study. Patients were given conservative therapy with or without ivabradine 5 mg bid for 30 days. A decrease in HR was better in the Ivabradine group (33 bpm) compared to the control group (24 bpm, $p = 0.023$) after 96 hours.[65]

HR >90 bpm shows a poor diagnosis for patients with MODS. The study performed by Nuding S et al. determined the effect of Ivabradine on HR, hemodynamics, and disease severity in patients with MODS (MODIfY Trial). In this two-arm phase II trial, 70 patients with MODS were included. Patients were prescribed standard treatment ± Ivabradine (5 mg bid) for 96 hours through the enteral route. The percentage of patients with a decrease in HR at least 10 bpm after 96 hours were considered as the primary outcome. The daily median HR was decreased by 7 bpm in the control group and by 16 bpm in the ivabradine group ($p = 0.014$) after 96 hours. The outcomes of the trial showed that the number of patients with MODS and a sinus rhythm of at least 90 bpm that experienced a decrease in HR after oral ivabradine did not vary considerably among groups.[66]

Patients with MODS typically present with an elevated HR that accompanies a highly impaired autonomic dysfunction with depressed parasympathetic control of the heart. A rise in HR increases the occurrence of cardiac events in critically ill patients. Also, raised HR in the early phase of MODS was an independent interpreter of increased 28-day mortality. De Santis V et al. performed a case study to determine the initial results of ivabradine use in three patients who had sepsis-related MODS after cardiac surgery. All evaluations were performed using the SAS Statistical Package, Release 9.2. All the patients established sinus tachycardia (HR >90 bpm). Mean arterial pressure (MAP) was continuous with norepinephrine support. MODS established at the third postoperative day in patients 1 and 2, while in patient 3 during the fourth postoperative day. Ivabradine was administered twice daily through a nasogastric tube for 18 hours. HR (mean difference –27.6) and cardiac index (CI) reduced after ivabradine administration, whereas End-Diastolic Volume Index (EDVI), stroke volume index (SVI), MAP, and SvO_2 increased. The study determined that ivabradine was well-tolerated and reduced HR in MODS patients.[67]

Chronic Obstructive Pulmonary Disease (COPD)

COPD is defined clinically as the occurrence of increasing respiratory symptoms, particularly dyspnea, cough and sputum production, and increased sputum purulence. COPD can disturb the QoL of patients, accelerate disease progression, and can lead to hospital admissions and death.[68]

Significance of HR Modulation in COPD

Increased sympathetic tone and usage of bronchodilators increase HR. It may deteriorate functional capacity in patients with COPD.[69]

Co-occurrence of HF and COPD is common, particularly in the elderly, and both share tobacco smoking as a strong risk factor. Both diseases share essential pathophysiological pathways, such as systemic inflammation, activation of the neurohumoral system, and metabolic modulation. Identifying COPD in patients with HF is complex due to the same clinical presentation and the risk of false-positive consequences with spirometry. Pulmonary function testing should be performed when HF patients are stable and euvolemic. Clinicians should recommend the same HF drugs to HF and COPD patients as in patients without COPD.

HF is a disorder with a considerable influence on pulmonary function. A main pulmonary effect of HF is phases of increased PCWP and pulmonary congestion with interstitial and peribronchiolar edema. It results in the reduction of diffusion capacity and initiation of pulmonary vascular bed "remodeling" in the long-term resulting in pulmonary arteriolar wall hypertrophy. In stable HF, pulmonary function testing exposes mostly variations in restrictive nature. A decrease of 20% as compared to age-, sex-, and height-matched controls in forced expiratory volume in 1 second (FEV1) and forced vital capacity (FVC) can be expected to be caused by HF. Thus, the ratio of FEV1/FVC (both around 20% reduction) is not essentially affected by the presence of HF when spirometry is performed in a stable phase of the disease.[70]

There is important proof that HR is a powerful predictor of mortality in both normal individuals and patients with CVD. The use of beta-adrenoceptor antagonists (BBs) has established the importance of lowering elevated HR in a patient's diagnosis. However, these agents are not prescribed to patients with obstructive airway disease as they can have unwanted adverse effects.[71]

European Respiratory Society/American Thoracic Society guidelines provided recommendations linked with corticosteroid therapy, antibiotic therapy, non-invasive mechanical ventilation, home-based management, and early pulmonary rehabilitation in patients having a COPD exacerbation.[68] In some clinical studies, ivabradine showed a positive effect on clinical status in COPD patients by decreasing HR, though currently it was only indicated only in the treatment of CHF and chronic stable angina pectoris. Mahmoud K et al. in 2016 performed the study to determine the short-term effect of the HR lowering drug ivabradine on clinical status in COPD patients. Patients ($n = 80$) were either taking ivabradine 7.5 mg twice per day or placebo for two weeks and also evaluated all patients. Results confirmed that the ivabradine group showed momentous improvement in 6-minute walk distance (from 192.6 ± 108.8 m at baseline to 285.1 ± 88.9 m at the end of the study) compared with the control group (230.6 ± 68.4 at baseline and 250.4 ± 65.8 m at the end of study) ($p <0.001$). This improvement in the drug group was related to the substantial improvement of dyspnea on the modified Borg scale ($p = 0.007$). Ivabradine can improve exercise capacity and functional class in COPD patients with RHR >90 bpm.[69]

Selective HR reduction with ivabradine is effective in patients with asthma and COPD, with no alteration in respiratory function or symptoms throughout the study. Ivabradine offers an interesting alternative, as an HR-lowering agent, in patients with respiratory disease and contraindications to BBs. Majewski S et al. performed a randomized, single-center, double-blind trial in an ambulatory setting. A total of 40 patients were enrolled in the study. All patients were prescribed ivabradine 7.5 mg bid for 5-day and placebo twice daily for 5-day. Ivabradine produced significantly lower mean HR than placebo in both groups of patients: asthma 67.4–8.38 vs 82.85–11.19 bpm ($p <0.001$) and COPD 69.75–8.9 vs 81.05–9.75 bpm ($p <0.001$).[71]

Moreover, in patients with moderate-to-very-severe COPD and coronary heart disease (CHD) comorbidity, ivabradine does not influence lung function. Whereas, inhaled salbutamol has side effects such as accelerated sinus rhythm, which is dangerous in patients with COPD and CHD. Therefore, to determine this, a cross-over, randomized, open-label study was performed. A total of 20 patients with COPD stage II-IV and comorbid CHD NYHA class I–III were enrolled. Spirometry with 400 mg salbutamol inhalation was performed on two sequential days of the study. Patients in group I was given 5 mg ivabradine per os 3 hours before salbutamol inhalation, and patients in group II were given 5 mg ivabradine on the second day of the study. The increased HR by 5.5 bpm (95% CI: 0.8; 10.2, p <0.03) was observed in the case of Salbutamol. After Ivabradine, there was no considerable change in HR by –2.4 bpm (–7.0; 2.3, p = 0.33) was observed through salbutamol. The attenuation of HR elevation by ivabradine was substantial, p <0.01. Ivabradine 5 mg per os inhibits HR increase after inhalation of 400 mg salbutamol.[72]

Pulmonary Arterial Hypertension (PAH)

PAH is defined as increased arterial pressure and pulmonary vascular resistance, which affects approximately 15–60 per million of the population. It is more frequently detected in females. PAH is related to considerable morbidity and mortality initiated by the progressive nature of the disease, which ultimately leads to HF and death. Various nonspecific symptoms are associated with PAH, such as breathlessness, fatigue, chest pain, and weakness. The patient's physical mobility and emotional state are affected by these symptoms and undesirably disturbs health-related quality of life (HRQoL).[73]

Significance of HR Modulation in PAH

BBs are generally used to improve the diagnosis of patients with left HF as lower HR at rest is favorable for the long-term diagnosis. Indeed, BBs are not indicated for pulmonary hypertension (PH) patients, as these agents possess possible negative effects on hemodynamics and exercise capacity. The negative inotropic and hypotensive effects of BBs are particularly the main concerns because PH patients are probably to be hypotensive with vasodilator therapies.[74]

Two possible mechanisms are there for the enhancement of the diagnosis of PH patients with BBs (Fig. 6.4). The first one is its direct influence on the pulmonary artery. The second possible mechanism is the influence of the development of biventricular dysfunction via HR decrease by adrenergic receptor blockade. PH causes not only RV dysfunction but also LV dysfunction.[74]

Pharmacological therapies for PAH, such as phosphodiesterase-5 inhibitors (PDE-5i), endothelin receptor antagonists, prostacyclin analogs, and lung transplantation are used to alleviate disease symptoms and slow disease progression, treatment-related adverse events. But the side effects of some routes of drug administration can negatively influence patients' daily life.[51] Ivabradine may be beneficial to improve biventricular dysfunction in PAH. It can decrease HR without any negative inotropic effects on the heart.[74] Though it is currently indicated only in the treatment of chronic heart failure and chronic stable angina pectoris; its effect has also been studied in PAH. Tytova G *et al.* in 2017 examined the effect of ivabradine on structure-functional peculiarities of the right ventricle, HR, and QoL in patients with chronic cor pulmonale (CCP). A total of 72 patients (38 men, 34 women,

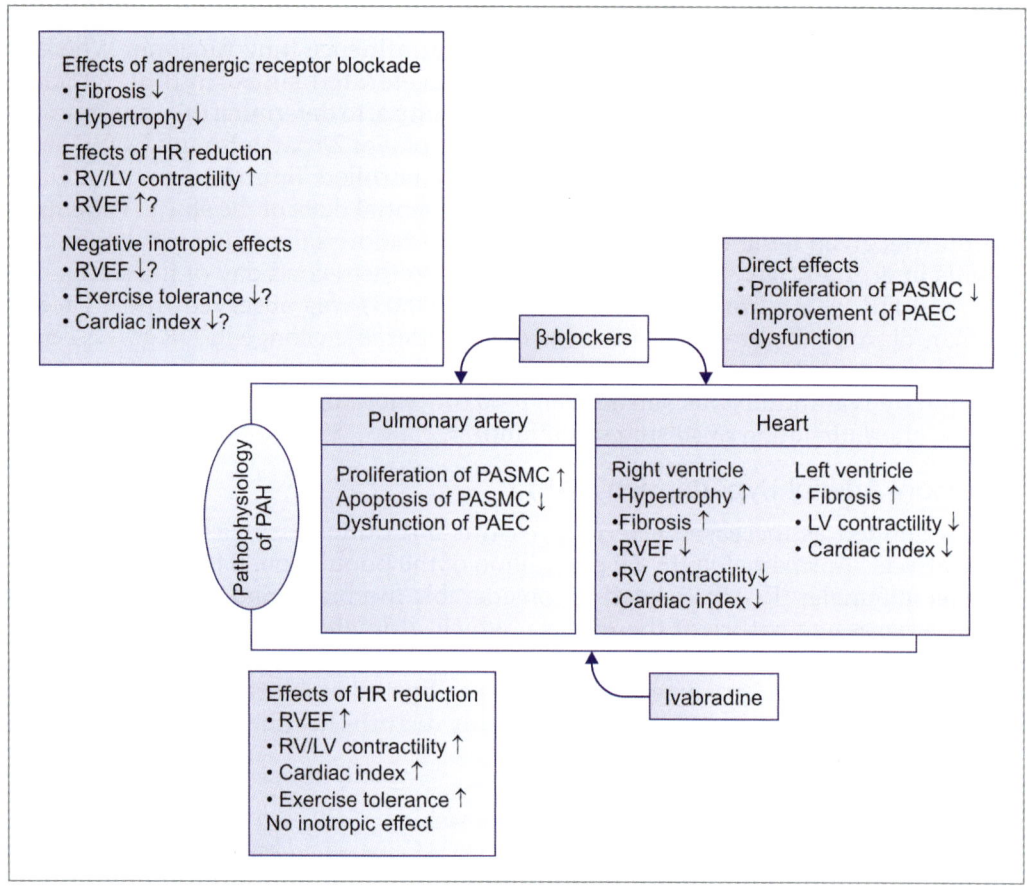

Fig. 6.4: Potential effects of BBs and ivabradine in PAH

and 41.3 ± 3.8 years) with CCP on a background of COPD and bronchial asthma (non-severe) without IHD were enrolled. Patients were allocated into two groups because of the prescription of ivabradine along with the basic cure. All patients underwent transthoracic echocardiography in 12 weeks. QoL was assessed based on SF-36. Outcomes showed that patients of the 2nd group had a more significant tendency to normalize of structure-functional data of the right heart chambers because of a considerable reduction in HR. Early administration of ivabradine inhibits the deteriorating of RHF, improving the structural-functional data of the right heart chambers, which has a positive effect on the QoL of these patients.[75]

PAH is a disabling chronic disorder indicated as increased pulmonary artery pressure due to increased pulmonary vascular resistance. Combination therapy is beneficial to improve pulmonary arterial pressure. Lately, HR reduction with ivabradine has been reported to be safe in a case series of PAH patients. The study performed by Correale M *et al.* evaluate the clinical effect of treatment with ivabradine in PAH patients. From July 1, 2009, to July 1, 2013, a total of 10 patients with PAH and right HF were included in the study. HR, echocardiography with an estimation of the pulmonary arterial systolic pressure (PASP), and functional capacity as per 6MWT were evaluated. Ivabradine was added to all patients with

HR >100 bpm or symptomatic for palpitations. After 3 months usage with ivabradine, HR was considerably decreased (75 ± 11 bpm *vs* 90 ± 10 bpm; *p* <.01), 6MWT performance was considerably increased (338 ± 95 m *vs* 288 ± 111 m; *p* <.05), and mean New York Heart Association (NYHA) functional class was considerably improved (2.4 ± 0.5 *vs* 3.3 ± 0.7). Outcomes revealed patients with PAH may be safely cured with ivabradine.[76]

Erectile Dysfunction (ED)

ED is the main health concern that can considerably disturb a man's psychosocial well-being. ED has usually been considered a disease of old age, though current proof proposes a growing occurrence of ED in men younger than 40 years.[77] Improvements in diagnostic and treatment options provide various chances to detect and treat young men with ED. After diagnosis, doctors have numerous choices for management, including behavioral therapy, oral medical therapy, ICI therapy, intraurethral suppository, penile revascularization, inflatable penile prosthesis, hormone supplementation therapy, and stem cell (SC) therapy. Oral treatment with PDE5 inhibitors is the most commonly used therapy with a high success rate due to its efficiency and ease of use. The four essential PDE5 inhibitors that are presently marketed include sildenafil, tadalafil, vardenafil, and avanafil. Alprostadil, a synthetic form of prostaglandin E1, is the only injectable drug for ED approved by the Food and Drug Administration (FDA).[77]

Significance of HR Modulation in ED

ED is related to various CV risk factors such as raised SBP, high RHR, and endothelial dysfunction and foresees CV events. Though, the relation between high HR and SBP and the development of ED is not clear. Kratz MT *et al.* examined 1,015 male patients included in the ED substudy of ONTARGET and TRANSCEND, determined the effect of mean HR and mean SBP and their relations with ED. Elevated HR had no add-on effect in patients with preceding ED. Also, high SBP had no effect after adjustment for covariates (OR: 1.03, 95% CI: 0.66–1.59, *p* = 0.91). Increased HR is related to ED in patients who are at risk for CV events. Elevated RHR might signify a CV risk indicator.[78]

HF is a predominant disorder that shares numerous risk factors with ED, for instance, atherosclerosis and endothelial dysfunction, and commonly happens concomitantly. ED considerably and adversely distresses QoL in patients with HF. Moreover, several factors such as depression, an imbalance of circulating vasomodulators, neurohormonal changes, decreased cardiac capacity, and potential adverse effects of HF medical therapy can cause ED in patients with HF. As endothelial dysfunction is the pathophysiologic sign of both ED and HF, thus the occurrence of concomitant ED with HF is not shocking. Also, current data have shown HR as an independent risk factor for ED. Ivabradine is used for the management of HF, decreases resting, and exercise HRs without disturbing cardiac contractility or BP. Though ivabradine is currently indicated only in the treatment of chronic heart failure and chronic stable angina pectoris, it was confirmed that ivabradine usage can improve endothelial function and ED in experimental models. Therefore, Mert KU *et al.* evaluated the effect of ivabradine treatment on ED in patients with HF via the International Index of Erectile Function (IIEF-5) questionnaire with 5 questions to assess erectile function quality on the last 6-month period. Accordingly, 29 patients, between 18 and 70 years of age, male with CHF known for at least 1 year, the NYHA functional class I–II, LVEF less than 40%, in sinus rhythm with RHR of at least 70 bpm, who were intended to be treated with Ivabradine according to the decision of their physicians were assessed to define ED. With ivabradine treatment, IEFF-5 questionnaire scores increased considerably (p = .003), in contrast, a major reduction in HR was shown as expected. HR is decreased progressively after ivabradine usage, and the mean reduction in HR was 11.5 ± 9.4. Similarly, a negative correlation was confirmed between a reduction in HR (p <.001) and an increase in IEFF-5 scores (p = .003).[79] Initial outcomes of this study revealed that ivabradine has positive effects on ED. These results were assumed to be dependent entirely on HR reduction. As a consequence, the cardiologist should elude neglecting ED to develop medical compliance and QoL in patients with HF.[79]

Take Home Pearls

- Patients with MODS normally present with an increased HR and extremely damaged autonomic dysfunction with depressed parasympathetic regulation of the heart.
- A raised HR may damage LV diastolic filling, increase myocardial oxygen demand, and compromise coronary blood flow.
- Decreasing HR with ivabradine can improve exercise capacity and functional class in COPD patients with RHR >90 bpm.
- In PAH patients, ivabradine may lessen HR without any negative inotropic effects like β-blockers, for instance, hypotension or a decrease in cardiac output.
- Erectile dysfunction is related to CV risk factors such as high RHR, endothelial dysfunction, and raised SBP, which predicts CV events.

TAKE HOME SUMMARY

HR is controlled by the ANS and reveals the metabolic demands of the body. It is related to CV consequences in all the phases of the CV continuum and patients with other CV disorders such as supraventricular tachycardia, valvular diseases, cardiogenic shock, and non-CV conditions, such as pulmonary, cerebrovascular, renal disease, sepsis, cancer, and erectile dysfunction. Numerous studies presented that ivabradine improved QoL and HR normalization in patients with these conditions. Though ivabradine is currently indicated only in the treatment of chronic heart failure and chronic stable angina pectoris, its effect has also been studied in other conditions. Pure HR decrease with ivabradine without any unwanted side effects associated with BBs may be better for symptomatic perfection in MS patients with NSR. HR regulation improves the image quality and analytic precision of CCTA. Various studies discovered that ivabradine is a possibly attractive substitute to presently used medications for the decrease in HR in patients undergoing CCTA. An enhancement in the clinical and biochemical considerations of tissue perfusion was detected with the use of ivabradine in patients in shock and tachycardia, independently of changes in cardiac output. The selective decrease in HR with ivabradine is effective in patients with asthma and COPD, with no modification in respiratory function. Ivabradine is an interesting substitute, as an HR-decreasing agent, in patients with respiratory disease and contraindications to BBs. Ivabradine also revealed substantial perfections in the functional capacity of PAH patients and patients with erectile dysfunction.

REFERENCES

1. Vukadinoviæ AN, Vukadinoviæ D, Borer, J, *et al*. Heart rate and its reduction in chronic heart failure and beyond. *Eur J Heart Fail*. 2017 Oct;19(10):1230–41.

2. van den Berg MP, Haaksma J, Brouwer J, *et al*. Heart rate variability in patients with atrial fibrillation is related to vagal tone. *Circulation*. 1997 Aug;96:1209–16.

3. Al-Hazim A, Al-Ama N, Marouf M, *et al*. Heart rate variability in patients with mitral stenosis: A study of 20 cases from King Abdulaziz University Hospital. *Annals of Saudi Medicine*. 2002; 22(3–4).

4. Zhang J, Fletcher JG, Harmsen WS, *et al*. Analysis of heart rate and heart rate variation during cardiac CT examinations. *Acad Radiol*. 2008 Jan;15(1):40–8.

5. Bedet A, Voiriot G, Ternacle J, *et al*. Heart rate control during experimental sepsis in mice: Comparison of ivabradine and β-blockers. *Anesthesiology*. 2020 Feb;132:321–9.

6. Rudiger A, Jeger V, Arrigo M, *et al*. Heart rate elevations during early sepsis predict death in fluid- resuscitated rats with fecal peritonitis. *Intensive Care Med Exp*. 2018 Dec;6:28.

7. Yang LT, Enriquez-Sarano M, Pellikka PA, *et al*. Resting heart rate and outcomes in patients with hemodynamically significant aortic regurgitation. *Journal of the American College of Cardiology*. 2019 Mar;73 (9_Supplement 1):1959.

8. Perna GP, Vagnarelli F, Volterrani M, *et al*. Heart rate modulation in stable coronary artery disease without clinical heart failure: What we have already learned from SIGNIFY?. *Contemp Clin Trials Commun*. 2016 Jun 23;4:58–63.

9. Supraventricular tachycardia (SVT). Available from: https://www.umcvc.org/conditions-treatments/supraventricular-tachycardia-svt

10. Gunduz H, Arinc H, Kayardi M, *et al*. Heart rate turbulence and heart rate variability in patients with mitral valve prolapse. *Europace*. 2006 Jul;8(7):515–20.

11. Brugada J, Katritsis DG, Arbelo E, *et al*. 2019 ESC Guidelines for the management of patients with supraventricular tachycardia The Task Force for the management of patients with supraventricular tachycardia of the European Society of Cardiology (ESC) Developed in collaboration with the Association for European Paediatric and Congenital Cardiology (AEPC). *European Heart Journal*. 2019 Sep;1–65.

12. Page RL, Joglar JA, Caldwell MA, *et al*. 2015 ACC/AHA/HRS guideline for the management of adult patients with supraventricular tachycardia: Executive summary: A report of the American College of Cardiology/American Heart Association task force on clinical practice guidelines and the Heart Rhythm Society. *Circulation*. 2016 Apr 5;133(14):e471–e505

13. Hellenbart EL, Griffin T, DiDomenico RJ. Beyond heart failure and ischemic heart disease: A scoping review of novel uses of ivabradine in adults. *Pharmacotherapy*. 2020 Apr 5;40(6):544–64.

14. Yusuf S, Camm AJ. The sinus tachycardias. *Nature Clinical Practice Cardiovascular Medicine*. 2005 Jan;2(1):44–52.

15. Pellegrini CN, Scheinman MM. Epidemiology and definition of inappropriate sinus tachycardia. *J Interv Card Electrophysiol*. 2016 Jun;46(1):29–32.

16. Ruzieh M, Moustafa A, Sabbagh E, *et al*. Challenges in treatment of inappropriate sinus tachycardia. *Curr Cardiol Rev*. 2018 Mar 14;14(1):42–4.

17. Still AM, Raatikainen P, Ylitalo A, *et al*. Prevalence, characteristics and natural course of inappropriate sinus tachycardia. *Europace*. 2005;7(2):104–12.

18. Olshansky B, Sullivan RM. Inappropriate sinus tachycardia. *J Am Coll Cardiol*. 2013 Feb 26;61(8):793– 801.

19. Benezet-Mazuecos J, Rubio JM, Farre J, *et al*. Long-term outcomes of ivabradine in inappropriate sinus tachycardia patients: Appropriate efficacy or inappropriate patients. *Pacing Clin Electrophysiol*. 2013 Jul;36(7):830–6.

20. Calo L, Rebecchi M, Sette A, *et al*. Efficacy of ivabradine administration in patients affected by inappropriate sinus tachycardia. *Heart Rhythm*. 2010 Sep;7(9):1318–23.

21. Gopinathannair R, Olshansky B. Management of tachycardia. *F1000Prime Rep*. 2015;7:60.

22. Mizumaki K. Postural orthostatic tachycardia syndrome (POTS). *Journal of Arrhythmia*. 2011;27(4):289– 306.

23. Anjum I, Sohail W, Hatipoglu B, *et al*. Postural orthostatic tachycardia syndrome and its unusual presenting complaints in women: A literature minireview. *Cureus*. 2018 Apr;10(4): e2435.

24. Barzilai M, Jacob G. The effect of ivabradine on the heart rate and sympathovagal balance in postural tachycardia syndrome patients. *Rambam Maimonides Med J*. 2015 Jul;6(3):e0028.

25. Ruzieh M, Sirianni N, Ammari Z, *et al*. Ivabradine in the treatment of postural tachycardia syndrome (POTS), a single center experience. *Pacing Clin Electrophysiol*. 2017 Nov;40 (11):1242–5.

26. Supino PG, Borer JS, Preibisz J, *et al*. The epidemiology of valvular heart disease: A growing public health problem. *Heart Fail Clin*. 2006 Oct;2(4):379–93.

27. Bhalavi V, Yadav BS. Distribution and pattern of valvular heart diseases by echocardiography: A tertiary care center study. *Journal of Evolution of Medical Dental Sciences*. 2016 Apr;5(27): 1394–9.

28. Rosano GM. Valvular heart disease in heart failure. *International Cardiovascular Forum Journal*. 2017;10:70–2.

29. Maganti K, Rigolin VH, Sarano ME, *et al*. Valvular heart disease: Diagnosis and management. *Mayo Clinic Proceedings*. 2010 May;85(5):483–500.

30. Brinkley DM, Gelfand EV. Valvular heart disease: Classic teaching and emerging paradigms. *American Journal of Medicine*. 2013 Dec 1;126(12):1035–42.

31. Cupido BJ, Peters F, Ntusi NA. An approach to the diagnosis and management of valvular heart disease. *South African Medical Journal*. 2016 Jan;106(1):39–42.

32. Echeverría JC, Avila N, Springall R, *et al*. Inflammation and reduced parasympathetic cardiac modulation in aortic-valve sclerosis. *Applied Sciences*. 2019 Sep;9(19):4020.

33. Oliveira MS, Muzzi RA, Araujo RB, *et al*. Heart rate variability and arrhythmias evaluated with Holter in dogs with degenerative mitral valve disease. *Arq. Bras. Med. Vet. Zootec*. 2014; 66(2):425–32.

34. Zheng KH, Tzolos E, Dweck MR. Pathophysiology of aortic stenosis and future perspectives for medical therapy. *Cardiol Clin*. 2020 Feb;38(1):1–12.

35. Cortez-Quiroga G, Mansilla CR, Torralba MD, *et al*. PW073 Is it better ivabradine than beta blockers in symptomatic severe aortic stenosis with coronary artery disease?. *Global Heart*. 2014 Mar;9(1):e275.

36. Marquis-Gravel G, Redfors B, Leon MB, *et al*. Medical Treatment of Aortic Stenosis. *Circulation*. 2016;134(22):1766–84.

37. Amosova E, Andrejev E, Zaderey I, *et al*. Efficacy of ivabradine in combination with beta-blocker versus uptitration of beta-blocker in patients with stable angina. *Cardiovascular Drugs and Therapy*. 2011 Dec;25(6):531–7.

38. Cortez-Quiroga GA, Mansilla CR, Torralba MD, *et al*. PS240 Clinical and hemodynamic analysis of the treatment with ivabradine in severe aortic stenosis. *Global Heart*. 2016 Jun;11:e54.

39. Cortez-Quiroga GA, Torralba MD, Mansilla CR. PO620 Reduction of heart rate with ivabradine in severe aortic stenosis: Clinical, echocardiographic and hemodynamic effects. *Global Heart*. 2018 Dec;13(4):513.

40. Shah SN, Sharma S. Mitral Stenosis. In: StatPearls [Internet]. Treasure Island (FL): StatPearls Publishing; 2020 Jan. Available from: https://www.ncbi.nlm.nih.gov/books/NBK430742/

41. Armstrong GP. Mitral valve prolapse (MVP). *MSD Manual Professional Version*; Feb 2020.

42. Agrawal V, Kumar N, Lohiya B, *et al*. Metoprolol vs ivabradine in patients with mitral stenosis in sinus rhythm. *Int J Cardiol*. 2016 Oct 15;221:562–6.

43. Parakh N, Chaturvedi V, Kurian S, *et al.* Effect of ivabradine vs atenolol on heart rate and effort tolerance in patients with mild to moderate mitral stenosis and normal sinus rhythm. *Journal of Cardiac Failure.* 2012 Apr;18(4):282–8.

44. Dhanger MK, Isser HS, Bansal S, *et al.* Comparative study of ivabradineversus atenolol in symptomatic mitral stenosis patients. *Indian Heart Journal.* 2014 Nov;66(S2):S133.

45. Saggu DK, Narain VS, Dwivedi SK, *et al.* Effect of ivabradine on heart rate and duration of exercise in patients with mild-to-moderate mitral stenosis: A randomized comparison with metoprolol. *Journal of Cardiovascular Pharmacology.* 2015 Jun;65(6):552–4.

46. Rajesh GN, Sajeer K, Sajeev CG, *et al.* A comparative study of ivabradine and atenolol in patients with moderate mitral stenosis in sinus rhythm. *Indian Heart Journal.* 2016;68(3):311–5.

47. Cicek D, Eldem HO, Kalay N, *et al.* Effects of a novel I(f) inhibitor; ivabradine, on the biochemical, hemodynamic, and electrophysiological parameters in symptomatic patients with mitral valve prolapse. *Acta Cardiol Sin.* 2010;26:253–8.

48. Japp AG, Gulati A, Cook SA, *et al.* The diagnosis and evaluation of dilated cardiomyopathy. *J Am Coll Cardiol.* 2016 Jun 28;67(25):2996–3010.

49. Clements IP, Miller WL, Olson LJ. Resting heart rate and cardiac function in dilated cardiomyopathy. *International Journal of Cardiology.* 1999 Dec 15;72(1):27–37.

50. Patel PA, Ali N. An Overview of Dilated Cardiomyopathy. *Annals of Cardiovascular Diseases.* 2018;3(1):1022.

51. Raja DC, Kapoor A, Sinha A, *et al.* Heart rate manipulation in dilated cardiomyopathy: Assessing the role of Ivabradine. Indian Heart Journal. 2018 Mar;70(2):246–251.

52. Mansour S, Youssef A, Rayan M, *et al.* Efficacy of ivabradine in idiopathic dilated cardiomyopathy patients with chronic heart failure. *Egyptian Heart Journal.* 2011;63(2): 79– 85.

53. Bonnet D, Berger F, Jokinen E, *et al.* Ivabradine in children with dilated cardiomyopathy and symptomatic chronic heart failure. *J Am Coll Cardiol.* 2017 Sep 5;70(10):1262–72.

54. Türker FS. Cardiogenic shock. Available from: https: www.intechopen.com/ books/advances-in-extra-corporeal-perfusion-therapies/cardiogenic-shock-1

55. Kosaraju A, Pendela VS, Hai O. Cardiogenic shock. StatPearls [Internet]. *Treasure Island (FL): StatPearls Publishing.* 2020 Jan. Available from: https://www.ncbi.nlm.nih.gov/books/NBK482255/

56. Hollenberg SM, Kavinsky CJ, Parrillo JE, *et al.* Cardiogenic shock. *Ann Intern Med.* 1999 Jul 6;131(1):47– 59.

57. Chiu MH, Howlett JG, Sharma NC. Initiation of ivabradine in cardiogenic shock. ESC Heart Failure. 2019 Oct;6(5):1088–91.

58. Chiu MH, Howlett JG, Sharma NC. Abstract 17278: Concomitant use of ivabradine in the setting of cardiogenic shock: A case series. *Circulation.* 2018 Nov 5;138(Suppl_1):A17278.

59. Adile KK, Kapoor A, Jain SK, *et al.* Safety and efficacy of oral ivabradine as a heart rate- reducing agent in patients undergoing CT coronary angiography. *Br J Radiol.* 2012 Aug;85(1016):e424–e428.

60. Guler EC, Yam Y, Jia K, *et al.* Effectiveness of point-of-care oral ivabradine for cardiac computed tomography. *Journal of Cardiovascular Computed Tomography.* 2020 Oct 6.

61. Metra M, Zaca V, Parati G, *et al.* Cardiovascular and noncardiovascular comorbidities in patients with chronic heart failure. *J Cardiovasc Med (Hagerstown).* 2011 Feb;12(2):76–84.

62. Gyawali B, Ramakrishna K, Dhamoon AS. Sepsis: The evolution in definition, pathophysiology, and management. *SAGE Open Medicine.* 2019;7:2050312119835043.

63. Muller-Werdan U, Stockl G, Werdan K. Advances in the management of heart failure: The role of ivabradine. *Vascular Health and Risk Management.* 2016;12:453–70.

64. ESICM LIVES 2018: Paris, France. 20-24 October 2018. *Intensive Care Medicine Experimental.* 2018;6(Suppl 2):40.

65. Value of heart rate control using ivabradine in patients with MODS self funding. Adapted from: https://www.cochranelibrary.com/central/doi/10.1002/central/CN-01959615/full

66. Nuding S, Schröder J, Presek P, *et al*. Reducing elevated heart rates in patients with multiple organ dysfunction syndrome with the If (funny channel current) inhibitor ivabradine. *Shock*. 2018 Apr;49(4):402–11.

67. De Santis V, Frati G, Greco E, *et al*. Ivabradine: A preliminary observation for a new terapeutic role in patients with multiple organ dysfunction syndrome. *Clin Res Cardiol*. 2014 Oct;103 (10):831–834.

68. Wedzicha (ERS co-chair) JA, Miravitlles M, Hurst JR, *et al*. Management of COPD exacerbations: A European Respiratory Society/American Thoracic Society guideline. *European Respiratory Journal*. 2017;49:1600791.

69. Mahmoud K, Kassem HH, Baligh E, *et al*. The effect of ivabradine on functional capacity in patients with chronic obstructive pulmonary disease. *Clinical Medicine (London)*. 2016 Oct;16(5):419–22.

70. Güder G, Rutten FH. Comorbidity of heart failure and chronic obstructive pulmonary disease: More than coincidence. *Curr Heart Fail Rep*. 2014 Sep;11(3):337–46.

71. Majewski S, Slomka S, Zielinska-Wyderkiewicz E, *et al*. Heart rate-lowering efficacy and respiratory safety of ivabradine in patients with obstructive airway disease: A randomized, double-blind, placebo-controlled, crossover study. *American Journal of Cardiovascular Drugs*. 2012 Jun 1;12(3):179–88.

72. Zulkarneev R, Zagidullin N, Abdrahmanova G, *et al*. Ivabradine prevents heart rate acceleration in patients with chronic obstructive pulmonary disease and coronary heart disease after salbutamol inhalation. *Pharmaceuticals (Basel)*. 2012 Apr;5(4):398–404.

73. Delcroix M, Howard L. Pulmonary arterial hypertension: The burden of disease and impact on quality of life. *European Respiratory Review*. 2015;24:621–9.

74. Yaoita N, Shimokawa H. Effect of heart rate reduction in pulmonary arterial hypertension. *American Journal of Physiology: Heart and Circulatory Physiology*. 2018 May 1;314(5):H889–H891.

75. Tytova G, Liepieieva O, Al-Karawi A, *et al*. P13371 Ivabradine in patients with chronic cor pulmonale and right heart failure. *European Heart Journal*. 2017 Aug;38(Suppl_1):ehx504.P3371.

76. Correale M, Brunetti ND, Montrone D, *et al*. Functional improvement in pulmonary arterial hypertension patients treated with ivabradine. *J Card Fail*. 2014 May;20(5):373–5.

77. Nguyen HM, Gabrielson AT, Hellstrom WJ, *et al*. Erectile dysfunction in young men-A review of the prevalence and risk factors. *Sex Med Rev*. 2017 Oct;5(4):508–20.

78. Kratz MT, Schumacher H, Sliwa K, *et al*. Heart rate and blood pressure interactions in the development of erectile dysfunction in high-risk cardiovascular patients. *European Journal of Preventive Cardiology*. 2014 Mar;21(3):272–80.

79. Mert KU, Dural M, Mert GÖ, *et al*. Effects of heart rate reduction with ivabradine on the international ýndex of erectile function (IIEF-5) in patients with heart failure. *The Aging Male*. 2018 Jun;21(2):93–8.

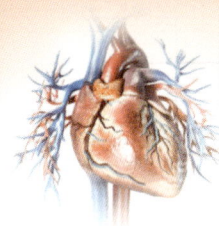

Index